Silent Ischemia
Current Concepts and Management

Workshop in Rottach-Egern
March 5—7, 1987

HERZ/KREISLAUF

Bayer

Th. v. Arnim / A. Maseri (Eds.)

Silent Ischemia

Current Concepts and Management

Springer-Verlag Berlin Heidelberg GmbH

PD Dr. Th. v. Arnim
Medizinische Klinik I
Klinikum Großhadern
Marchioninistraße 15
8000 München 70, F.R.G.

A. Maseri M.D., F.R.C.P.
Cardiovascular Unit,
Royal Postgraduate Medical School,
Hammersmith Hospital
Ducane Road,
London W 12 OHS, U.K.

CIP-Kurztitelaufnahme der Deutschen Bibliothek

Silent ischemia: current concepts and management; [Workshop, Rottach-Egern, March 5—7, 1987]
Th. v. Arnim; A. Maseri (eds.). — Darmstadt: Steinkopff; New York : Springer, 1987.
ISBN 978-3-662-12999-9 ISBN 978-3-662-12997-5 (eBook)
DOI 10.1007/978-3-662-12997-5
NE: Arnim, Thomas von [Hrsg.]

Originally published by Dr. Dietrich Steinkopff Verlag GmbH & Co. KG, Darmstadt in 1987.
Medical Editorial: Juliane K. Weller — Production: Heinz J. Schäfer

Preface

"Silent Ischemia, Current Concepts and Management" contains the proceedings of a conference held in Rottach-Egern, West Germany, March 5 to 7, 1987. We are most grateful to the authors for the effort to provide manuscripts before the meeting, to the sponsor, Bayer AG, for their generous support and to the publishers for their efficient collaboration, all of which have made the appearance of this book possible.

When discussing silent myocardial ischemia, the first question is: "why is it silent?". To approach this question, a deeper look has to be taken into the pathophysiology of cardiac pain and the excitatory and inhibitory mechanisms involved. It has to be borne in mind that – in contradiction to what the poets have told us so beautifully for many centuries – the heart is a visceral and not a sensitive organ.

If asymptomatic ischemia did not carry prognostic significance comparable to the symptomatic manifestations of ischemia, then the problem of silent ischemia would be very academic and without consequences for treatment. Therefore studies on prognosis of silent ischemia are of great importance, as their results should indicate how aggressively patients are to be managed.

Silent ischemia can be detected by the same techniques used to identify the presence of symptomatic ischemia. Exercise testing, nuclear medical techniques, two dimensional echocardiography and angiography represent the main basis for demonstration of silent ischemia in a laboratory. Ambulatory Holter monitoring provides information on episodes of silent ischemia occurring throughout ordinary daily life and on the relationship to the different levels of activity of the patients.

"What is the prevalence of silent ischemia in different patient groups? Are there special characteristics of patients prone to develop silent ischemia? Which are the most practical means of detecting silent ischemia in large numbers of people at risk?" These questions should to be answered in order to establish rational guidelines for clinical practice. If silent ischemia is a precursor of acute coronary events, like acute myocardial infarction or sudden death, then its detection would suggest appropriate interventions, designed to modify the course of the disease.

The management of silent ischemia has to find its place between the extremes of a very conservative approach, reluctant to intervene before any symptoms occur and an aggressive approach. The trend seems to favor the approach of treating ischemia in the same way whether it is symptomatic or asymptomatic. However the demonstration, that treatment of silent ischemia will improve the prognosis of the patients is still uncertain. The demonstration of silent ischemia depends on objective means of documenting ischemic changes. The demonstration of success of any treatment therefore also depends on the same objective methods, which may be time consuming, or on the documentation of an improved prognosis, which is certainly even more time consuming.

The issues are presented in the book by the distinguished investigators and clinicians who assembled in Rottach-Egern for the conference. We hope that the readers will find in the book useful guidelines for current practice and for future research.

Th. v. Arnim
A. Maseri

Munich, March 1987

Contents

Management

The discussions have been edited by Th. v. Arnim.

Central mechanisms of pain control: a survey

M. J. Millan

Department of Neuropharmacology, Max-Planck-Institut für Psychiatrie, Planegg-Martinsried, F.R.G.

The nature and problem of pain

Pain is a subjective experience reflecting actual, assumed or potential tissue damage, variable in intensity and, in general, localizable in space and in time. It is comprised of not only a sensory/perceptive but also of an emotional/affective and cognitive/conscious component. Though of limited utility, such a characterization has the virtue of drawing attention to the complexity of pain and to the fact that it is a phenomenon which can be monitored from its inception in sensory nerve endings, via the spinal cord and brainstem, to the highest levels of the CNS, the limbic system and cortex. At each level of this hierarchy of processing and integration, mechanisms for its modulation are operative and each level offers the possibility of therapeutic intervention in pain control.

It is our regrettable inability to satisfactorily manage (in particular chronic) pain which lies at the heart of the continuing intensive interest in mechanisms of pain and pain control. Perhaps paradoxically, a further clinical problem relates to the insufficiencies (and idiosyncracies) of acute pain as a warning system, and its occasional failure to alert in, for example, heart malfunction and disease.

The purpose of this article is to introduce certain aspects of the processing and control of pain and the complexities encountered in its study. The subject of pain is no less massive than that of, for example, vision or the cardiovascular system. Correspondingly, this can only be an outline sketch. However, the citations offered are predominantly recent, extensive review articles (e.g. 1, 2, 10, 12, 17, 21, 22, 24) which treat in depth both of those issues raised here and those for which space was insufficient to allow for their consideration. For illustrative purposes, emphasis is afforded to the opioids: this is not for parochial reasons but since opioidergic mechanisms of pain modulation are by far the most diverse, widespread and the best-understood. Furthermore, synthetic opioids remain of inestimable importance in the therapeutic treatment of many types of pain in man.

The transmission and processing of noxious information

i) Sensory nerve endings (see refs. 2, 3, 4, 8, 19, 22, 24)

Noxious information is initiated in (structurally unspecialized) specific nerve endings external to the CNS (in skin, skeletal muscle and the viscera). These are normally silent and are differentially sensitive to intense mechanical, thermal and chemical stimuli: two important types are polymodal C and mechanical Aδ. The sensitivity of these terminals can be greatly (and synergistically) facilitated by the local release of chemicals derived from neighbouring tissue (e.g. serotonin, histamine, prostaglandins) and plasma (e.g. bradykinin). Substance P (which is present in primary afferent neurones and may transmit noxious information in the spinal cord) is also liberated from terminals themselves upon tissue damage and, in causing extravasation, it indirectly sensitizes terminals by encouraging access thereto of the agents mentioned above. This peripheral part of the neuroaxis is very much the domain of non steroidal anti-inflammatory aspirin-like drugs which inhibit the synthesis of prostaglandins (6). However, the multiplicity of the factors involved in determining the sensitivity and activity of these nerve endings and the recent detection of many novel peptides in primary afferent neurones (16, 18, 24) suggests scope for the future discovery of novel classes of analgetic agents active in the periphery. Further, there are reports that actions of opioidergic substances in the periphery, probably directly upon nerve endings, may inhibit the transmission of noxious information to the spinal cord (8, 12). A characterization of the biochemical and pharmacological properties of these opioid or opioid-like receptors may prove fruitful: the advantages of an opioid analgetic not susceptible to abuse nor inducing dependence and devoid of other CNS side-effects are obvious. Finally, it may be noted that the activity of these terminals can be indirectly modified by agents not directly interacting therewith. For example, in ischemic pain, an improvement in local blood flow and oxygen supply induced by a non-analgetic vasodilator would evidently be effective.

ii) Primary processing in the spinal cord (1, 2, 3, 4, 7, 11, 19, 22, 24)

Small calibre Aδ myelinated and C unmyelinated afferents bearing noxious information travel to the dorsal horn of the spinal cord (or trigeminal nucleus) wherein they transmit the noxious signal mono- or poly-synaptically to neurones projecting to the brain. The major target for noxious information in the brain is the thalamus which receives this primarily via the spinothalamic tract. However, it is important to note that there are additional sites of termination of projection neurones in the medulla (reticular nuclei), mesencephalon (central and periaqueductal grey) and, via the thalamus, the somatosensory cortex and limbic system; in each case, these structures are also of significance in mechanisms of pain control (1, 5, 10, 11, 14, 15, 21). There are, essentially, two major types of neurone which receive noxious input in the spinal cord and relay this to the brain: nociceptive-specific (high-threshold) neurones and wide-dynamic range neurones which also respond strongly to low intensity (non-noxious) stimuli.

There is limited evidence that there is a pre-synaptic inhibition of those primary afferent fibers carrying noxious input to the spinal cord, and opioids may be involved in any such mechanism (11, 16, 24). However, it is primarily a post-synaptic action to suppress the activity of brain projection neurones excited by incoming noxious stimuli which can diminish the flow of noxious information to the suprasegmental level. This inhibition can be effected either directly or indirectly (via local interneurones) and is exerted by two different neuronal sources.

Firstly, neurones in the brainstem (primarily noradrenergic and serotoninergic), projecting to the dorsal horn (1, 4, 5, 10, 11, 15, 24). These are activated by, for example, opioidergic systems in the periaqueductal grey and rostral, ventral medulla and are thought to underlie the ability of stimulation of brainstem structures to induce an analgesia against visceral and somatic pain in animals and man. Interestingly, noxious stimuli may also engage these centrifugal pathways, representing a mode of negative feedback mediated ultimately at the spinal level.

Secondly, primary afferent fibers themselves can inhibit the activity of brain projection neurones in the dorsal horn (2, 3, 19, 22, 24). This includes those actually conveying the noxious message which may, in addition to directly exciting the projection neurones, indirectly inhibit these via interneurones in the dorsal horn: a fraction of these interneurones are probably opioidergic. Similarly to the activation of descending inhibitory pathways, this may represent a mode of negative feedback. Furthermore, large diameter, low threshold afferents *not* carrying noxious information can inhibit (largely via interneurones) the excitations of the brain projection neurones elicited by noxious stimuli. Such an action probably relates to the familiar experience that rubbing an injured area can help moderate the pain and also to the analgetic of low threshold, non-painful, transcutaneous electrical stimulation.

Both of the above-described mechanism of inhibition of brain projection neurones by primary afferent (non-noxious) input were key elements in the "gate" model of pain-control conceptualized by Melzack and Wall (19). It should be mentioned that there is considerable convergence of primary afferent input from various body regions in the spinal cord. For example, it is probable that there are no spinal neurones receiving an input from visceral organs which do not also receive a somatic input. This intra- (and inter-)segmental convergence not only helps explains referred pain and secondary hyperalgesia, but also why stimulation of remote tissues (e.g. mustard plaster or rubbing of the stomach) may relieve pain in other tissues. Further, the ability of noxious input to activate inhibitory descending pathways is not restricted in its actions to the particular regions affected but more widespread in its effects ("diffuse") and can elicit an analgetic action in remote body regions. It is possible that is possible that such a mechanism relates to many models of acute stress-induced analgesia (1, 9, 12, 13, 20, 24). For example, the ability of noxious foot-shock applied to the paws of rats to evoke an analgetic response as quantified on the tail. Finally, it should be noted that non-noxious stressful stimuli can also elicit such an analgesia. The biological significance of such mechanisms of environmentally-induced analgesia (in, for example, fights with other conspecifics) are discussed elsewhere (9, 12).

iii) Brain (1, 3, 4, 11, 15, 17, 23, 24)

Concerning mechanisms of pain control in the brain, we have already considered the engagement of inhibitory descending pathways. There is little doubt that there exist complementary mechanisms within the brain itself and involving the ascending (from the brainstem) noradrenergic, serotoninergic (and other types of) input to the thalamus, limbic system and cortex. Our knowledge of these is profoundly limited. However, at the sites of termination and synapse formation of the spinal projection neurones transmitting noxious information to the brain, the target neurones excited must also be subject to modulation; there is evidence that opioids are involved in such a function, e.g. in the thalamus (11, 24). Further, it is generally assumed that not only can the transmission of noxious information from the thalamus (and other sites) to the cortex and limbic system be suppressed but that there are also mechanisms active within these structures themselves. These higher centres are responsible for the conscious/cognitive and emotional appreciation and differentiation of pain and the assessment of its significance. Mechanisms operative therein remain largely unexplored. Nevertheless, that there is an involvement of opioid in such processes seems certain in view of their ability to relieve the distress associated with pain and their anxiogenic and mood-improving properties (11, 14, 21). In discussions of the nature of spinal processing and other neuronal mechanisms of pain control such a role should not be forgotten.

The complexity of the neurochemistry of pain modulation

In the above lines, little commentary was made concerning the neurochemistry of the various pathways involved in the transmission and modulation of pain. In the majority of cases this is simply not known. Notably, the identity of the primary afferent transmitters of noxious information from the periphery to the spinal cord remains obscure (7, 16, 18, 22, 24): though glutamate and substance P are promising candidates, there is a multiplicity of other neuropeptides present therein and this fundamental question remains in urgent need of resolution. In addition to noradrenaline and serotonin (which have been mentioned above) other classes of classical transmitter (GABA, acetylcholine, glutamate), various putative neurotransmitters or neuromodulators (e.g. histamine) and a multitude of neuropeptides may play a role in the modulation of pain (1, 4, 15, 16, 17, 18, 23, 24). They are all broadly and differentially distributed in various regions of the brain, including these structures discussed above which are implicated in pain modulation, and are also found in the dorsal horn of the spinal cord. Furthermore, their application directly into discrete regions of the brain or spinal cord results in a modulation of nociceptive thresholds, generally an analgesia (15, 23). This vast array of endogenous substances of potential physiological or therapeutic importance in pain control currently presents a major challenge. It also draws attention to the complexity of the issue of pain control.

This complexity is further exemplified by a brief consideration of the opioids, the natural counterparts of morphine, which certainly do fulfil a decisive role in pain control at various levels of the neuroaxis (1, 10, 11, 12, 15, 20, 24). The opioids optimally illustrate the complexity of the problem: indeed, the apparently straight forward question of "What is the role of opioids in pain control" is by no means so simple.

Firstly, there exists a great number (in excess of 25) of opioid peptides which are proteolytically processed from three precursors encoded by three independent genes (12). Each of these families (represented by β-endorphin, enkephalin and dynorphin) are broadly and differentially distributed throughout the CNS in regions involved in pain control and may be found in the systemic circulation; moreover, there is evidence for their occurrence in primary afferent fibers and that they may be synthesized in the periphery (8, 12, 16, 18). Clearly, one must distinguish both between the particular opioid peptides and also the particular pools; that is, not only β-endorphin vs dynorphin but also dynorphin in the thalamus vs dynorphin in the dorsal horn of the spinal cord. Further, there is a multiplicity of opioid receptor types (μ, δ, κ) in the CNS (12). Since there is *no* direct correspondence between the peptides and the receptor types this represents a further complication. One must clearly consider the (contrasting) roles of the various receptor types. This question points to a further element of complexity and there are two critical factors of importance as regards the function of these receptors types. Firstly, spinal, as compared to cerebral, pools of the receptors; secondly, the nature of the nociceptive stimulus, whether thermal or non-thermal (pressure and chemical). Table 1 summarizes the action of the various receptor types at the segmental and suprasegmental level.

Table 1. Suspected roles of various opioid types in pain control.

	Brain		Spinal Cord	
	thermal	non-thermal	thermal	non-thermal
μ	major	major	major	major
δ	minor	minor	major	minor
κ	none	none	minor	major

A final variable to consider as regards the role of opioids in the control of pain is as to the nature of the response evaluated. Thus, the spinally, initiated reflex withdrawal of a limb is to be distinguished from the cerebrally-integrated vocalization response and co-ordinated whole-body escape. These can be differentially modulated and correspond to the difference between the perceptive/sensory and affective/emotional component of pain. A drug can affect the experience of pain without greatly modifying its intensity and vice versa. Clinically, under treatment with morphine, patients often assert that though the pain is still there, it ceases to bother them; morphine primarily (though not exclusively) increases the ability to tolerate the pain and reduces its unpleasantness, actions related to its anxiolytic properties and positive influence on mood (14, 21). Morphine will of course increase the vocalization threshold to pain in animals. Interestingly, an agonist at κ-opioid receptors (which do not mediate positive but rather aversive effects on mood) does not increase vocalization thresholds though it will suppress the withdrawal reflex to pain via an action in the spinal cord (12).

In conclusion, though this is by no means a exhaustive discussion of relevant parameters, these observations should serve to illustrate the complexity of the study and mechanisms for the modulation of pain. In addition, it is evident that a great deal more remains to be learned, and from an enhanced understanding, it is to be hoped that novel insights and opportunities for the improved therapy of pain may be won.

Acknowledgement

The author was supported by the Deutsche Forschungsgemeinschaft.

References

1. Basbaum A, Fields HL (1984) Endogenous pain control systems. Ann Rev Neurosci 7: 309–338
2. Brown AG (1981) Organization in the spinal cord. Springer Verlag, Berlin

3. Dubner R, Bennett GJ (1983) Spinal and trigeminal mechanism of nociception. Ann Rev Neurosci 6: 381—418
4. Fields HL, Dubner R, Cervero F (1985) (eds) Advances in Pain Research and Therapy, Vol 9, Raven Press, New York
5. Fitzgerald M (1986) Monoamines and descending control of nociception. Trends Neurosci 7: 5—7
6. Goodman GA, Goodman LS, Rall TW, Murad F (1985) The pharmacological basis of experimental therapeutics. MacMillan, New York
7. Iggo A, Streedman WM, Fleetwood-Walker B (1986) Spinal processing: anatomy and physiology of spinal nociception, Phil Trans R Soc Lond B 308: 235—252
8. Inoki R and Kudo T (1986) Enkephalins and bradykinin in dental pulp, Trends Pharm 7: 275—279
9. Kelly DJ (1986) (ed) Stress-induced analgesia, Ann NY Acad Science, vol 467
10. Mayer DJ (1980) Centrifugal central of pain. In: Ng, LL, Bonica J (eds) Pain, Discomfort and humanitarian care. Elsevier Press, Amsterdam, pp 83—105
11. Millan MJ (1982) Endorphins and nociception: an overview, Meth Find Exp Clin Pharmacol 4: 445—462
12. Millan MJ (1986) Multiple opioid systems and pain, Pain 27: 303—349
13. Millan MJ (1981) Stress and endogenous opioid peptides; a review. Mod Probl Pharmacopsychiat 17: 49—67
14. Millan MJ, Duka Th (1981) Anxiolytic properties of opiates and endogenous opioid peptides and their relationship to the action of benzodiazepines, Mod Probl Pharmacopsychiat 17: 123—141
15. Pert A (1980) Psychopharmacology of analgesia and pain. In: Ng LL and Bonica J (eds) Pain, Discomfort and Humanitarian Care, Elsevier Press, Amsterdam, pp 139—191
16. Ruda MA, Bennett GJ, Dubner RJ (1986) Neurochemistry and neural circuitry in the dorsal horn, Prog Brain Res 66: 219—268
17. Siggins GR, Gruol DL (1986) Mechanisms of transmitter action. In: Mountcastle VB, Bloom FE and Geiger SR (eds) Handbook of Physiology — The Nervous System, vol. IV, Williams and Wilkins, Baltimore, pp 44—114
18. Tohyama M, Shiotani M (1986) Neuropeptides in spinal cord. Prog Brain Res 66: 177—218
19. Wall P (1980) The substantia gelatinosa; A gate control mechanism set across a sensory pathway, Trends Neurosci 3: 221—224
20. Watkins LR, Mayer DJ (1982) Organization of endogenous opiate and non-opiate pain control systems, Science 216: 1185—1192
21. Wikler A (1980) Opioid Dependence, Plenum Press, New York
22. Yaksh TL, Hammond DH (1982) Peripheral and central substrates involved in the rostral transmission of nociception information. Pain 13: 1—85
23. Zadina JE, Banks WA, Kastin AJ (1986) Central nervous system effects of peptides, 1980—1985, Peptides 7: 497—537
24. Zieglgänsberger W (1986) Central control of nociception. In: Mountcastle VB, Bloom FE and Geiger SR (eds) Handbook of Physiology — The Nervous System, Vol IV, Williams and Wilkins, Baltimore, pp 581—645

Author's address:
Dr. M. J. Millan
Dept. of Neuropharmacology
Max-Planck-Institut für
Psychiatrie
Am Klopferspitz 18a
8033 Planegg-Martinsried
F.R.G.

Peripheral innervation of the heart

E. Weihe

Anatomisches Institut der Johannes Gutenberg-Universität Mainz

Summary

The present immunohistochemical study demonstrates the multiplicity, histotopography and origin of peptidergic innervation in the mammalian heart. Neuropeptide Y (NPY) is the major representative of peptides in cardiac sympathetic efferents. Sympathetic afferents are characterized by the presence of tachykinins, calcitonin gene-related peptide and apparently also some opioid peptides. Predominant peptides of the vagal system are tachykinins. The intrinsic peptidergic system predominantly consists of vasoactive intestinal polypeptide/peptide histidine isoleucine. Paracrine systems are merely opioidergic. Target relations of extrinsic and intrinsic peptidergic nerves were found to be more differentiated than currently believed. The different peptidergic neuronal pathways were not strictly separated. The chemical phenotype of the different neuronal pathways and paracrine systems seems to be more complex than presently known. The detailed chemoanatomical data presented here should be a good basis for further clarifying the suggested physiological and pathophysiological roles of multiple cardiac peptide- and non-peptide messenger systems.

Introduction

The innervation of the mammalian heart comprises extrinsic and intrinsic components. Extrinsic cardiac innervation consists of vagal preganglionic (cholinergic) and sympathetic postganglionic (noradrenergic) efferent neurones and of primary afferent neurones derived from vagal and spinal sensory ganglia. Intrinsic innervation is delivered by intracardiac ganglia of various locations which, albeit not exclusively, contain cholinergic neurons (cf. 7). Beyond this classical view, the development of knowledge in the recent years of the "peptide revolution" points to a more complex chemical heterogeneity of cardiac innervation. A varied plethora of peptidic messenger candidates have been localized immunohistochemically to cardiac nerves (6—8, 15, 17, 20—22) and characterized in cardiac extracts by combining chromatography with radioimmunoassay or bioassay (1, 24). Since knowledge about the chemical multiplicity, origin, interspecies variations and exact histotopography of peptidergic cardiac innervation is still fragmentary the present study will address some of these open questions by a sensitive light microscope (LM) immunohistochemical approach. The possibly fundamental significance of peptides in cardiac physiology and pathophysiology will be discussed on the basis of these novel chemoanatomical constellations of cardiac innervation.

Material and Methods

Tissue-processing for immunocytochemistry

Hearts, stellate ganglia, dorsal root ganglia of lower cervical and upper thoracic segments, and vagal nerves of adult mammalian species (ten guinea-pigs, five rats, four cats, two dogs, and three rabbits) were fixed by perfusion with Bouin's solution (22). One isolated pig heart was perfused with Bouin's fixative. Human atrial tissue was obtained during open heart surgery for valve replacement and fixed by immersion in Bouin. One human stellate ganglion was obtained by therapeutic stellatectomy carried out on an adult male patient suffering ischemic disease of the upper limbs. Tissues were processed for LM immunohistochemistry using immunoenzymatic methods based on streptavidin-biotin kits (25, 26). Immunoreacted sections were analyzed and photographed in a Leitz-Orthoplan light microscope.

Antisera

A plethora of commercial (Peninsula, Immunonuclear, Amersham, Serotec) and donated antisera were used:
1. Rabbit polyclonal antisera against non-opioid peptides, neuropeptide Y (NPY), calcitonin gene-related peptide (CGRP), the tachykinin substance K (SK), neurotensin (NT), vasoactive intestinal polypeptide (VIP), peptide histidine isoleucine (PHI), atrial natriuretic factor (ANF), neurotensin (NT) 2. Rat monoclonal antibody (ascites) against the tachykinin substance P (SP) 3. Rabbit polyclonal antisera against proenkephalin-derived opioid sequences Met-enkephalin (ME), Met-enkephalyl-Arg-Gly-Leu (ME—RGL); amidorphin (AMIDOR) crossreacting with peptide F, metorphamide (METOR); against prodynorphin-derived opioid sequences, dynorphin A 1—17 (DYN A), dynorphin A 1—8 (DYN 1—8), alpha-neoendorphin (NEO), dynorphin B (DYN B); against Leu-enkephalin (LE) which can be processed from both proenkephalin and prodynorphin; and against proopiomelanocortin-derived β-endorphin (β-END) and alpha-melanocyte-stimulating-hormone (MSH).
Polyclonal antisera were used in dilutions ranging from 1 : 6.000 to 1 : 80.000. Monoclonal antibodies were applied in a dilution range of ascites from 1 :100 to 1 : 800. Specificities of antisera were as described (2, 22, 23, 25, 26).

Results

Peptides, (ir) opioid and non-opioid, were found to be differentially distributed in intracardiac and extracardiac nerves and ganglia known to project to the heart. However, varying degrees of overlapping patterns were also observed.

Sympathetic ganglia

The distribution of (ir) peptides was extensively studied in stellate ganglia of guinea-pig (Table 1). The predominant (ir) peptide in the sympathetic system was NPY which was

present in many principal ganglionic cells. In comparison, (ir) VIP, coexisting with (ir) PHI, was present in only a minority of postganglionic neurons. A few NEO (ir) principal neurons were found to be faintly stained by antisera against CGRP.
The other (ir) peptides investigated were restricted to varicose and non-varicose fibers and some of them were also present in paraganglionic cells. Apparently, the bulk of codistributed fibers containing (ir) SP, SK, or CGRP were non-varicose and seemed to trespass the ganglion. MSH (ir) fibers were exclusively non-varicose and trespassing; their diameter was in the larger myelinated range whereas all other (ir) peptides were in fibers of smaller diameter (C, A delta range).
Apart from quantitative differences, the constellation observed in guinea-pig was principally the same in the other animal species investigated. NPY was generally the preponderant peptide in postganglionic neurons. Interestingly, a few principal ganglionic cells of human stellate ganglion contained (ir) LE and CGRP.

Vagal nerve

As regards projecting fibers within the vagal nerve, (ir) tachykinins and CGRP were predominant peptides. Of minor frequency was the (ir) opioid peptide LE whereas other opioids were not unequivocally visible. Immunoreactivities of these peptides were all present in small diameter fibers intermingled with non-(ir) fibers and the impression of substantial overlap was obtained. Interestingly, (ir) NPY was absent from projecting fibers whereas a few VIP (ir) fibers were seen. However, some NPY (ir) vasomotor fibers to vasa nervorum were present. Again, (ir) MSH was present in larger myelinated fibers. Except for quantitative differences, the situation was similar in all species investigated.

Spinal ganglia

Dorsal root ganglia of guinea-pig were extensively studied (see Table 2). Preponderant primary sensory peptides were the tachykinins with the main representative SP and the non-tachykinin CGRP. Immunoreactivities of these two peptides were found to coexist not only in the guinea-pig but also in the rat, cat and rabbit, where they were equally frequent. Evidence for primary sensory opioid peptides (apparently exclusively derived from prodynorphin) were obtained in guinea-pig, cat and less clearly in rabbit, but not in rat. VIP/PHI (ir) perikarya and fibers were only sporadically encountered. The situation in dog, pig and human could not be clarified. There was no evidence for the presence of NPY in primary sensory afferents. MSH (ir) material was in the majority of large and also of some intermediate ganglionic cells and myelinated fibers.

Histotopography of (ir) peptides in the heart

a) Neuronal systems

The overall constellation is exemplified for the guinea-pig heart (see Table 3). According to these results, NPY is the major (ir) peptide present in nerves supplying all cardiac key-

Table 1. Immunoreactive peptides in stellate ganglia of guinea-pig.

	principal ganglionic cells	nerve fibres		paraganglionic cells
		trespassing	varicose	
NPY	++++	++	++	—
SP/SK/CGRP	—	+++	+	—
VIP/PHI	+	+	+	—
LE/ME	—	+	+++	++
AMIDOR	—	+	++	—
ME-RGL	—	+	+++	+
METOR	—	+	++	—
DYN A/B/1-8	—	+	+	+
NEO	+	+	+	+
MSH	—	++	—	—
ß-END	—	+	++	—

Subjective rating scale of immunoreactive fibres or cells: - absent: + infrequent: ++ frequent: +++ very frequent: ++++ abundant

Table 2. Immunoraective peptides in lower cervical and upper thoracic dorsal root ganglia of guinea-pig.

	ganglionic cells			nerve fibers		
	small	intermediate	large	C	A delta	larger
SP	++++	+++	+	++++	++	+/—
SK	++	++	—	++	++	—
CGRP	++++	+++	+	++++	++	+
VIP/PHI	+	+	—	+	+	—
ME, ME-RGL	—	—	—	—	—	—
METOR	—	—	—	—	—	—
AMIDOR	—	—	—	—	—	—
LE	++	+	—	++	+	—
DYN A/B	++	+	—	++	+	—
NEO	++	+	—	++	+	—
MSH	—	—/+	++++	—	—	++++

Subjective rating of immunoreactive fibers and cells — absent; + infrequent; ++ frequent; +++ very frequent; ++++ abundant

areas rather homogeneously (Fig. 1). The presence of (ir) NPY in some intracardiac ganglionic cells is indicative of the fact that NPY is not only extrinsic but also intrinsic. Except for its absence in intrinsic neurons, NT is similarly distributed but less frequent than NPY. Tachykinins and CGRP had a wide but less homogeneous distribution than NPY (Fig. 4a, b). There was clear preponderance of this group of peptides in nerves to the coronary vasculature (Fig. 2) and in non-neuroeffector constellation (Fig. 4b).

The prevalent (ir) form of opioid peptides in the heart was that of LE (Fig. 3). We also observed (ir) NEO in many cardiac nerves but the visualization was somewhat hampered by a relatively high background-staining of interstitial and perivascular tissues. The distribution of (ir) LE nerve fibers somewhat resembled that of (ir) tachykinins and CGRP but their density was lower. Some (ir) DYN B or DYN A fibers were detected in atria and ventricles, merely restricted to the vasculature. Again, relatively high background

staining may have caused underestimation of dynorphinergic/neoendorphinergic neuronal systems.
With the exception of MSH, all (ir) peptides were localized in small diameter fibers of C and A delta class. MSH was restricted to large diameter myelinated fibers and absent from neuroeffector junctions.
For further details and differential distribution of (ir) peptides in nerves supplying the different segments of coronary vasculature, see Table 3.

b) Paracrine systems

Opioid peptides were the predominant (ir) peptides in paracrine systems of the heart as revealed by the presence of (ir) LE in paraganglionic cells (Table 3) of intracardiac ganglia (in the sinuatrial junction, in the interatrial septum, along coronary arteries in coronary sulci and coronary sinus) and of cardiac chemoreceptor glomera (in aortopulmonary and pericoronary areas). DYN 1—8 was another (ir) form of opioid peptides present in paraganglionic cells. Cardiac glomera were extensively innervated by fibers containing the majority of the (ir) peptides investigated.

c) Interrelation of peptidergic innervation to the endocrine heart

By analyzing consecutive sections of right and left atria and auricles alternately stained for (ir) ANF and (ir) peptides it was observed that NPY was the prevailing neuronal cardiac peptide which had widespread interrelation to endocrine atrial cells of the heart containing (ir) ANF (Table 3, Fig. 1), whereas nerves containing other peptides had indirect and rare contacts to myoendocrine cells (Table 3, Fig. 5).

d) Interspecies variations

With the exception of the opioid peptides and minor quantitative differences, the pattern of peptidergic innervation described for the guinea-pig heart was essentially representative for all species investigated. The density of (ir) NPY innervation was higher in the dog and cat than in guinea-pig heart.
Interestingly, human atria contained all the neuronal peptides found in the guinea-pig, except for opioid peptides, which could not be investigated because of high background staining due to immersion fixation. Also in the human heart, there was close interrelation of NPY-containing nerves to atrial myoendocrine cells. Immunoreactivities for opioid peptides were present in dog, pig and cat hearts in similar locations to the guinea-pig but could not be identified in rat or rabbit heart.

Discussion

The present immunohistochemical study has extensively characterized the multiplicity, differential histotopography and neuroeffector relations of peptidergic innervation in the

Table 3. Histotopography of selected immunoreactive peptides in the guinea-pig heart.

	SP	SK	CGRP	NPY	VIP/PHI	LE
intrinsic cardiac ganglia						
ganglionic cells	—/+	—	—/+	+/++	++	—/+
varicose fibers	+++	+++	+++	++++	++	++
paraganglionic cells	—/+	—	—	—	—	++
cardiac glomera						
paraganglionic cells	—/+	—	—	—	—	++
varicose fibers	++	+	++	++	++	+
neuroeffector junctions						
SA-node	+	+	++	+++	++	+
AV-node	+	+	++	+++	++	+
atrial muscle and endocrine cells	—/+	—	++	++++	+	—/+
ventricular muscle cells	—	—	+	+++	—	—
neuroeffector junctions with coronary vasculature						
epicardial arteries	+++	++	+++	++++	+	+
intramural arteries	+++	++	+++	++++	++	+
arterioles	++	+	++	++++	++	+
capillaries	—/+	—	+	++	+	+
venules	+	—	+	++	+	+
veins	++	+	++	+	+	+
interstitial nerves						
myocardium	+++	+	+++	+++	+	+
conduction system	++++	++	++++	++++	++	++
endocardium	++++	++	++++	+++	+	++
valves	++++	++	++++	+++	+	++
epicardium	+++	++	+++	++	+	++
pericardium	+++	++	+++	++	+	++

Subjective rating scale of immunoreactive varicose nerve fibers or cells: — absent; + infrequent; ++ frequent; +++ very frequent; ++++ abundant

mammalian heart. By having monitored the extracardiac distribution of peptides in neurons which have connections to the heart, some conclusions can be drawn about the origin, interrelation to classical sympathetic/parasympathetic systems, and function of cardiac neuronal peptides.

Sympathetic cardiac efferents

Extrinsic cardiac NPY, absent from spinal sensory ganglia and vagal nerve, is apparently of exclusive postganglionic sympathetic origin (1, 6, cf. 15). In the vicinity of cardiac ganglia, where NPY is found in some ganglionic cells, it is impossible to differentiate intrinsic and extrinsic NPY fiber systems. Because of its high concentration in the heart of several species (1), reflected in the high density of fibers containing NPY, it has to be

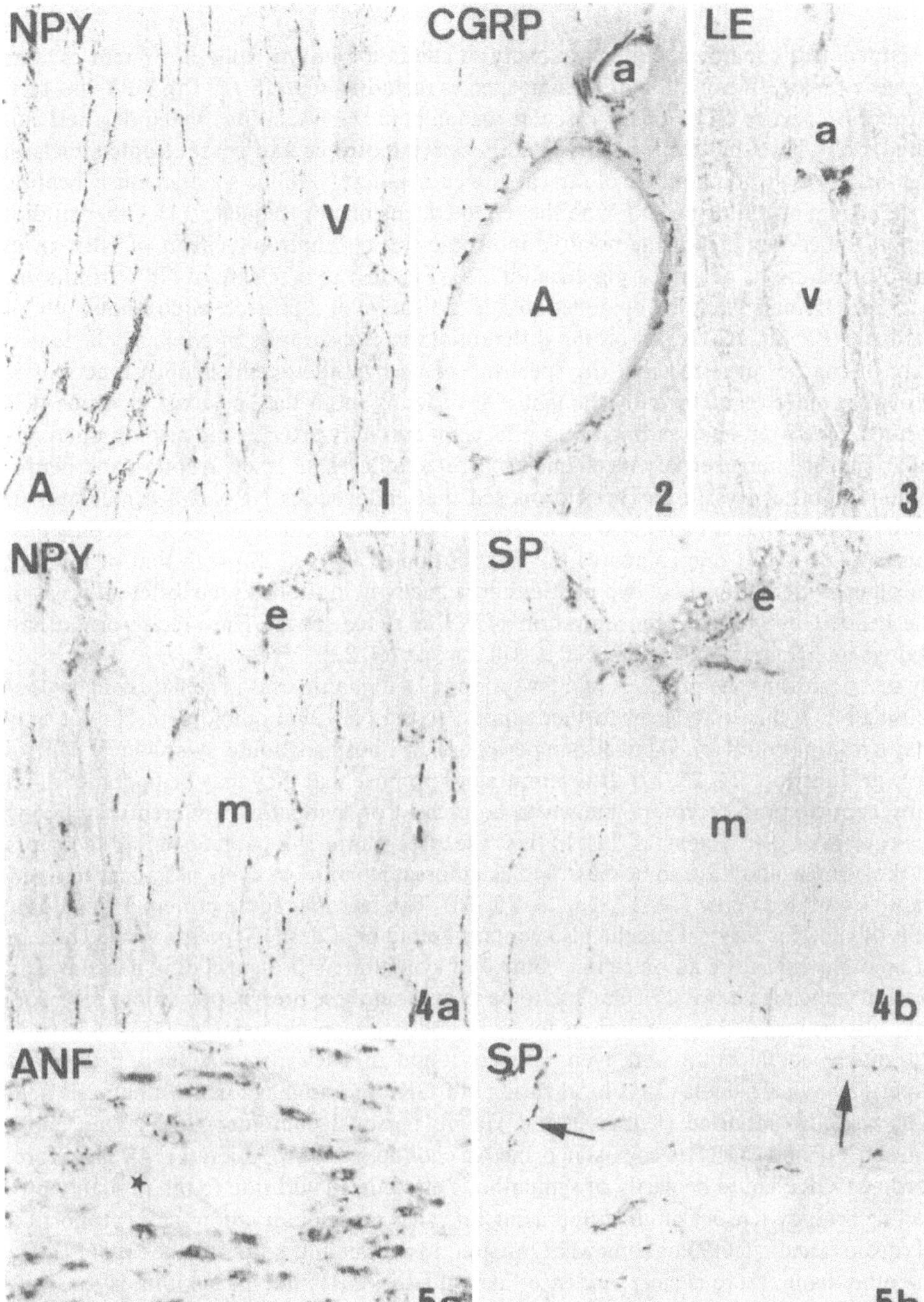

Distribution of (ir) peptides in different areas of the mammalian heart. **Fig. 1.** Right atrium of cat. Numerous varicose fibers in contact with myocardiocytes, capillaries and a branching intramural artery (A). A few fibers innervating a small vein (V) (× 500). **Fig. 2.** Dog ventricle. Neuroeffector junctions to intramural artery (A) and arteriole (a) (× 500). **Fig. 3.** Right atrium of guinea-pig; arteriole (a), venule (v) (× 1250). **Fig. 4.** Distribution of (ir) peptides in adjacent longitudinal sections of juxtaendocardial papillary muscle of guinea-pig. Note differential densities of varicose nerve fibers in muscular (m) vs. endocardial (e) parts (× 800). **Fig. 5.** Distribution of (ir) peptides in consecutive sections of right auricle of guinea-pig. SP in perivascular regions where no myoendocrine cells are present (*) and in loose connection to myoendocrine cells (arrows) (× 500).

regarded as the major peptide cotransmitter candidate in sympathetic efferent cardiac nerves of many, if not all, mammalian species including man (6, cf. 15). NPY has constrictor properties on coronary vascular segments in the intact innervated dog and isolated rabbit heart but lacks positive and negative inotropic and chronotropic effects in papillary muscle preparations of rat, cat and guinea-pig (1). In the spontaneously beating right atrium of guinea-pig, NPY neither effected tension nor frequency (1). Other studies report the contrary, showing positive inotropic and chronotropic effects of NPY in in vitro preparations of guinea-pig atria (cf. 15). The fact that release of NPY from sympathetic efferents could be demonstrated is indicative of a possible endogenous role of cardiac NPY (cf. 15). Based on the differential histotopography of NPY, as elucidated here, it can be suggested that the spectrum of its hypothetic endogenous functions is probably wider than currently thought if it is acting in all the key areas in which it is located. One would expect prevailing effects on coronary arteries and also on microcirculation, peripheral sensory mechanisms, cardiac reflexes, chemoperception and neuroendocrine influences. It has been proposed that endogenous NPY is a comediator of noradrenaline, but it could also be a cardiac candidate for non-adrenergic neurotransmission (cf. 15). If one compares the distribution of NT (cf. 22) with that of NPY, it becomes evident that these two peptides are equally ubiquitous in the different areas of the heart. However, the concentration of NT is much lower. The precise origin and endogenous function of cardiac NT is still unclear (cf. 22).

By demonstrating the presence of a few principal ganglionic cells in stellate ganglia containing NEO, this study gives further support to the view that opioid peptides not only play a role in central (cf. 9) but also in peripheral, i.e. postganglionic, sympathetic control of heart function (24, 25, 27). It is tempting to propose that they may be operational on presynaptic opioid receptors, known to be present on sympathetic efferents supplying the cardiovascular system (cf. 11). In this case, presynaptic sympathetic opioid receptors in the heart would have to be classified as autoreceptors, most likely of kappa, but perhaps also of delta type (11, 12, 16, 24, 25, 26). The fact that some principal ganglionic cells of superior cervical ganglia also contain opioid peptides (13) points to the concept of opioid presynaptic autoreceptor control of sympathetic postganglionic neurons as a general principle (cf. 11, 25). One has to be aware that these presynaptic opioid receptors may also be targeted by the various forms of endocrine opioid peptides (16).

Puzzlingly, somatostatin and even SP were found in a few postganglionic neurons of superior cervical ganglia (3). A localization of CGRP in postganglionic sympathetic neurons was also reported (Kummer and Heym, personal communication). One paper showed VIP and CGRP to coexist in principal cholinergic neurons of rats (14). Therefore, cardiac CGRP could be partly of sympathetic efferent, in addition to the probably prevailing primary sensory origin. Supporting this view is the observation that a proportion of cardiovascular CGRP is somewhat resistant to capsaicin treatment in the rat (17). On the other hand, there is clear evidence that cardiac CGRP, like tachykinin, is sensitive to capsaicin and therefore sensory (8, 15). In this context it is necessary to point out that this study showed the presence of CGRP in a few postganglionic sympathetic neurons in man but not in other species. Taken altogether, this indicates that the chemical phenotype of sympathetic neurons and, consequently, of cardiac sympathetic efferents, is not yet completely understood. We have to consider the transmitter- or neuromediator-candidacy of other peptides and of non-peptidic substances like ATP (cf. 5, 15). The same is probably true of sympathetic cardiac afferents.

Sympathetic cardiac afferents

Cardiac neuronal opioids (24) could stem from primary sensory neurons of cervical and thoracic dorsal root ganglia which project to the heart via sympathetic nerves, since the presence of prodynorphin-opioid peptides in primary afferents was demonstrated in some species (23, 26). Interestingly, these opioid peptides were shown to coexist with SP and CGRP in a subpopulation of primary afferents (cf. 25, 26). Since retrograde tracing and capsaicin depletion clearly have shown that SP is present in cardiac sympathetic afferents which have their perikarya in dorsal root ganglia (6) it is argued that the same constellation is true for those opioid peptides (26). It is suggested that tachykinins, CGRP and opioid peptides serve nociceptive/antinociceptive mechanisms in cardiac sympathetic afferents. This is a novel hypothesis in the search for the cardiac nociceptor (4). Although coexisting, tachykinins and CGRP probably fulfill differential roles in the peripheral cardiac endings of these afferents (cf. 15). CGRP seems to have cardioexcitatory effects and increases cardiac muscle tension. This effect is not shared by tachykinins. On the other hand, tachykinins and CGRP could be synergistic in their antidromic effects on coronary circulation including microcirculatory events, such as plasma extravasation, which may play a neglected role in pathophysiology. Reflex loops of these afferents to cardiac and sympathetic ganglia are also conceivable. It has been argued that endogenous opioid peptides could inhibit the release of co-existing mediators, like tachykinins and CGRP, via presynaptic autoreceptors of the kappa and delta type, on both their cardiac and spinal endings (26). This could be a primary sensory mechanism which may explain some of the relationships between cardiovascular and pain regulatory systems (25, 28 and Millan, this volume). In principle, any of the growing number of mediator candidates detected in perikarya of spinal ganglia (cf. 5, 15, 25) which give rise to C or A delta fibers is a potential cardiac sensory messenger. In contrast, MSH which is absent from varicose fibers, is a candiate for mediating trophic rather than transmitter or neuromodulator functions (cf. 25), a role which, however, may also be shared by some of the other cardiac peptides (5, 15, 25).

Vagal cardiac efferents and afferents

Retrograde tracing and immunohistochemistry have demonstrated that SP and other tachykinins are contained in vagal cardiac afferents with perikarya in the nodose ganglion and projecting centrally to the nucleus of the solitary tract (6, 15). It remains to be established whether opioid peptides are following the same pattern. It will be also mandatory to unequivocally differentiate these and other peptides as regards their location in afferent vs efferent vagal cardiac fibers. In principle, this has to be done with any cardiac peptide which is also present in the vagal nerve. Vagal cardiac afferents containing tachykinins probably play a crucial role in chemo- and baroafferent functions of the heart (6, 22) and, like sympathetic afferents, could link their afferent information via reflex collaterals to intrinsic and sympathetic ganglia (22).

Intrinsic cardiac neurons

The first peptide detected in intrinsic cardiac neurons was VIP (20) which was confirmed in this study and complemented by the demonstration of coexisting PHI which is related to the VIP precursor (15). It remains to be established whether intrinsic cardiac VIP/PHI neurons are cholinergic. VIP/PHI intracardiac fibers can be intrinsic and/or extrinsic. In the latter case, they could stem from sympathetic efferents or afferents. A vagal origin is also conceivable (cf. 22). The interrelation to intrinsic NPY neurons also needs to be further investigated. It is not unlikely that other peptidergic intrinsic neurons will be detected with even more sensitive methods than employed here.

Paracrine and endocrine cardiac systems

The paraganglionic cells of the heart may represent a so far neglected source of cardiac peptides. It would be not surprising if future studies could find more peptides in this disseminated system of APUD cells (cf. 25) than shown in this study. Preliminary observations in my laboratory indicate that neurotensin, tachykinins and others are cardiac paracrine candidates. Most interestingly, the concentration of messenger RNA for proenkephalin is higher in the rat heart than in the brain (10). These authors argued that paraganglionic cells could be a source, to which this and another study by us (25) give support. The interrelation of peptidergic nerves to paraganglionic cells of cardiac ganglia and of chemoreceptor glomera indicate that paracrine functions of the heart are under extensive neuronal control and vice versa. It remains to be established whether there is also a peptidergic nervous control of the release of ANF from endocrine atrial cells. In this respect, the present study points to the possible contribution of NPY and perhaps also of VIP/PHI (Table 3), but less likely of tachykinins or of CGRP because varicose nerve fibers containing the latter form only irregular neuroeffector junctions with endocrine cells producing ANF. Interrelations of sympathetic innervation with the role of cardiac ANF have been recently reported (19).

General functional implications and future perspectives

Cardiac peptides have to be generally regarded as important novel mediator candidates contributing to multiple neuronal cybernetics of the heart. The chemoanatomical pattern indicates that they are not merely acting independently from, but in concert with, each other and with classical transmitters (cf. 15). On the other hand, an independent non-adrenergic non-cholinergic transmitter function cannot be excluded. The great multiplicity of peptides would allow a sophisticated "fine tuning" of a variety of functions which can be expected to be even more complex than described here since the list of potential neuromediators is still growing and now also includes substances like ATP and even leukotrienes (5, 15).
From what is known about the distinct neuropharmacological profiles of the peptidic messengers investigated in this study, it appears deducible that they may serve distinct physiological and, perhaps more importantly, pathophysiological functions. In this context, it is paticularly noteworthy that the human heart was also found to be extensively innervated by peptidergic nerves. Therefore, it seems appropriate to suggest that disturbances in neuronal peptide metabolism combined with malproportions in cardiac mediator "cocktails" may have etiological significance in clinical situations such as silent

ischemia, coronary spasm, coronary heart disease without occlusion (syndrome X; cf. 18) and certain forms of arrhythmias. Peptides like SP and CGRP are good candidates for the mediation of cardiac pain in man which, speculatively, may be suppressed peripherally by an endogenous opioid system of the heart itself; a hypothesis, which points to the relationship between cardiovascular and pain regulatory systems (25, 28; Millan, this volume). Such mechanisms may even be important in the pathophysiological events accompanying coronary heart disease or heart attack. Clearly, the pathophysiological and clinical significance of peptides and other novel cardiac mediators needs further experimental elucidation which may lead to the development of new cardiac therapeutics.

Acknowledgements

For donation of some of the antisera I would like to thank A. Herz and coworkers D. C. Liebisch, B. Seizinger, R. M. Arendt (Munich) and E. Weber, Oregon. The technical assistance of Mrs. A. Leibold and critical reading of the manuscript by D. Nohr are gratefully mentioned.

References

1. Allen JM, Gjörstrup P, Björkman JA, Ek L, Abrahamsson T, Bloom SR (1986) Studies on cardiac distribution and function of neuropeptide Y. Acta Physiol Scand 126: 405—411
2. Arendt RM, Stangl E, Zähringer J, Liebisch DC, Herz A (1985) Demonstration and characterization of alpha-human atrial natriuretic factor in human plasma FEBS Lett 189: 57—61
3. Ariano MA, Kenney SL (1985) Peptide coincidence in rat superior cervical ganglion. Brain Res 340: 181—185
4. Baker DG, Coleridge HM, Coleridge JCG, Nerdrum T (1980) Search for a cardiac nociceptor: Stimulation by Bradykinin of sympathetic afferent nerve endings in the heart of the cat. J Physiol 306: 519—536
5. Burnstock G (1986) The changing face of autonomic neurotransmission. Acta Physiol Scand 126: 67—91
6. Dalsgaard C, Franco-Cereceda A, Saria A, Lundberg JM; Theodorsson-Norheim E, Hökfelt T (1986) Distribution and origin of substance P- and neuropeptide Y-immunoreactive nerves in the guinea-pig heart. Cell Tissue Res 243: 477—485
7. Forssmann WG, Reinecke M, Weihe E (1982) Cardiac innervation. In: Bloom SR, Polak JM, Lindenlaub E (eds) Systemic role of regulatory peptides. Schattauer, Stuttgart, New York, p 329—349
8. Gibbins IL, Furness JB, Costa M, MacIntyre I, Hillyard CJ, Girgis S (1985) Co-localization of calcitonin gene-related peptide-like immunoreactivity with substance P in cutaneous, vascular and visceral sensory neurons of guinea pigs. Neurosci Lett 57: 125—130
9. Holaday JW (1983) Cardiovascular effects of endogenous opiate systems. Ann Rev Pharmacol Toxicol 23: 541—594
10. Howells RD, Kilpatrick DL, Bailey LC, Noe M, Udenfriend S (1986) Proenkephalin mRNA in rat heart. Proc Natl Acad Sci USA 83: 1960—1963
11. Illes P, Bettermann R, Ramme D: Sympathoinhibitory opioid receptors in the cardiovascular system. In: Buckley JP, Ferrario C (eds) Brain Peptides and Catecholamines in Cardiovascular Regulation in normal and disease states. Raven Press, Oxford (in press)
12. Kosterlitz HW (1985) Opioid peptides and their receptors. Proc R Soc Lond B 225: 27—40
13. Kummer W, Heym C, Colombo M, Lang R (1986) Immunohistochemical evidence for extrinsic and intrinsic opioid systems in the guinea pig superior cervical ganglion. Anat Embryol 174: 401—405

14. Landis SC, Fredieu JR (1986) Coexistence of calcitonin gene-related peptide and vasoactive intestinal peptide in cholinergic sympathetic innervation of rat sweat glands. Brain Res 377: 177—181
15. Lundberg JM, Hökfelt T (1986) Multiple co-existence of peptides and classical transmitters in peripheral autonomic and sensory neurons — functional and pharmacological implications. In: Hökfelt T, Fuxe K, Pernow B (eds) Progress in Brain Research Vol 68, Elsevier Amsterdam, New York, Oxford, p 241—262
16. Millan MJ, Herz A (1986) The endocrinology of the opioids. Int Rev Neurobiol 26: 1—84
17. Mulderry PK, Ghatei MA, Rodrigo J, Allen JM, Rosenfeld MG, Polak JM, Bloom SR (1985) Calcitonin gene-related peptide in cardiovascular tissues of the rat. Neuroscience 14: 947—954
18. Opherk D, Zebe H, Weihe E, Mall G, Dürr C, Gravert B, Mehmel H, Schwarz F, Kübler W (1981) Reduced coronary dilatory capacity and ultrastructural changes of the myocardium in patients with angina pectoris but normal coronary arteriograms. Circulation 63: 817—825
19. Sasaki A, Kida O, Kangawa K, Matsuo H, Tanaka K (1986) Involvement of sympathetic nerves in cardiosuppressive effects of alpha-human atrial natriuretic polypeptide (alpha-hANP) in anesthetized rats. Eur J Pharmacol 120: 345—349
20. Weihe E, Reinecke M (1981) Peptidergic innervation of the mammalian sinus nodes: Vasoactive intestinal polypeptide, neurotensin, substance P. Neurosci Lett 26: 283—288
21. Weihe E, Reinecke M, Opherk D, Forssmann WG (1981) Peptidergic innervation (substance P) in the human heart. J Mol Cell Cardiol 13: 331—333
22. Weihe E, Reinecke M, Forssmann WG (1984) Distribution of vasoactive intestinal polypeptide-like immunoreactivity in the mammalian heart: interrelation with neurotensin- and substance P-like immunreactive nerves. Cell Tissue Res 236: 527—540
23. Weihe E, Hartschuh W, Weber E (1985) Prodynorphin opioid peptides in small somatosensory primary afferents of guinea-pig. Neurosci Lett 58: 347—352
24. Weihe E, McKnight AT, Corbett AD, Kosterlitz HW (1985) Proenkephalin- and prodynorphin-derived opioid peptides in guinea-pig heart. Neuropeptides 5: 453—456
25. Weihe E, Hartschuh W, Gauweiler B, Fink T, Nohr D: Multiplicity of opioidergic pathways related to cardiovascular innervation: differential contribution of all three opioid precursors. In: Stumpe KO, Kraft K (eds) Proceedings of the Satellite Symposium to the 11th Scientific Meeting of ISH 1986, Opioid Peptides and Blood Pressure Control. Springer Berlin-Heidelberg-New York (in press)
26. Weihe E, Leibold A, Nohr D, Fink T, Gauweiler B. Coexistence of prodynorphin-opioid peptides and substance P in primary sensory afferents of guinea-pigs. NIDA Monograph (in press)
27. Xiang JZ, Archelos J, Lang RE (1984) Enkephalins in the heart. Clin and Exper Theory and Practice A6 (10&11): 1883—1888
28. Zamir N, Maixner W (1986) The relationship between cardiovascular and pain regulatory systems. In: Kelly DD (ed) Stress induced analgesia. The New York Academy of Sciences, New York, pp 371—384

Author's address:
Prof. Dr. E. Weihe
Anatomisches Institut der
Johannes Gutenberg-Universität
Saarstraße 19—21
6500 Mainz

Pathophysiology of ischemic cardiac pain

A. Malliani

Istituto Ricerche Cardiovascolari, CNR; Patologia Medica, Centro "Fidia", Ospedale "L. Sacco", University of Milan, Italy

In recent years experimental models have provided crucial data for choosing between "intensity" or "specificity" as the property for characterizing the basic afferent code transmitting cardiac nociception: a choice that is fundamental to our interpretation of the mystery that in clinics still envelops the elusive link between myocardial ichemia and pain (12).

The characteristics of these two hypotheses have already been summarized (13, 14). In short, the intensity mechanism, the most obvious to be formulated, assumes that pain results from an excessive stimulation of receptive structures. Alternatively, pain may be conceived of as a specific sensation, that is the product of the excitation of a well-defined nociceptive apparatus, the functional characteristics of which make it responsive only to a limited class of events, the stimuli that are "noxious", the term used by Sherrington (20). On the somatic side there are findings suggesting that both certain primary afferent units and certain higher order cells to which they project are excited solely or most effectively by stimuli strong enough to threaten the integrity of tissue (3, 22). However, these facts do not deny the fundamental importance played by other modulatory mechanisms upon nociceptive information (29).

From a conceptual point of view, over these theories another traditional general principle seems to reign, assigning to pain a protective or self-preserving value to the organism. Extrapolated to the viscera, and in particular to the heart, this view implies the existence of a "warning system" (4). In this article I should like to make the following points, based on experimental data:

1. Specific cardiac nociceptors are unlikely to exist.
2. The peculiarities of the afferent code transmitting nociception are still a matter for hypotheses; however, the incapability of this afferent information to signal damage and danger constantly and without ambiguity, suggests that the "warning" reflects a subsidiary rather than a fundamental function.

Do specific cardiac nociceptors exist?

This question can be explored experimentally. Peripheral sensors purely nociceptive in function should have no background discharge (3) as a consequence of their high threshold, which renders them unresponsive to normal events and excitable only with strong stimuli: those which are likely to be noxious. Thus, the recruitment of their silent fibers by a peripheral stimulus could represent an unambiguous signal to the centers. As was briefly recalled above, there are some findings, on the somatic side, which could be interpreted along these lines.

Recently, an intense electrophysiological investigation was carried out into the properties of either the small myelinated or unmyelinated ventricular sympathetic afferent fibers, i.e. the afferent fibers that are more likely to convey cardiac nociception. In our hands these fibers always appeared to possess a mechanosensitivity that makes them responsive to normal hemodynamic events. Coronary occlusion or intracoronary administration of bradykinin, i.e. possible algesic stimuli, increased markedly their tonic impulse activity, but a recruitment of silent afferent fibers could not be appreciated (11, 13, 14).

Thus it seemed to us that ventricular sympathetic sensory endings behaved like low-threshold polymodal receptors. This matter, however, is under debate. Uchida and Murao (28) and Coleridge and his colleagues (1, 18) maintain that some afferents appear exquisitely sensitive to chemicals, like bradykinin, and thus particularly apt to function as pure nociceptors. In our opinion, this population of so-called primarily chemosensitive receptors is only an extreme of a continuum spectrum: what is crucial is that they generate a spontaneous impulse activity and display some sensitivity to mechanical events. Given the complexity of the relationship between receptive endings and the ventricular muscle it should not be surprising to find a whole spectrum of possibilities, having on one side prevalent mechanosensitivity and on the other chemosensitivity. However, the artificial distinction of a continuum in two populations seems to provide a rather sterile tool.

Moreover, some of the experimental results that we will report cannot be reconciled with the hypothesis of the existence of primarily chemosensitive cardiac nociceptors.

Experimental preparations and adequacy of the stimulus

Pain is a conscious experience that can be explored only indirectly with experimental preparations; accordingly, different opinions on peripheral nociceptive mechanisms are often the result of different preparations.

In lightly anesthetized animals or those recovering from anesthesia, it is quite easy to obtain behavioral reactions by applying stimuli likely to be noxious to the heart. Decades ago, Sutton and Lueth (27) observed that traction on a ligature placed around a coronary artery could elicit "evidence of severe pain" after a very few seconds, this latency suggesting a mechanical nature of the stimulus. On the contrary, in long-term experiments, coronary occlusion performed through implanted occluders does not produce pain reactions, at least during the initial minute of occlusion. Clearly, in all these cases it is difficult to quantify how noxious the stimulus is.

The nonapeptide bradykinin was likely to furnish a remarkable tool for the experimental analysis of this subject, since it could be quantified when used as a stimulus. Indeed, the initial observation by Guzman et al. (8) appeared extremely sound and easy to interpret, describing how intracoronary injections of bradykinin produced overt pain reactions in dogs recovering from recent surgery.

However, when the intracoronary injections of bradykinin were administered to conscious dogs after full recovery from the operation necessary for their instrumentation, a marked pressor sympathetic reflex was elicited but in the absence of pain reaction (20). Similarly, the injection of bradykinin into the pericardial sac induced a pressor reflex in absence of signs of pain.

The importance of recovery from anesthesia and recent surgery in explaining these apparent discrepancies, was explored in a few experiments by injecting bradykinin during the first week after surgery. At that time the animals' recovery was still incomplete and some animals exhibited vocalisation and agitation suggesting a pain reaction. This behavioral response was no longer present when the same animals were tested again, later on, at a time of complete recovery. Thus, a similar stimulus appears algogenic or not, depending exclusively on the specific experimental set.

A new hypothesis

The observation that, under appropriate experimental conditions, an excitation of the cardiac sensory supply, likely to be massive, did not elicit signs of pain appears to represent a total defeat for the specificity theory, at least if nociceptors were postulated to be exquisitely sensitive to algogenic substances (1, 18, 28).

On the other hand, the intensity theory also appears, as such, too naive. As a working hypothesis we proposed (11) a modified version of the intensity mechanism. Cardiac pain would result from the extreme excitation of a spatially restricted population of afferent sympathetic fibers: hence from an afferent code based on a peculiar spatio-temporal pattern. Hence, an intense excitation of afferent sympathetic fibers would be more likely to reach the effectiveness of a nociceptive code when characterized by spatial heterogeneity. Therefore, besides the extension and severity of ischemia, which would determine the background of the afferent excitation, further crucial stimulations of the sensory endings could occur in those regions where mechanical stretching is maximal, or where an abnormal vasomotion or a distortion of a highly innervated vascular structure takes place. Indeed, in the course of one experiment, a peculiar position maintained by the coronary cannula, lying just outside the wall of the vessel and below the adventitia, determined that each minute injection distended a very limited portion of the vessel. In this case, injections of saline and not only of bradykinin evoked a pain reaction, even after full recovery from surgery (15).

The implications of this hypothesis could be relevant. When the activation of the cardiac sympathetic afferent fibers is widely and homogeneously distributed, as in the case of intracoronary injection of bradykinin or, more currently, during a marked increase in arterial pressure, central inhibitory modulations (29) would prevent the onset of pain. Conversely, recent thoracic surgery, by inducing a localized somatic afferent barrage, could decisively contribute, through mechanisms of convergence at the spinal level, to genesis of the algogenic code. As to the heart, to reiterate this point, a spatially restricted mechanical abnormality localized in the myocardium or in the abundantly innervated coronary arteries could lead to pain more efficiently than a more widely distributed myocardial ischemia with its chemical component. Along this line of reasoning, one could also explain why even a restricted coronary denervation accompanying by-pass interventions could produce a strategic interruption of the afferent channel, thus leading to the disappearance of pain in the absence of improvements in ventricular function.

Clinical observations

In recent years, monitoring of patients exhibiting spontaneous and reversible electrocardiographic changes typical of episodes of transient myocardial ischemia, has offered a powerful tool for investigating the clinical consistence of the symptom cardiac pain. It was soon recognized that the hemodynamic profile of the crises could appear substantially similar, whether or not accompanied by pain (7, 16). Quite often, hypertension and tachycardia occurring during the episode, unrelated to pain, appeared to represent a pressor reflex from the heart (11, 20) rather than a "vasomotor storm" (9). However, it was also clear that there was no way of predicting whether or not pain would accompany the episode. More recently (17) it was recognized that several factors are likely to be implicated in the genesis of pain, such as the duration of the episode or the severity of ischemia. For instance, ischemic episodes were usually painless when shorter than 3 minutes and associated with increases in left ventricular filling pressure smaller than 7 mm Hg. However, above these values the onset of pain was unpredictable. In short, duration and severity of ischemia appeared necessary but not sufficient factors. On the other hand, angioplasty in humans, a sort of acute experimental ischemia, induces pain only in a variable manner (26).

In the current clinical debate on the causes of the exclusiveness of cardiac pain (12), factors like subjective pain threshold (5, 24) and peripheral neuropathies (19), are surely worth a detailed analysis, as much as the controversial role of the endorphines (30).

However, it should be appreciated that the most crucial model is not offered by the asymptomatic patients, but by the asymptomatic episodes. Indeed, the temporal sequence of ischemic episodes, sometimes more than one per hour, about 70% of which are unaccompanied by pain (2, 17), seems to furnish a most intriguing clinical puzzle in which what appears to be a stochastic absence of pain cannot be attributed to peripheral neuropathies or to any other stable functional condition of the individual, such as high pain threshold.

It is our hypothesis that the site of this elusiveness could be in the heart, where apparently similar ischemic episodes could in fact activate quite different afferent codes as a result of the extreme complexity of the mechanical and chemical events. Unfortunately, even the most careful measurements at the level of the heart are unlikely, at the moment, to give a key in terms of the afferent nociceptive code.

Still, many more attempts are necessary in order to correlate what can be measured at the periphery with the onset of pain. In this regard it could be very interesting to monitor also the newly individuated indexes of sympathetic and vagal activities (21). In considering all this, it should be borne in mind that pain is not an all or nothing sense but embraces a whole spectrum of sensations (24).

In this article I am not equating pain in the course of transient myocardial ischemia and in the course of myocardial infarction, when the accumulation of chemicals is likely to be massive, and the destruction of nerve terminals is also likely to contribute to an intense and spatially heterogenous afferent excitation; yet reports on myocardial infarction pioneered as early as the 'thirties (6) the clinical suspicion that cardiac pain could fail to signal myocardial necrosis.

A few conclusions

The "spatio-temporal pattern" hypothesis explains why no stimulus acting on the heart should be expected, because of its quality, to elicit pain as a rule.

There is little question that malignant arrhythmias are among the most important risk factors for sudden death (10): the severity of arrhythmias can often be appreciated by a patient, such an appraisal being totally independent of pain but rather dependent on the degree of awareness and culture.

Thus the "warning system" does not signal appropriately either damage or danger: this porosity seems to denote a different biological purpose for the afferent cardiac fibers and in particular for their sympathetic contingent. This could well be their participation in the neural regulation of circulation (11).

Clinicians know how to use a symptom when present; the question is also how to accept its absence. Pathophysiology, based on recent findings, can appreciate, as one face of reality, what appears to be a failure with respect to a more protective pathophysiological doctrine.

References

1. Baker DG, Coleridge HM, Coleridge JCG, Nerdrum T (1980) Search for a cardiac nociceptor: stimulation by bradykinin of sympathetic afferent nerve endings in the heart of the cat. J Physiol 306: 519—536
2. Biagini A, L'Abbate A, Emdin M, Testa R, Mazzei MG; Carpeggiani C, Michelassi C, Andreotti F, Marchesi C, Benassi A (1986) Electrocardiographic monitoring: temporal versus spatial information and data processing. Can J Cardiol (suppl A): 142A—148A
3. Burgess PR, Perl ER (1973) Cutaneous mechanoreceptors and nociceptors. In: A Iggo (ed), Handbook of Sensory Physiology; Vol 2, Somatosensory System, Springer-Verlag, Berlin, pp 29—78
4. Cohn PF (1980) Silent myocardial ischemia in patients with a defective anginal warning system. Am J Cardiol 45: 697—702
5. Droste C, Greenlee MW, Roskam H (1986) A defective angina pectoris pain warning system: experimental findings of ischemic and electrical pain test. Pain 26: 199—209
6. Gorham LW, Martin SJ (1938) Coronary occlusion with and without pain. Arch Int Med 62: 821—839
7. Guazzi M, Polese A, Fiorentini C, Magrini F, Bartorelli C (1971) Left ventricular performance and related haemodynamic changes in Prinzmetal's variant angina pectoris. Brit Heart J 33: 84—94
8. Guzman F, Braun C, Lim RKS (1962) Visceral pain and the pseudoaffective response to intra-arterial injection of bradykinin and other algesic agents. Arch Inter Pharmacol, 136: 353—384
9. Lewis T (1931) Angina pectoris associated with high blood pressure and its relief by amyl nitrate; with a note on Nothnagel's syndrome. Heart, 15: 305—327
10. Lown B (1979) Sudden cardiac death: the major challenge confronting contemporary cardiology. Am J Cardiol 43: 313—328
11. Malliani A (1982) Cardiovascular sympathetic afferent fibres. Rev Physiol Biochem Pharmacol 94: 11—74
12. Malliani A (1986) The elusive link between transient myocardial ischemia and pain. Circulation 73: 201—204

13. Malliani A, Lombardi F (1982) Consideration of the fundamental mechanisms eliciting cardiac pain. Am Heart J 103: 575—578
14. Malliani A, Pagani M, Lombardi F (1984) Visceral versus somatic mechanisms. In: Wall PD, Melzack A (eds) Textbook of Pain, Churchill Livingstone, Edinburgh, pp 100—109
15. Malliani A, Lombardi F, Pagani M (1986) Sensory innervation of the heart; In: Cervero F, Morrison FB (eds) Progress in Brain Research, Vol 67, pp 39—58
16. Maseri A, Severi S, De Nes M, L'Abbate A, Chierchia S, Marzilli M, Ballestra AM, Parodi O, Biagini A, Distante A (1978) "Variant" angina: one aspect of a continuous spectrum of vasospastic myocardial ischemia. Am J Cardiol 42: 1019—1035
17. Maseri A, Chierchia S, Davies G, Glazier J (1985) Mechanisms of ischemic cardiac pain and of silent myocardial ischemia. Am J Med 79: 7—11
18. Nerdrum T, Baker DG, Coleridge HM, Coleridge JCG (1986) Interaction of bradykinin and prostaglandin E_1 and cardiac pressor reflex and sympathetic afferents. Am J Physiol 250: R815—R822
19. Nesto RW, Phillips RT (1986) Asymptomatic myocardial ischemia in diabetic patients. Am J Med 80 (suppl 4c): 40—47
20. Pagani M, Pizzinelli P, Furlan R, Guzzetti S, Rimoldi O, Sandrone G, Malliani A 1985 Analysis of the pressor sympathetic reflex produced by intracoronary injections of bradykinin in conscious dogs. Circ Res 56: 175—183
21. Pagani M, Lombadi F, Guzzetti S, Rimoldi O, Furland R, Pizzinelli P, Sandrone G, Malfatto G, Dell'Orto S, Piccaluga E, Turiel M, Baselli G, Cerutti S, Malliani A (1986) Power spectral analysis of heart rate and arterial pressure variabilities as a marker of sympatho-vagal interaction in man and conscious dog. Circ Res 59: 178—193
22. Perl ER (1971) Is pain a specific sensation? J Psychiatr Res 8: 273—287
23. Procacci P, Zoppi M, Padeletti L and Maresca M (1976) Myocardial infarction without pain. A study of the sensory functions of the upper limbs. Pain 2: 309—313
24. Procacci P, Zoppi M (1984) Heart Pain. In: Wall PD, Melzack R (eds) Textbook of Pain, Churchill Livingstone, Edinburgh, pp 309—318
25. Sherrington CS (1906) The integrative action of the nervous system. Yale University Press, New Haven
26. Sigwart V, Grbic M, Payot M, Goy J-J, Essinger A, Fischer A (1984) Ischemic events during coronary artery balloon obstruction. In: Rutishauser, W., Roskamm H (eds) Silent myocardial ischemia. Springer-Verlag Berlin, pp 29—36
27. Sutton DC, Lueth HC (1930) Experimental production of pain on excitation of the heart and great vessels. Archs Intern Med 45: 827—867
28. Uchida Y, Murao S (1974) Bradykinin induced excitation of afferent cardiac sympathetic nerve fibers. Jpn Heart J 15: 84—91
29. Wall PD Melzack R (eds) (1984) Textbook of pain. Churchill Livingstone, Edinburgh
30. Weidinger F, Hammerle A, Sochor H, Smetana R, Frass M, Glogar D (1986) Role of beta-endorphins in silent myocardial ischemia. Am J Cardiol 58: 428—430

Author's address:
A. Malliani, M.D.
Istituto Ricerche Cardiovascolari
via Bonfadini 214
20138 Milano
Italy

Alpha-receptors and transient ischemia

S. Chierchia

Cardiovascular Unit, Hammersmith Hospital, London, U.K.

Introduction

A series of studies based on ambulatory ECG and arterial pressure monitoring in patients with chronic stable, predominantly effort-related angina and severe coronary artery disease have shown that the majority of ischemic events which occur during normal unrestricted daily activity, are not preceded by an increase in the major determinants of myocardial oxygen consumption (1—4). They occur at levels of heart rate or rate-pressure product well below those observed at the beginning of exercise-induced ST-segment depression. These findings imply that in these patients, ischemia is often the consequence of transient active impairment of regional myocardial perfusion, rather than of an increase in myocardial oxygen demand exceeding the residual coronary flow reserve.
Clinically, the extent by which transient impairment of coronary flow is responsible for these patients' symptoms can be gathered from the frequency of "spontaneous" episodes of angina and by the magnitude of variability in their exercise capacity from time to time, or day to day. Obviously, this evidence would be clearer in patients with a reasonably good maximal residual coronary flow reserve than in those who can never tolerate even a minimal effort without developing myocardial ischemia.
In this article, we will briefly review the evidence supporting the role of changes in coronary vasomotor tone in the pathophysiology of chronic, effort-related angina. We will mainly concentrate on the aspects related to the effects of the sympathetic nervous system on the coronary circulation.

Evidence for the role of vasoconstriction in chronic stable angina

Epicardial coronary arteries

A large body of evidence now indicates that most atheromatous segments of epicardial coronary arteries still retain the capability of undergoing significant changes in the lumen due to active vasoconstriction. An increase in stenosis severity has been observed at angiography during physical manoeuvres such as isometric and dynamic exercise (5—6), and the cold pressor test. These changes can be prevented or reversed by administration of nitrate or calcium channel blockers. Unlike spasm, the observed vasoconstriction is never occlusive nor does it impair distal filling and run-off of the involved coronary vessel. In actual fact, the changes in stenosis diameter are usually rather subtle and difficult to detect unless quantitative angiographic techniques are employed. In most instances, they are not associated with subjective symptoms and/or electrocardiographic changes suggestive of acute myocardial ischemia; these may occur, at the side of a subocclusive organic lesion and are represented by ST-segment depression and never elevation. Even if powerful vasoconstrictors, such as ergonovine, are used, their administration usually results in diffuse vasoconstriction with increased severity of epicardial coronary lesions and not in interruption of flow, as is typically the case in variant angina.

Constriction of "small vessels" and collaterals

Apart from the effect on epicardial coronary lesions, physiological changes in coronary vasomotor tone can also involve coronary collaterals as well as small "resistive" vessels. The established belief that the vascular territory distal to a "critical" lesion is, by definition, "maximally vasodilated", probably only applies to some animal models. There is evidence to suggest that, also in the presence of hemodynamically significant structures, the distal, resistive component still retains the capability of vasodilating and vasoconstricting.

A recent animal experiment, showed that cardiac sympathetic stimulation can elicit an increase in distal coronary resistance, which is inversely correlated to the severity of the stenosis applied to the epicardial coronary artery (7). The more the reactive hyperemic response (a physiological index of stenosis severity) is impaired, the more constriction is observed following sympathetic stimulation. The response is partially abolished by phentolamine, but not by prazonin, suggesting that the effect is mediated by post-synaptic receptors of the alpha 2 sub-type.

Persistence of an ischemic response to exercise testing is not uncommon after successful angioplasty. Although this observation is often attributed to angiographic underestimation of diffuse disease or to distal embolisation, the possibility that "small vessel" constriction could limit adequate supply, despite removal of epicardial lesions, should be kept in mind. In fact, objective measurements obtained with Doppler flow velocity probes show, in some patients, residual limitation of regional vasodilatory reserves despite successful removal of epicardial coronary lesions by angiography (Dr. C. White, personal communication).

In the individual patient, the likelihood of changes in coronary vasomotor tone to involve "resistive" vessels or collaterals, can only be inferred from a combination of clinical and angiographic characteristics. Obviously, the possibility of changes in epicardial stenosis severity cannot be considered if, for instance, the patient presents with complete occlusion of one vessel only and yet exhibits a large variability in effort tolerance and/or attacks of angina for no apparent reason.

The sympathetic nervous system in the regulation of coronary blood flow and epicardial coronary arterial tone

All coronaries, down to the smallest arterioles, have extensive adrenergic innervation (8). Histochemical studies have shown a preponderance of alpha receptors in the larger epicardial vessels, while beta receptors predominate in small arteries (8). In various animal preparations, stimulation of cardiac sympathetic nerves invariably causes the coronary blood flow to increase (9). However, a reduction in flow is observed if the chronotropic and inotropic effects of adrenergic stimulation are prevented by beta blockade and ac-

tivation of alpha receptors is unmasked (9). Coronary vasoconstriction mediated by stimulation of alpha receptors has also been obtained with stimulation of the posterior hypothalamus (10) and with baroreceptor hypotension after beta blockade (11).
A tonic alpha-adrenergic coronary vasoconstrictor activity has been shown in the dog both at rest and during exercise (12—13); this can be reflexly reduced by carotid sinus nerve stimulation or by phentolamine (12—13). Similar findings have been obtained in man by Orlick et al. (14); these authors measured coronary blood flow by thermodilution and found evidence for a basal coronary constrictor tone which was reduced by phentolamine and absent in patients with transplanted, denervated hearts.
Injection of noradrenaline into vein grafts at coronary bypass surgery resulted in a large, transient reduction of coronary flow, due to activation of alpha-adrenergic receptors (15). The same receptors probably mediate the reduction in coronary blood flow observed in patients with coronary artery disease during the cold pressor test (16). Coronary arteriography during "cold pressor" reveals only minimal changes in the diameter of epicardial arteries (17); the observed changes in coronary vascular resistance and flow are thus likely to be consequent to constriction of the small resistance vessels which are not visualized at angiography.
In several animal species, including man, alpha receptor mediated constriction of large epicardial arteries has been convincingly demonstrated in vitro (18—20). Barbour (21) obtained human coronary arteries soon after death and produced strong constrictions after adding adrenaline to the organ bath. Kountz (22) using a similar technique, showed that low concentrations of adrenaline produced contraction, while higher concentrations caused relaxation. More recently, Ginsburg et al. (23) studied the effects of various vasoactive drugs on fresh human arteries from heart transplant recipients and found that their basal tone was not affected by alpha or beta blockade. The arteries responded to alpha and beta stimulation, but the magnitude of alpha constriction was comparatively small when compared to beta dilatation.
Constriction of large epicardial arteries in response to intravenous methoxamine, a powerful alpha-adrenergic agonist, has been described in conscious, chronically instrumented dogs (24). The reduction in coronary diameter occurred in the presence of a marked increase of aortic pressure and hence of coronary distending pressure; however, coronary blood flow was apparently not affected. Minor reductions in coronary diameter have also been reported in man, at coronary arteriography, during handgrip and after administration of epinephrine following beta blockade.

Alpha adrenergic receptors and effort angina

All physiological conditions which are known to increase the sympathetic outflow to the heart, result in the release of active mediators from sympathetic nerve endings which are located on both the myocardium and the coronary smooth muscle. Although the effects of beta receptor stimulation in both physiological and pathological conditions are relatively well known, those of alpha-stimulation, especially in the setting of coronary artery disease, are less clear. Moreover, growing evidence suggests that substances other than catecholamines could contribute to sympathetic transmission in the heart, and receptors different from the classic ones could mediate physiological responses to adrenergic stimulation (see chapter 2, this book).

A decrease in coronary sinus flow, often associated with angina and ST-segment depression, was observed with cardiac sympathetic stimulation induced by the cold pressor test in anginal patients with severe coronary atheroma (16). As the authors pointed out, in the presence of critical coronary disease and severe impairment of vasodilatory reserve, alpha-mediated coronary vasoconstriction, unopposed by metabolically-mediated dilatation, is probably sufficient to impair regional myocardial perfusion and to cause ischemia.

More recent observations also indicate that coronary vasoconstriction resulting from sympathetic stimulation could play a relevant pathophysiological role in patients with chronic effort angina. Studies based on ambulatory ECG monitoring during normal, unrestricted daily activities, have shown that, in these patients, transient ischemic events predominate in the daytime (between 6 a.m. and 9 p.m.), when the resting levels of heart rate, an index of cardiac sympathetic activation, are higher (3—4). Although the majority of these events are not preceded by an increase of the major hemodynamic determinants of myocardial oxygen consumption they are, almost invariably, associated with an increase in heart rate and blood pressure which parallels the development of ST-segment depression. Although it is possible that the hemodynamic pattern here described simply results from reflex activation of sympathetic afferences to the heart caused by ischemia, it is also possible that primary adrenergic stimulation of the cardiovascular system could, on the one hand, increase myocardial demand and, on the other, limit or reduce supply by alpha-mediated constriction.

Constriction of atheromatous segments of epicardial coronary arteries following reflex or pharmacological adrenergic stimulation is now well documented (see previous sections). Whether or not the same may occur at the level of smaller "resistive" vessels is not yet clear.

We recently tested this hypothesis in a group of eight patients with effort angina, severe limitation of exercise capacity and complete proximal occlusion of the left anterior descending coronary artery (25). In all, we could document by angiography the presence of visible collaterals supplying the myocardium distal to the occlusion. Patients underwent supine bicycle-ergometer exercise in control conditions and after administration of the alpha-adrenergic blocking agent phentolamine. The drug was selectively infused, over five minutes, in the coronary artery supplying collaterals to the occluded LAD. The electrocardiogram, left ventricular pressure and the oxygen saturation in the great cardiac vein were continuously monitored throughout the study.

During control, exercise induced in all patients diagnostic ST-segment depression, increase in left ventricular end-diastolic pressure and decrease in great cardiac vein oxygen saturation. After phentolamine, exercise-induced ischemia was less severe, as shown by the lesser increase in end-diastolic pressure, myocardial oxygen extraction and ST-segment depression.

The increase in rate-pressure product induced by exercise was similar during control and after phentolamine, indicating that the improvement observed after treatment was related to improved myocardial perfusion, rather than reduction in metabolic demand. This interpretation is further supported by the angiographic observation that, after phentolamine, the collateral circulation to the ischemic myocardium was markedly improved. It therefore appears reasonable to conclude that, at least in some patients with effort angina, alpha-mediated constriction of coronary collaterals supplying the myocardium distal to an occluded epicardial vessel, could play a relevant role in limiting residual coronary flow reserve and in contributing to the development of ischemia induced by cardiac sympathetic stimulation. It is also possible that constriction of small, "resistive" vessels, distal to a critical epicardial lesion, is an important pathophysiological factor in effort angina.

References

1. Schang SJ Jr, Pepine CJ (1977) Transient asymptomatic ST segment depression during daily activity. Am J Cardiol 39: 396—402
2. Deanfield JE, Maseri A, Selwyn AP, Ribeiro F, Chierchia S, Krikler S, Morgan M (1983) Myocardial ischaemia during daily life in patients with stable angina: its relation to symptoms and heart rate changes. Lancet, October 1: 753
3. Chierchia S, Gallino A, Smith G, Maseri A, Deanfield J, Morgan M, Croom M (1984) The role of heart rate in the pathophysiology of chronic stable angina. Lancet, December 15: 1353
4. Chierchia S, Balasubramanian V, Muisen L, Sonecha T, Davies G, Maseri A, Raftery J (1984) Transient impairment of coronary flow: a frequent cause of ischaemia in chronic stable angina during normal daily life. J Am Coll Cardiol 3 (2): 579
5. Brown BG, Bolson E, Frimer M, Dodge HT (1978) Angiographic distinction between variant angina and non-vasospastic chest pain. (Abstr) Circulation 57 & 58 (Suppl II) II: 122
6. Hattenhauer M, Neill WA (1975) The effect of cold air inhalation on angina pectoris and myocardial oxygen supply. Circulation 51: 1053
7. Heusch G, Deussem A (1983) The effects of cardiac sympathetic nerve stimulation of perfusion of stenotic coronary arteries in the dog. Circ Res 53 (1): 8—15
8. King MP, Angelalsos ET, Uzgiris I (1971) Innervation of the coronaries. (Abstr) Fed Proc 30: 613
9. Feigl EO (1967) Sympathetic control of coronary circulation. Circ Res 20: 262
10. Alanis J, Lopes E, Rosas O (1962) Changes in dog's coronary circulation by hypothalamic stimulation. Arch Inst Cardiol Mex 22: 743
11. Hacket JG, Abboud FM, Mark AL, Schmid PG, Heistad DD (1972) Coronary vascular responses to stimulation of chemoreceptors and baroceptors. Circ Res 31: 8
12. Murray PA, Vatner SF (1979) Alpha-receptor attenuation of the coronary vascular response to severe, spontaneous exercise in the conscious dog. Circ Res 45: 654
13. Vatner SF, Franklin D, Van Citters RL (1970) Effects of carotid sinus nerve stimulation on the coronary circulation of the conscious dog. Circ Res 27: 11
14. Orlick AE, Ricci DR, Alderman EL, Stinson EB, Harrison DC (1978) Effects of alpha-adrenergic blockade upon coronary hemodynamics. J Clin Invest 62: 459
15. Greenfield JC, Rembert JC, Young JG Jr, Oldham NH Jr, Alexander JA, Sabiston DC (1972) Studies of blood flow in aorta to coronary venous bypass grafts in man. J Clin Invest 51: 2724
16. Mudge GH, Grossman W, Mills RM, Lesch M, Braunwald E (1976) Reflex increase in coronary vascular resistance in patients with ischemic heart disease. N Engl J Med 295: 1333
17. Raizner AE, Chahine RA, Ishimori T (1980) Provocation of coronary artery spasm by the cold pressor test. Hemodynamic, arteriographic and quantitative angiographic observations. Circulation 62: 925
18. Bayer BL, Mentz P, Forster W (1974) Characterization of the adrenoreceptors in coronary arteries in pigs. Eur J Pharmacol 29: 58
19. Bohr DF (1967) Adrenergic receptors in coronary arteries. Ann NY Acad Sci 139: 799
20. Zuberbuhler RC, Bohr DR (1965) Responses of coronary smooth muscle to catecholamines. Circ Res 16: 431
21. Barbour HG (1912) The constricting influence of adrenalin upon the human coronary arteries. J Exp Med 15: 404
22. Kountz WB (1932) Studies on the coronary arteries of the human heart. J Pharmacol Exp Ther 45: 65
23. Ginsburg R, Bristow ME, Harrison DC, Stinson EB (1980) Studies with isolated human coronary arteries: some general observations, potential mediators of spasm, role of calcium antagonists. Chest 78 (Suppl): 180

24. Vatner SF, Pagani P, Manders WT, Pasipoularides F (1981) Alpha-adrenergic control of large coronary arterial resistance and elastic stiffness in the conscious dog. In: Les Alphabioquants; Masson, Paris, pp 167—178
25. Chierchia S, Pratt T, De Coster P, Maseri A (1985) Alpha-adrenergic control of collateral flow: another determinant of coronary flow reserve. Circulation 72 (111): 190

Author's address:
Sergio Chierchia, M.D., F.A.C.C.
Cardiovascular Unit
Royal Postgraduate Medical School
Hammersmith Hospital
Ducane Road
London, W12 OHS
UK

Experimental approach to painful and painless ischemia

C. Droste and H. Roskamm

Rehabilitationszentrum für Herz- und Kreislaufkranke (Medical Director: Prof. Dr. H. Roskamm) Bad Krozingen, West Germany

Introduction

In asymptomatic myocardial ischemia, from the point of view of pain research, we face the situation that the nociceptive stimulus is present and can be objectively demonstrated, but the nociceptive answer (angina pectoris pain) is missing. Consequently there must be reasons on the various levels of pain development, conduction or processing which explain why many people with myocardial ischemia have no or next to no pain (asymptomatic patients); why in many patients myocardial ischemia is sometimes accompanied by pain and sometimes not (asymptomatic episodes).
The neurophysiology of pain in its fundamental principles is the same for every pain. The following levels exist:

1. Pain receptors

Paravascular free nerve endings in the myocardium are identified as pain receptors (27, 31, 34, 44). Via various intermediate steps, myocardial ischemia activates nociceptive stimuli which in turn are able to stimulate receptors so that these pass on pain impulses. In heart pain little is known about these mechanisms. Chemical and mechanical stimuli seem to participate in pain development, possibly in a complex interaction (15).

2. Afferent nerve pathways

The free nerve endings collect in different plexus, run to the sympathetic trunck ganglia and enter the posterior horn of the spinal cord via the ramus communicans albus (36, 44, 54) (Fig. 5).

3. Spinal cord and supraspinal regulation

After entering the posterior horn, the fibers cross and run upwards in the tractus spinothalamicus to the center, where they are passed on via intermediate stages in the thalamus to the cortex. Here the pain is perceived consciously.

Reasons for pain absence even when a pain stimulus is present should be found in these different levels of pain perception.

Destruction of afferent nerves

One idea is that the pain is interrupted somewhere, for example, because of polyneuropathia, diabetes mellitus or diffuse coronary heart disease with a large loss of myocardium. This factor may well be relevant in single cases, but is not the most important explanation for asymptomatic myocardial ischemia.
Studies comparing patients with and without asymptomatic myocardial ischemia found that diabetes was not increased (10) and that coronary heart disease was not more diffuse in asymptomatic patients (16). Studies conducted on diabetes mellitus found only a slightly higher percentage of silent ischemia (1, 8).

Neuronal encoding of peripheral painful stimuli

In pain research, three fundamental principles are known according to which peripheral painful stimuli are coded and modified on their way to the center (26) (Fig. 1).
The *specificity theory* assumes that there are specific nociceptive neurons which conduct pain only (A in Fig. 1).
The *intensity theory* is based on the idea that the question of whether a peripheral stimulus is actually experienced as painful is decided not by the kind of receptor but by the intensity of the stimulus (B in Fig. 1).
The *gate control theory* assumes that whether, or how intensively, pain is felt is a result of a balance between the activity of large and small diameter afferent fibers and of central impulses. These impulses function as an inhibitory control in the posterior horn of the spinal cord or in higher centers.
These three theories are of importance for nociception, especially for visceral nociception and it is to be assumed that the reasons for pain absence in asymptomatic myocardial ischemia can be found here.
For coronary pain the specificity theory is probably not valid, even though some investigators (4, 23, 51) have found indications of specific cardiac nociceptors. Studies by Malliani and coworkers (36) show that heart pain is more likely to be connected with the intensity theory. This would mean that the intensity of the peripheral stimulus is an important factor in heart pain.
One reason for pain absence in asymptomatic myocardial ischemia is therefore that the peripheral pain stimulus is not intensive enough. This can be caused, for example, by a low grade of myocardial ischemia. The results from some studies point in this direction and have found, for example, that ischemic episodes are shorter and less pronounced in asymptomatic myocardial ischemia or that exercise-induced myocardial ischemia is more accompanied by pain when left ventricular filling pressure is increased (9, 14).
This factor is significant, especially when in the same person ischemia is sometimes combined with angina pectoris and sometimes not (asymptomatic ischemic episodes). Not all authors indicate differences in intensity of ischemia (3, 6, 11, 32, 50) and some of those who do, do so only very discretely. There are cases where even with very pro-

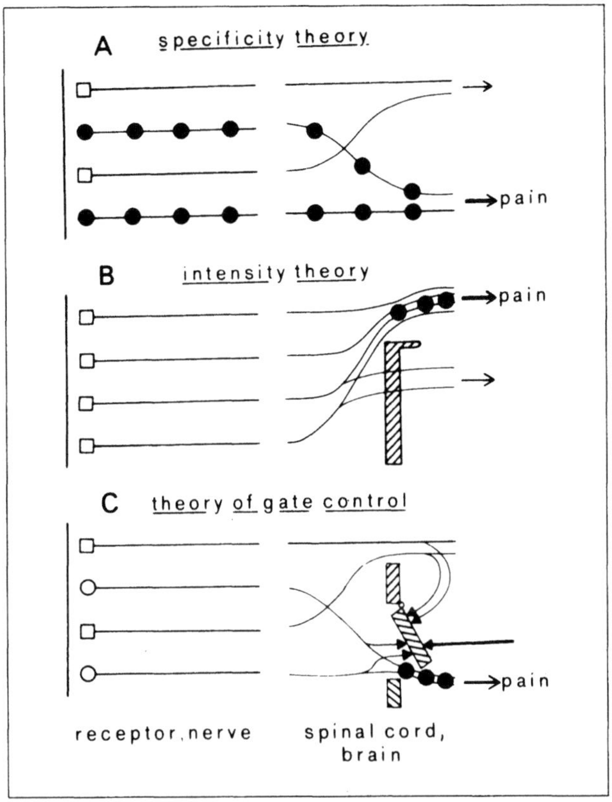

Fig. 1. Theories of neuronal encoding of peripheral painful stimuli (with permission from Handwerker, see [26]).

nounced objective ischemia no pain is present and also cases in which patients feel absolutely no pain in spite of distinct objective ischemia (asymptomatic ischemic patients). Here it must be assumed that one more factor is responsible: a varying central pain level, as postulated for the intensity theory, with different influences on pain modification processes in the posterior horn of the spinal cord and higher up.

In an experimental study we have tried to follow up these latter factors.

Methods

Subjects

We studied a group of 30 patients with a very extreme type of asymptomatic myocardial ischemia and compared them to 30 patients with a consistently reproducible symptomatic myocardial ischemia (16). Symptomatic and asymptomatic patients had angiographically proven severe coronary artery disease, defined as a diameter reduction of more than 75% in at least one coronary artery.

We selected our 30 asymptomatic patients over a period of 3 years from a pool of more than 3200 patients who had undergone coronary angiography. All had reproducible

asymptomatic manifestation of ischemia in several exercise tests. They exhibited a significant ST-segment depression in an average of 2.7 examinations without any signs of angina pectoris. The mean ST-segment in these tests was substantial at 0.38 mV. Other factors that could have indicated false positive ST-segment depression in these patients (digitalis medication, hypopotassium levels, mocardial hypertrophy, valvular disease) were excluded.
In addition to the ST-segment depression a second independent sign of ischemia was present in most of our investigated patients. In the symptomatic and asymptomatic groups, 27 patients demonstrated a pathologically high pulmonary capillary pressure during exercise, as measured by a floating catheter examination.
Of our 30 asymptomatic patients, 24 also reported no angina pectoris during everyday life; the remaining six patients had only mild symptoms. Of the 30 asymptomatic patients, 25 exhibited electrocardiographic evidence of previous myocardial infarction. In five of these patients the infarction occurred silently. Another seven of these patients "noticed" their infarction but experienced no direct pain.

Procedures

Three different pain-receptive modalities were employed to measure pain experimentally: an electrical pain test, cold pressor test, and ischemic pain test (for details see ref. [16]).

Results

Symptomatic and asymptomatic patients did not show any significant difference in degree of vessel disease or ejection fraction. Also, in coronary risk factors (age, smoking, hypertension, diabetes, cholesterol, and triglycerides), no significant differences were found between the groups. Furthermore, there were no significant differences in parameters of exercise testing, such as maximum effort, maximum heart rate, and maximum systolic or diastolic blood pressure.
Significant differences were exhibited between the symptomatic and asymptomatic groups for all pain tests. Symptomatic patients demonstrated a mean electrical pain threshold of 0.55 mA. This finding agrees well with results of 4,000 measurements in normal subjects where a mean threshold of 0.55 mA was found. Asymptomatic patients indicated a significantly higher mean threshold of 1 mA ($p < 0.001$).
In the ischemic pain test (experimentally induced ischemia on the working muscle of the non-dominant arm) asymptomatic patients exhibited a higher pain threshold and pain tolerance, both values reaching a significant level. Whereas for the symptomatic patients, ischemic pain occurred after an average of 70 s, asymptomatic patients first reported pain after an average of 98 s ($p < 0.01$).
In the cold pressor test, pain tolerance showed significantly higher values in asymptomatic patients ($p < 0.01$).
In a further development of our method we have chosen experimentally induced ischemic skeletal muscle pain in the forearm of a patient with asymptomatic myocardial ischemia, as a model for studying processes of pain perception which cannot be examined directly

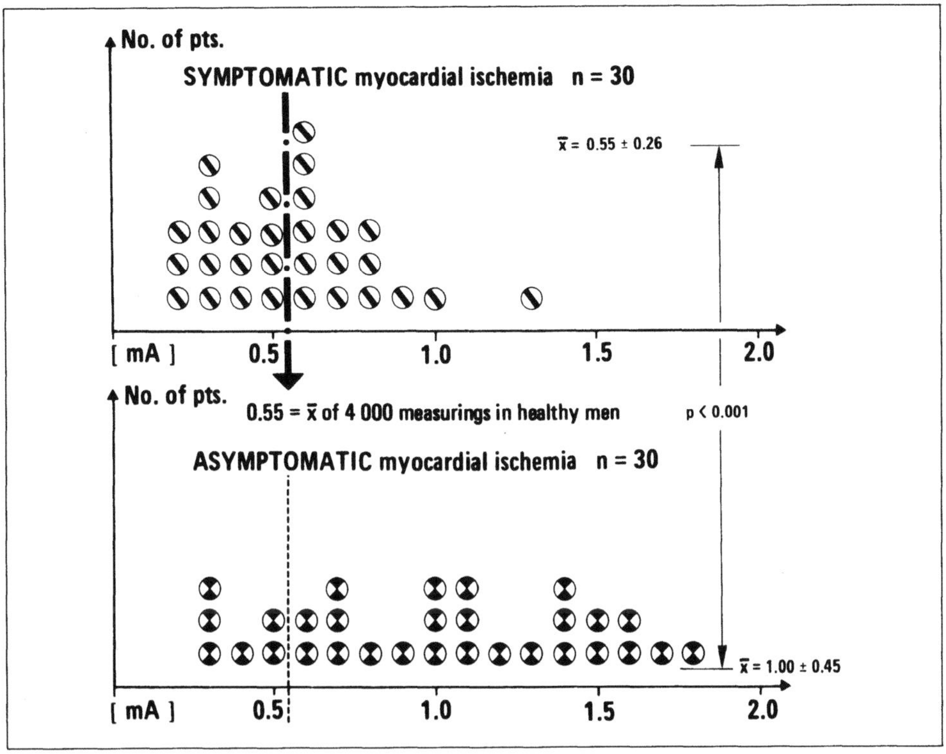

Fig. 2. Electrical pain threshold in symptomatic and asymptomatic patients (15).

in the heart (19). It is known from neurophysiology, that skeletal muscle pain and heart muscle pain have a lot of similarities.

Transcutaneous partial oxygen tension ($tcpO_2$) and skin blood flow (using heat clearance rate) were non-invasively monitored during the ischemic test using the Oxymonitor (Hellige Co.). This instrument consists of a polarographic sensor positioned on the skin surface of the forearm. Heart rate and respiration were simultaneously recorded, and the time elapsing to threshold and tolerance levels was assessed.

Figure 3 presents the mean values for $tcpO_2$ (upper trace) and heart rate (lower trace) for symptomatic (dashed lines) and asymptomatic (solid lines) groups. As is evident in this figure, the asymptomatic patients exhibited lower $tcpO_2$ levels at threshold and tolerance and needed more time to reach threshold and tolerance levels than did symptomatic patients.

Discussion

Our investigations show that patients with asymptomatic myocardial ischemia have a diminished sensitivity to noxious stimulation (hypoalgesia). Recently, Maseri et al. (37) have been able to reproduce these results. In patients with painless ischemia the same tests that we used were applied, and a higher threshold and tolerance were also found.

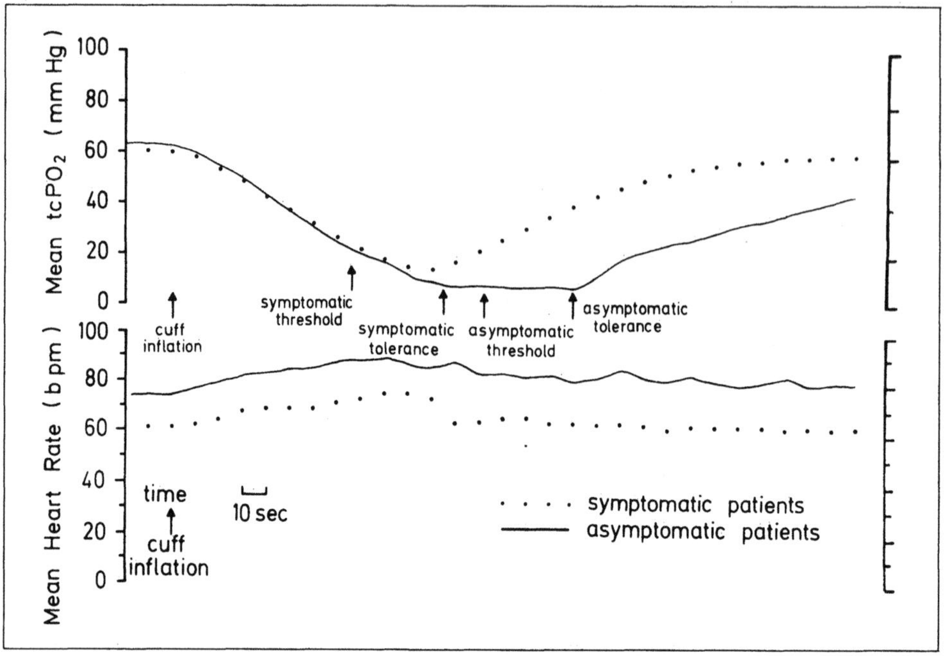

Fig. 3. Time course of mean values of $tcpO_2$ (upper traces) and heart rate (lower traces) for symptomatic (dotted lines; $n = 6$) and asymptomatic (solid lines; $n = 6$) patients. Time of cuff inflation denoted by arrows. Threshold and tolerance levels are depicted separately (arrows) for symptomatic and asymptomatic groups (19).

Recently Falcone et al. (21) using a good quality experimental pain test (dental pulp stimulation) has also been able to show that patients with asymptomatic myocardial ischemia have a significantly higher pain threshold compared to patients with symptomatic myocardial ischemia.

It is often noted that patients with symptomatic and asymptomatic myocardial ischemia overlap considerably in their threshold and tolerance rates. This, however, is because of the limited reliability of one pain test alone. When using a series of tests the groups can be more easily separated from each other (17). In three parallel pain tests 22 symptomatic patients had higher than normal results in only eight cases. No patient had a higher result in more than one test. On the other hand, out of 20 asymptomatic patients examined, all of whom had a very pronounced form of asymptomatic myocardial ischemia, 17 had a higher than normal result in one test or more, 11 patients in two tests or more, seven in three, and two in four pain tests.

The question arises of how this ascertained hypoalgesia in asymptomatic patients can be explained. The answer is not a general indifference to pain (analgesia), because all patients in our studies were able to experience pain and did not show any noticeable neurological deficiencies compared to symptomatic patients. It can be assumed that the differences in pain perception in these patients can be explained by the basic models for the coding and regulation of pain mentioned above (Fig. 1).

The intensity theory, which is probably valid for coronary pain, presumes a central pain threshold (B in Fig. 1). Consequently, hypoalgesia in patients with asymptomatic myo-

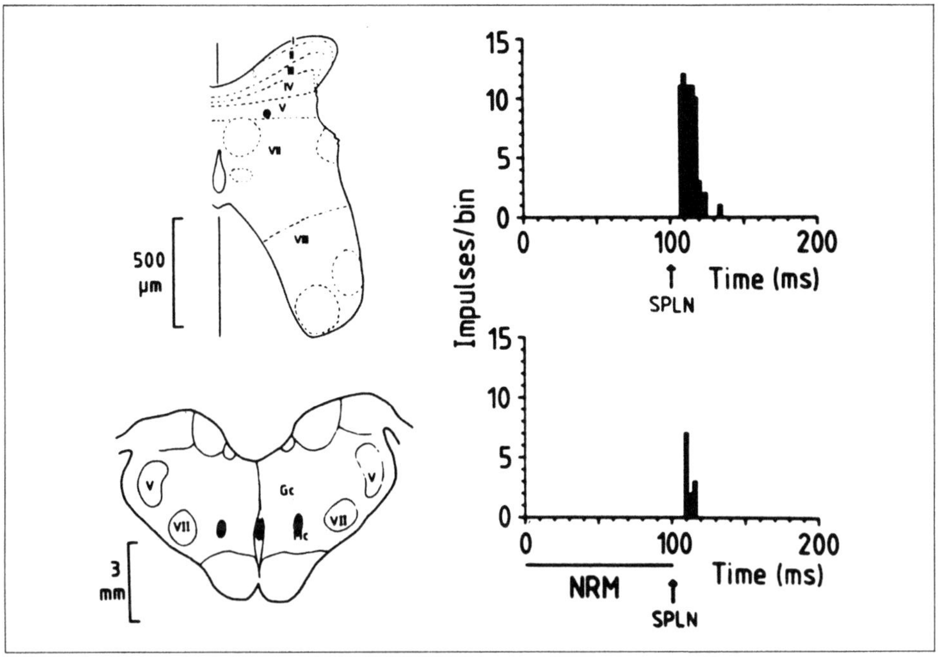

Fig. 4. Descending inhibitory control of visceral pain; for details see text (with permisson from Cervero et al., see [7]).

cardial ischemia can be interpreted as the effect of a higher central threshold. A further possible explanation could be found at the level of descending pain inhibition (C in Fig. 1). Each pain is subject to strong descending inhibition. This is accomplished by descending nervous pathways at the level of the spinal cord and at supraspinal levels.

Recently, it has been shown that visceral pain is also clearly subject to this inhibition (7, 35). This is shown in Fig. 4 in an animal experiment. On stimulation of the nervus splanchnicus and registration in the posterior horn of the spinal cord (Fig. 4, upper left side) the impulses shown on the upper right result. If the nucleus raphe magnus (known to be a pain inhibitory center) is then also stimulated (lower left; length of stimulation marked on the lower right hand side) with the stimulation of the nervus splanchnicus remaining the same, the impulses transmitted to the center are clearly inhibited (Fig. 4, lower right side).

Cardiac pain is also subject to this descending inhibition (Fig. 5). In this illustration, the left side shows the ascending nervous pathways of pain (white arrows) and the right side shows the descending inhibitory pathways (black arrows).

The nucleus raphe magnus, the formatio reticularis, and the periaqueductal grey have all been proved to be pain inhibitory centers (22). At the neural level, enkephalin, serotonin, and adrenalin are known to be active inhibitory substances within this inhibitory system (49).

As well as the neural system there is a humoral system in which mainly endorphins are involved.

In the neural and humoral systems there are parts which are conveyed by opioids, that is, blockade by naloxone, as well as non-opioid parts (38) (Table 1). The pain inhibitory

Fig. 5. Descending inhibitory control of cardiac pain (18).

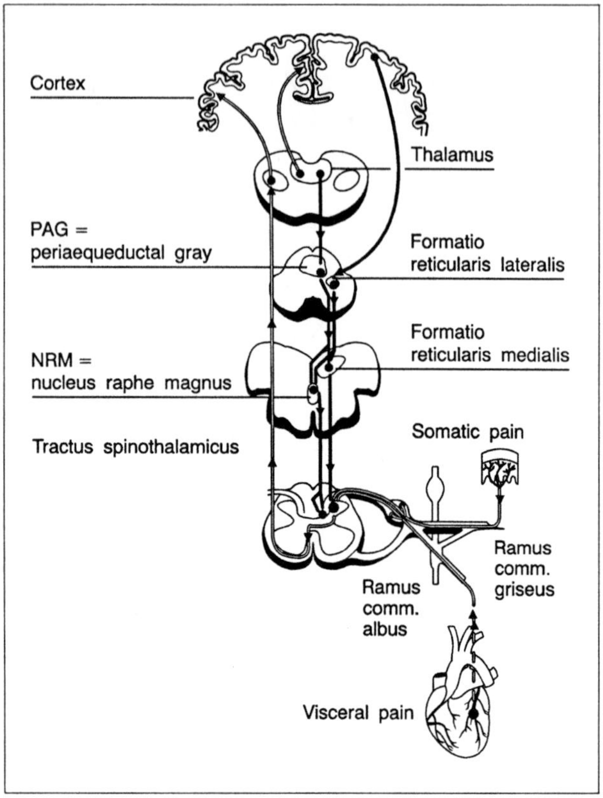

Table 1. Fundamental principles of multiple endogenous opiate and nonopiate analgesia systems.

Classes of Analgesia	Similarity to opiates (Naloxon)	Endocrine lesions (Hypophysectomy	Neural lesions (PAG lesion)
Neural/Opiate	↓	∅	↓
Neural/Nonopiate	∅	∅	↓
Hormonal/Opiate	↓	↓	∅
Hormonal/Nonopiate	∅	↓	∅

system has a low resting tone, which may possibly be permanently raised in certain individuals (5). There are also individuals with a raised concentration of endorphins in the liquor, so that they need less analgesic after an operation than others (47).

The pain inhibitory system is strongly activated by specific situations. Stimuli include pain itself (48), injury (40), stress (33), physical exercise (2, 24, 29, 30, 39), and other factors. There are also pronounced individual differences in the ability to activate the endogenous pain inhibitory system. One third of all individuals have absolutely no pain at the onset and minutes to hours after very severe partial injuries such as a fracture or an amputation, as Melzack et al. have been able to prove with patients from a surgical

admission center (40). It is a striking similarity that around one third of all myocardial infarctions occur painlessly.
The pain inhibitory system may be a phylogenetic relict which had a survival function in earlier times. It may even ensure the maintainance of vital functions in certain extreme situations (shock, exceptional psychophysiological stress, injury, dangerous situations, war, combat sports) even today.
With regard to the cardiological aspect, the activation of this system by physical exercise is especially interesting. For the activation of the humoral system with the possibility of tracing endorphins in the serum, a higher short-term exercise in the anaerobic range (lactate > 4—5 mmol/l) or long distance running is necessary (2, 13, 24, 29, 30, 39). In higher exercise regions the emitted endorphins can be blocked by naloxone, so that pain (2, 39) and also angina pectoris pain (19, 45, 52) is stronger. But the role of endorphins in asymptomatic myocardial ischemia is still contradictory.
The failure of naloxone to initiate pain in some studies with silent myocardial ischemia (12, 20, 53) suggests that the mechanism of the perception of coronary pain is more complex. Perhaps the dose of naloxone was inadequate, exercise stimulus was not intensive enough, or there may have been patients with endorphin-modulated angina and with nonendorphin modulation. Han has recently argued that not all opioid-dependent analgesic mechanisms can be influenced by low to moderate doses of naloxone (25). In these doses, naloxone is generally assumed to antagonize preferentially μ-opioid receptors. There are other opioid receptors (42) which can be antagonised by naloxone only in very high concentrations or which are naloxone-insensitive.
One should bear in mind that measurements of endorphins in the serum only give a limited idea of the endogenous processes; measurements inside the liquor would give a better picture of the modulatory role of endorphin systems in these patients. An activation of the humoral endogenous opioid system seems to be responsible for the pain intensity in myocardial infarction (46), even though these results are also still contradictory (43).
To summarize, the experimental approach to painful and painless ischemia shows that processes in the neural coding of peripheral painful stimuli play a considerable part in modifying coronary pain.
Explanations for missing pain in asymptomatic myocardial ischemia include an individually raised central pain level and higher activation capacity (there may also be raised resting tone) of an endogenous pain inhibitory system. This can be said especially of patients who have exceptionally little pain compared to others, or no pain at all in spite of objective myocardial ischemia (asymptomatic patients).
Diurnal variations in the individual pain threshold may possibly be involved in the distribution of painful and painless ischemic episodes during the day.

References

1. Abenavoli T, Rubler S, Fisher VJ, Axelrod HI, Zuckermann KP (1981) Exercise testing with myocardial scintigraphy in asymptomatic diabetic males. Circulation 63: 54—64
2. Arentz T, Meirleir K de, Hollmann W (1986) Die Rolle der endogenen opioden Peptide während Fahrradergometerarbeit. Dtsch Z Sportmed 7: 210—219
3. Arnim Th von (1985) ST-Segment-Analyse im Langzeit-EKG. Dtsch Med Wochenschr 110: 1047—1051

4. Baker DG, Coleridge HM, Coleridge HCG, Nerdrum T (1980) Search for a cardiac nociceptor: stimulation by bradykinin of sympathetic afferent nerve endings in the heart of the cat. J Physiol 306: 519—536
5. Buchsbaum MS, Davis GC, Bunner WE (1977) Naloxone alters pain perception and somatosensory evoked potentials in normal humans. Nature 270: 620—662
6. Cecchi AC, Dovellini V, Marchi F, Pucci P, Santoro CM, Fazzini PF (1983) Silent myocardial ischemia during ambulatory electrocardiographic monitoring in patients with effort angina. J Am Coll Cardiol 1: 934
7. Cervero F, Lumb BM, Tattersall JEH (1986) Supraspinal loops that mediate visceral inputs to thoracic spinal cord neurones: involvement of descending pathways from raphe and reticular formation. Neurosci Lett (in press)
8. Chiariello M, Indolfo C, Cotecchia MR, Sifola C, Romano M, Condorelli M (1985) Asymptomatic transient ST changes during ambulatory ECG monitoring in diabetic patients. Am Heart J 110: 529—534
9. Chierchia S, Lazzari M, Freedman B, Brunelli C, Maseri A (1983) Impairment of myocardial perfusion and function during painless myocardial ischemia. J Am Coll Cardiol 1: 924
10. Chipkin SR, Frid D, Alpert JS, Baker SP, Dalen JE, Aronin N (1986) Painless myocardial ischemia in diabetics and non-diabetics during exercise tolerance testing (Abstract). Clin Res 34: 879A
11. Cohn PF, Brown EJ, Wynne BL, Holman BL, Atkins HL (1983) Global and regional left ventricular ejection fraction abnormalities during exercise in patients with silent myocardial ischemia. J Am Coll Cardiol 1: 931
12. Cohn PF, Patcha R, Singh S et al. (1985) Studies on the pathophysiology of silent myocardial ischemia: effect of naloxone on pain threshold during exercise tests (Abstract). Clin Res 33: 177A
13. Colt EWD, Wardlaw SL, Frantz AG (1981) The effect of running on plasma β-endorphin. Life Sci 28: 1637—1670
14. Deanfield JE, Selwyn AP, Chierchia S, Maseri A, Ribiero P, Krikler S, Morgan M (1983) Myocardial ischemia during daily life in patients with stable angina: its relation to symptoms and heart rate changes. Lancet 2: 753
15. Droste C (1984) Neurophysiologie des Koronarschmerzes. In: Roskamm H (ed) Koronarerkrankungen, Handbuch der Inneren Medizin, Vol IX/3, Springer, Berlin Heidelberg New York, pp 157—174
16. Droste C, Roskamm H (1983) Experimental pain measurement in patients with asymptomatic myocardial ischemia. J Am Coll Cardiol 940—945
17. Droste, C, Roskamm H (1986) Interkorrelation verschiedener experimenteller Schmerzschwellenmeßwerte bei Patienten mit asymptomatischer Myokardischämie (Abstrakt). Z Kardiol 75: 75
18. Droste C, Roskamm H (1987) Variability in the perception of painful stimuli in patients with silent ischemia. In: Julian D et al. (eds) Mononitrates II, Berlin Heidelberg New York, Springer (in press)
19. Droste C, Greenlee MW, Roskamm H (1986) A defective angina pectoris pain warning system: experimental findings of ischemic and electrical pain test. Pain 26: 199—209
20. Ellestad MH, Kuan P (1984) Naloxone and asymptomatic ischemia: Failure to induce angina during exercise testing. Am J Cardiol 54: 982—984
21. Falcone C, Guasti L, Codega S, de Servi S, Ghio S, Specchia G, Montemartini C (1987) Pain threshold in patients with coronary artery disease. Poster presented at the International Symposium "Myocardial ischemia and exercise", Tutzing-Munich, 6—8 November 1986 (in press)
22. Fields HL, Basbaum AI (1984) Endogenous pain control mechanisms. In: Wall PD, Melzack R (eds) Textbook of pain. Churchill Livingston, Edinburgh London Melbourne New York, pp 142—152
23. Foreman RD, Blair RW, Ammons WS (1986) Neural mechanisms of cardiac pain. Prog Brain Res 67: 227
24. Fraioli P, Moretti C, Paolucci D, Alicicco E, Crescenzi F, Fortunio G (1980) Physical exercise stimulates marked concomitant release of β-endorphin and adrenocorticotropic hormone (ACTH) in peripheral blood in man. Experimentia 36: 987—989
25. Han JS (1985) Letter to the editor. Pain 21: 307—308

26. Handwerker HO (1984) Experimentelle Schmerzanalyse beim Menschen. In: Zimmermann M, Handwerker HO (eds) Schmerz, Springer, Berlin Heidelberg New York, pp 87—123
27. Hirsch EF, Nigh CA, Laye MP, Cooper T (1962) Terminal innervation of the heart. II. Studies of the perimysial innervation apparatus and of the sensory receptors in the rabbit and in the dog with the techniques of total extrinsic denervation, bilateral cervical vagotomy, and bilateral thoracic sympathectomy. Arch Pathol 77: 172—187
28. Hirzel HO, Leutwyler R, Krayenbuehl HP (1985) Silent myocardial ischemia: hemodynamic changes during dynamic exercise in patients with proven coronary artery disease despite absence of angina pectoris. J Am Coll Cardiol 6: 275—284
29. Howlett TA, Tomlin S, Ngahfoong L, Rees LH, Bullen BA, Skrinar GS, McArthur JW (1984) Release of β-endorphin and met-enkephalin during exercise in normal women: response to training. Br Med J 288: 1950
30. Janal MN, Colt EWD, Clark WC, Glusman M (1984) Pain sensitivity, mood, and plasma endocrine levels in man following long-distance running: effects of naloxone. Pain 19: 13—25
31. Katz LN, Mayne W, Weinstein W (1935) Cardiac pain: presence of pain fibres in the nerve plexus surrounding the coronary vessels. Arch Intern Med 55: 760—772
32. Kunkes SH, Pichard AD, Smith H, Gorlin R, Hermann MV, Kupersmith J (1980) Silent ST segment deviations and extent of coronary artery disease. Am Heart J 100: 813
33. Lewis JW, Terman GW, Shavit Y, Nelson LR, Liebeskind JC (1984) Neural, neurochemical, and hormonal bases of stress-induced analgesia. In: Kruger L, Liebeskind JC (eds) Advances in pain research and therapy, Vol. 6, Raven Press, New York, pp 277—288
34. Lim RKS, Liu CN, Guzman F, Braun C (1962) Visceral receptors concerned in visceral pain and the pseudoaffective response to intra-arterial injection of bradykinin and other algesic agents. J Comp Neurol 118: 269—294
35. Lumb BM (1986) Brainstem control of visceral afferent pathways in the spinal cord. Prog Brain Res 67: 279
36. Malliani A, Pagani M, Lombardi F (1985) Visceral versus somatic mechanisms. In: Wall PD, Melzack R (eds) Pain. Churchill Livingston, Edinburgh, pp 100—109
37. Maseri A, Chierchia S, Davies G, Glazier J (1985) Mechanisms of ischemic cardiac pain and silent myocardial ischemia. Am J Med 79 (Suppl 3A): 7—11
38. Mayer DJ, Watkins LR (1984) Multiple endogenous opiate and nonopiate analgesia systems. In: Kruger L, Liebeskind JC (eds) Advances in pain research and therapy, vol 6, Raven Press, New York, pp 523—576
39. Meirleir K de, Naaktgeboren N, Steirteghem A, van, Gorus F, Olbrecht J, Block P (1986) Beta-endorphin and ACTH levels in peripheral blood during and after aerobic and anaerobic exercise. Eur J Appl Physiol 55: 5—8
40. Melzack R, Wall PD, Ty TC (1982) Acute pain in an emergency clinic: latency of onset and descriptor patterns related to different injuries. Pain 14: 33—43
41. Pasi A, Meyer M, Boltshauser E, Foletta D, Gramsch C (1982) Failure of naloxone to reverse analgesia in congenital insensivity to pain, and variable plasma levels of β-endorphin-like activity (letter to the editor) Lancet 1: 622
42. Paterson SJ, Robson LE, Kosterlitz HW (1983) Classification of opioid receptors. Br Med Bull 39: 31—39
43. Pertovaara A, Koivula T, Leppäluoto J (1984) The magnitude of acute cardiac pain is dependent on the growth rate of infarction but not influenced by pituitary endorphins. Pain (Suppl 2): 299
44. Seagard JL, Pederson HJ, Kostreva DR, Van Horn DL, Kampine JP (1978) Ultrastructural identification of afferent fibres of cardiac origin in thoracic sympathetic nerves in the dog. Am J Anat 153: 217—232
45. Sheps DS, Adams KF, Price C, Orlando G, Margolis B, Koch G (1985) Endorphins are related to pain perception in patients with ischemic heart disease (Abstract). Clin Res 33: 748A
46. Stoupel E, Pinchas A, Gilad I, Laron Z, Agmon J (1987) Plasma β-endorphins are negative correlated with pain intensity in acute myocardial infarction (Abstract No. 559). X World Congress of Cardiology, Washington 14—19 September 1986 (in press)
47. Tamsen A, Sakurada T, Wahlström A, Terenius L, Hartvig P (1982) Postoperative demand for analgesics in relation to individual levels of endorphins and substance P in cerebrospinal fluid. Pain 13, 171—183

48. Terenius L., Tamsen A (1982) Endorphins and the modulation of acute pain. Acta Anaesthesiol Scand 74 (Suppl): 21–24
49. Terman GW, Lewis JW, Liebeskind JC (1984) Endogenous pain inhibitory substrates and mechanisms. In: Benedetti C, Chapman CR, Moricca G (eds) Advances in pain research and therapy, Vol 7, Raven Press, New York, pp 43–56
50. Tzivoni D, Benhorin J, Gavish A, Stern S (1985) Holter recording during treadmill testing in assessing myocardial ischemic changes. Am J Cardiol 55: 1200–1203
51. Uchida Y, Murao S (1974) Potassium-induced excitation of afferent cardiac sympathetic nerve fibers. Am J Physiol 226: 603–607
52. VanRijn T, Rabkin SW (1981) Effect of naloxone on exercise-induced angina pectoris: a randomized double blind crossover trial. Life Sci 38: 609–615
53. Weidinger F, Hammerle A, Sochor H, Smetana R, Frass M, Glogar D (1986) Role of beta-endorphins in silent myocardial ischemia. Am J Cardiol 58: 428–430
54. White JC (1957) Cardiac pain, Anatomic pathways and physiologic mechanisms. Circulation 16: 644–655

Authors' address:
Dr. med. Dr. phil. Dipl.-Psych. C. Droste
Benedikt Kreutz Rehabilitationszentrum
für Herz- und Kreislaufkranke
Südring 15
7812 Bad Krozingen

Discussion on Pathophysiology

Chairmen: G. Riecker and A. Malliani

The discussion started with the question of whether parallels can be drawn to ischemia from animal experiments where chronic pain activates opioid systems. Millan assented but mentioned the limited amount of experimental data, the difficulty in comparing human and animal experiments and the fact that no animal model existed for visceral pain (apart from the chronic dog model, Malliani).

Different groups had different experiences with the effect of naloxon on ischemic pain. Droste pointed out that in two of his patients the injection of naloxon unmasked angina on exercise. He mentioned two other studies with similar effects, while in a further two, naloxon was not effective. This may have been an effect of dosage or it may be that a battery of stimuli is necessary. Chierchia mentioned his negative results with naloxon in high doses in four patients with Prinzmetal angina. Naloxon has a different affinity to different types of receptors (Millan).

Therefore the absence of pain may be an opioidergic effect, even when it cannot be blocked by naloxon. Malliani rated the evidence of naloxon effects as as yet inconclusive.

To the question of the effect of exercise on opioid systems, Millan called for especially careful interpretation of plasma level studies. It is unproven whether endorphin plasma levels have any causal relation to analgesic effects. On the other hand, stressful stimulation in conflict situations with other species can activate the pain inhibitory systems. Another opioidergic effect may be reward, for example, the receipt of positive stimuli such as food or sex. Asked about of the influence of opioids on single, isolated sympathetic fibers. Millan mentioned direct inhibitory actions in opioid receptors on presynaptic adrenergic nerve terminals. These would also inhibit the release of noradrenaline and inhibit its constrictive action on coronary arteries. Morphine would probably not be useful in inhibiting this noradrenaline release. Substances working on the kappa receptor seem more promising but have not yet been tried clinically.

Asked why myocarditis with abcesses or sarcoid heart disease is not painful, Weihe pointed out, that the adequate stimulus for cardiac pain is unknown. This leads us to the question of whether pure nociceptive fibers exist in the heart and if so, what their distribution might be. Malliani reasoned that pure nociceptors do not exist, because all afferents from the heart have spontaneous impulse activity and all intensify the discharge with physiological stimuli. The definition of nociceptor theory would require that they have no background activity and are recruited only by a stimulus strong enough to be noxious to the tissue. There seems to be no purpose in animals possessing thousands of fibers to facilitate awareness of a coronary emergency. The heart does not have an alarm system that can be expected to give alarm, and therefore it is not defective when sometimes it does not give a warning.

Droste quoted histochemical studies in which free nerve endings have been demonstrated in the myocardium which could be pain receptors. Weihe, however, agreed with Malliani that viscera including the heart have no pure nociceptors.

Tzivoni asked for an interpretation of the findings of his own studies in which pain was less common in post-infarct ischemia than in patients who had not had an infarction. As explanations, the destruction of fibers (Malliani) or differences in the spatial distribution of ischemia (Droste) were offered. The notion that variant angina may be less painful than exercise-induced angina was questioned by Chierchia, who interpreted it by the fact that during exercise testing, one of the endpoints is to produce anginal pain. Chierchia opposed the over-simplistic equation that painless ischemia equals vasospastic ischemia and would therefore ask for therapy with vasodilators. He emphasized that silent ischemia has the same pathophysiological mechanism as painful ischemia. Silent ischemia may occur during acute myocardial infarction where thrombosis is the cause of ischemia, during exercise, where ischemia is caused by increased demand or during vasospastic ischemia, where decreased supply is the problem.

Rutishauser asked how, in chronic instrumented animals three days after thoracotomy, pain could be assessed. Malliani mentioned the differences between injections of bradykinin, which the dog does not feel and the injection of penicillin, during which the dog can very well show its pain.

Rafflenbeul reported his experience with intracoronary injections of bradykinin in patients. During these injections all patients have pain, which is a diffuse pain — unlike angina — all over the body. All patients experienced a fall in blood pressure. Malliani commented on the fact that this can appear with many drugs and that all nerve endings can be massively activated. If humans hearts had a specific sense of pain, then angioplasty should produce pain on 100% of occasions, which it does not. This shows an elusive link and should be one reason not to base treatment, prognosis or the follow-up of the patient merely on the presence or absence of cardiac pain.
Asked about the implications of his findings on alpha receptors affecting coronary sinus flow, Chierchia mentioned other experiments in which resting coronary sinus flow increased after administration of alpha-blockers. If alpha-mediated constriction is abolished, resting flow increases, as well as flow, during exercise. This might be a physiological explanation as to why the sympathetic nervous system constricts coronary arteries during sympathetic stimulation: it may be to avoid luxury perfusion and intramyocardial plethora which could in itself be harmful to the tissue.
Lichtlen pointed out the role that alpha tone has on the coronaries and which could be demonstrated by vasoconstriction after beta-blockade. Chierchia drew attention to the fact that there are probably many more substances involved in sympathetic stimulation and other receptors which are mediating coronary vasoconstriction. Acetylcholine, for instance, can induce coronary vasoconstriction directly, in the absence or in the presence of endothelium. It may not, therefore, be a specific marker of endothelial denudation. Both Chierchia and Riecker, in his final statement, commented on the importance of applying measurements of coronary blood flow in future studies. Not only should the epicardial coronary arteries be concentrated upon but also the small vessels, where the bulk of the resistance lies.

Silent myocardial ischemia in middle aged men: Long term clinical course

J. Erikssen[1], P. F. Cohn[2], E. Thaulow[3], P. Mowinckel[1]

[1] Med. Dept., Central Hospital of Akershus, Nordbyhagen, Norway.
[2] Cardiological Div., Dept. of Medicine, State University of New York at Stony Brook, USA (visiting professor, London)
[3] Dept. of Clinical Physiology, Ullevål Hospital, Oslo, Norway.

Subjects and methods

During the years 1972—1975, a group of 2014 apparently healthy men participated in a cardiovascular survey examination aimed at detecting subclinical CAD by means of a comprehensive, noninvasive test program (4). All worked in 5 companies in Oslo, Norway, preselected since they had been giving regular annual or biennial health checks to their employees for some years. All available health data were scrutinized prior to entry into the study, and all those who had had any of the diseases noted in Table 1 were primarily excluded, as were all men who on arrival for the survey examination, reported that any of these diseases/disorders had been diagnosed or suspected elsewhere, prior to the survey examination.

The examination program is apparent from Table 2 and the final subdivision of the total material from Table 3. Fifty men with a positive exercise ECG test result as the sole indicator of their asymptomatic CAD formed the basis of the present report (4).

All 50 have been followed closely until death or up to the present study examination. None were lost to follow-up. During the follow-up period, all had at least one annual examination, which included a complete examination, blood tests and a symptom-lim-

Table 1. Exclusion criteria applied when selecting the baseline population*

Exclusions were made primarily, and at attending the baseline examination, in all men with any of the following diseases/disorders:

1. Known or suspected coronary heart disease.
2. Other known heart disease.
3. Hypertension treated with drugs.
4. Known diabetes mellitus and clinical diabetes diagnosed for the first time at the baseline study.
5. Malignant disease (excluding skin cancer).
6. Disorders of the locomotor system preventing the conduction of a bicycle ergometer test.
7. Miscellaneous diseases (severe lung disease, liver disease, renal disease etc.).

* 86% of employees (see Subjects and methods section) eligible for the survey study participated (n = 2014 men, aged 40—59 years).

Table 2. Baseline examination program

1. Registration of a comprehensive case history (including World Health Organisation questionnaire on angina).
2. Complete physical examination.
3. A panel of laboratory tests, including a lipid profile, an intravenous glucose tolerance test, spirography study.
4. Resting 12-lead ECG and 6-lead monitored near maximal bicycle exercise ECG-testing.
5. X-ray of heart/lungs.
6. Phonocardiographic study.
7. Study of platelet adhesitivity.
8. Study of various coagulation factors.
9. Study of insulin response to the intravenous glucose tolerance test.
10. Selective coronary angiography in subjects with survery findings suggesting the presence of possible, latent coronary artery disease.

Table 3.

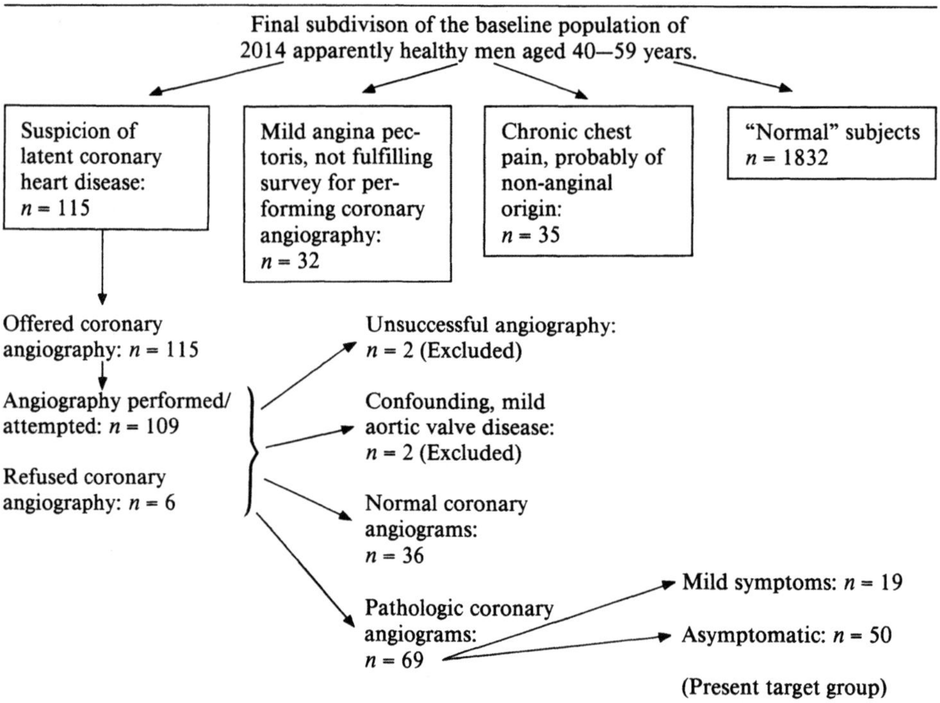

ited exercise ECG test using a technique identical to the baseline test (4). In addition all were given free access to medical aid, and were specifically asked to seek medical advice if they developed chest pain, severe, unexplained dyspnea or any symptom which they themselves thought warranted further scrutiny. Repeated angiographic studies and bypass operations during follow-up were only performed for clinical reasons. None had prophylactic bypass operations.

Follow-up events have been subdivided as follows:

1. Coronary deaths
2. Myocardial infarctions
3. Angina pectoris de novo

In addition we have also noted the presence or absence of a more pathologic exercise ECG during follow-up examinations. The criteria are reported in detail elsewhere (6). *Coronary angiographic progression* was diagnosed when: (a) an increased number of vessels were significantly stenosed (b) when a complete occlusion was detected in an area where a vessel had been observed on the first angiogram (c) when a vessel which was only partially obstructed during the first angiographic study had been increasingly stenosed by the second (or third) angiogram. The criterion was that the relation between stenosis diameter and the prestenotic vessel had decreased by $\geqq 25\%$ between two angiographic views.

Coronary artery disease progression was diagnosed in the presence of CHD events 1, 2 and 3 and/or angiographically verified progression (6). Data are given from the 8 year and 12.5 year follow-up.

Results

The time from the baseline study to the present last examination was 11—14 years (mean 12.5). The data on CHD events are given in Figs. 1, 2 and 3, in which data from the 8 years (A in each figure) and the 12.5 year (B in each figure) examinations are compared. On the first occasion, 3 subjects had died; additionally, 7 had had an MI, 16 had developed AP and 27 had developed a more pathologic exercise ECG. Only 17 were clinically unchanged from the baseline study. At 12.5 years, 11 had died; 8 of the remaining had had an MI, 18 had AP and 26 of the remaining men alive had angiographic signs of

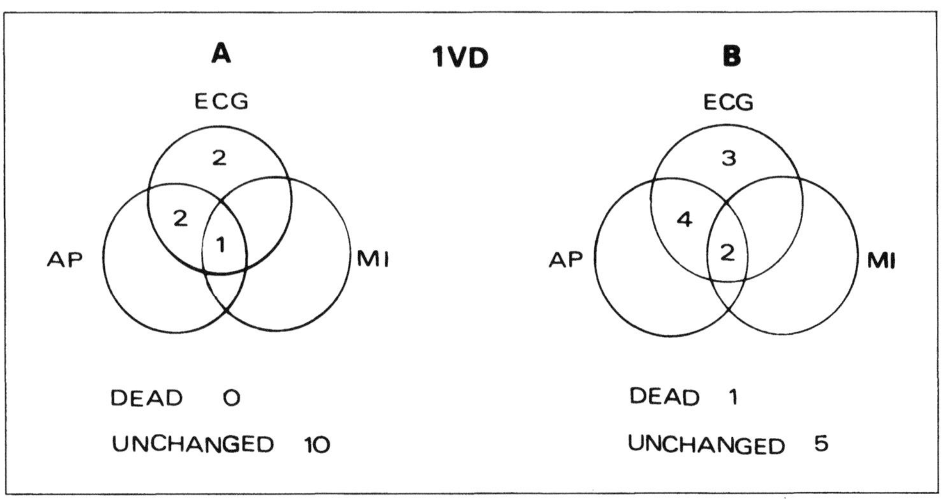

Fig. 1. Venn diagram showing the number of coronary events among men with IVD at the baseline examination. A: findings at 8 years, and B: findings at 12.5 years follow-up.

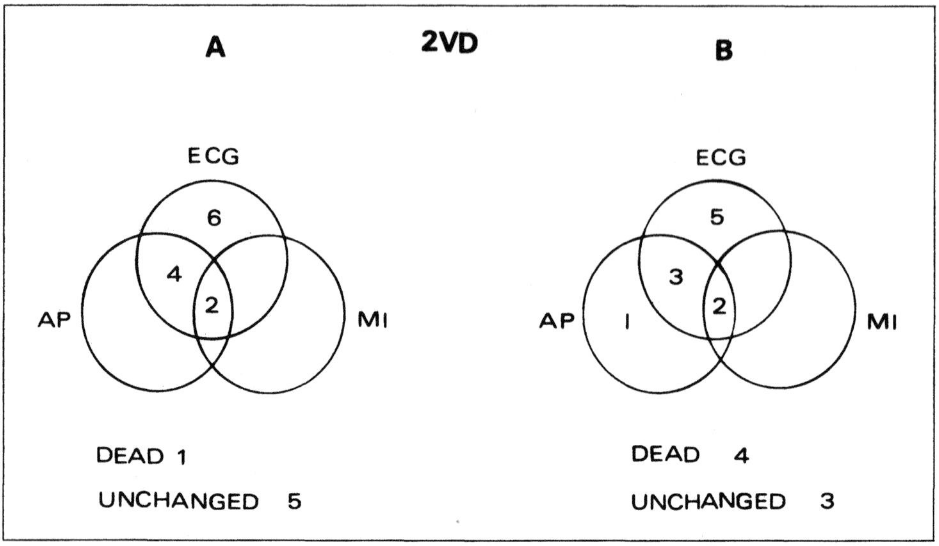

Fig. 2. Venn diagram showing the number of coronary events among men with 2VD at the baseline examination. A: findings at 8 years, and B: findings at 12.5 years follow-up.

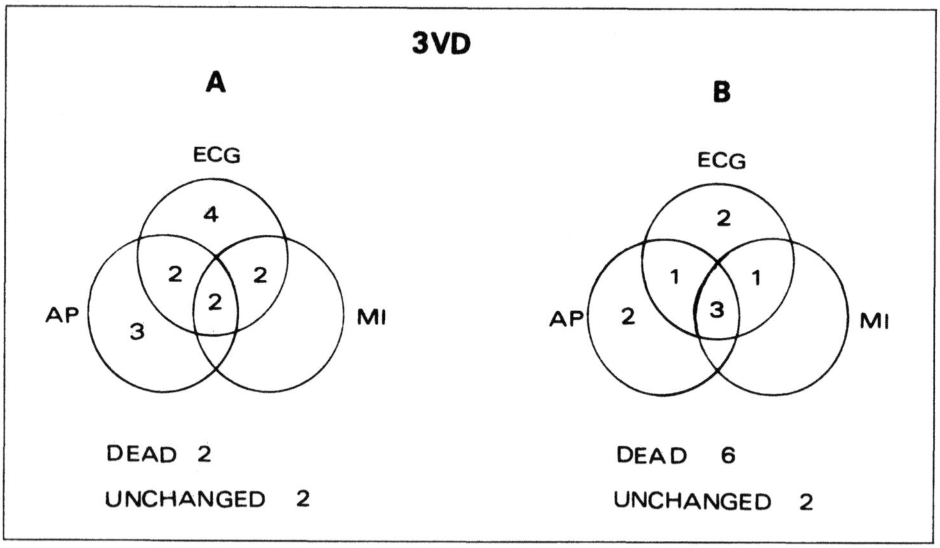

Fig. 3. Venn diagram showing the number of coronary events among men with 3VD at the baseline examination. A: findings at 8 years, and B: findings at 12.5 years follow-up.

exercise ECG deterioration. The various combinations of events are apparent from the Venn diagrams.

Of the 11 who died, 9 had died from CHD and 2 from cancer. The latter two probably had a progression of their CAD, according to the autopsy findings, at death 7 and 9 years after the baseline study, respectively; a second coronary angiographic study was not available in these 2 men.

Twenty-eight had at least one additional coronary angiographic study, but performed at considerably varying intervals: e.g., the first took place one year after the original study and the last was performed recently, i.e., 14 years after the original study. Four had unchanged angiographic findings after intervals of between 6 and 10 years, whereas 24 had evidence of CAD progression.

The mortality rate was 35% among those with a baseline 3VD, 22% among those with a baseline 2VD and only 7% among those with 1VD. Although suggestive, these differences do not reach statistical significance. As can be seen, mortality occurred mainly during the last few years of observation, i.e., mainly after 10 years of observation (Figs. 1, 2, 3). Only one subject died without having developed angina pectoris on MI prior to his death. Thus although 9 of the 11 deaths were related to CHD and 7 of the 9 were sudden and unexpected, only one had no angina pectoris prior to his death. He died during violent exertion after a heavy meal.

Discussion

Exercise ECG testing contributes independently of other so-called coronary risk factors to CHD risk prediction (5, 7). The main concern in using exercise ECG testing to diagnose CHD is the large number of false positive tests. Although the number of false positive diagnoses an be minimized by taking into consideration results from other non-invasive tests, such as thallium scintigraphy, isotope ventriculography at rest/during exercise, exercise echocardiography, electrokymography, etc., data from such validational studies are lacking in population studies. Moreover, all these non-invasive tests have their limitations. Hence, coronary angiography should therefore be considered the "gold standard" for the final diagnosis of coronary artery disease (CAD) so far.

Whereas repeated angiograms in patients with clinical disease suggest progression in most subjects tested (11), these materials are heavily biased. On the other hand, the knowledge of progression rate is almost nonexistent in asymptomatic subjects with proven CAD. The obvious reason is that very few authors have performed coronary angiography in asymptomatic subjects (1, 4, 8).

Our present data are reasonably representative of what can be detected by our baseline protocol (4). Thus, of 115 subjects with a baseline suspicion of previously undetected CAD, 109 gave their informed consent for the coronary angiographic evaluation (4). Of these, 105 had a complete examination, whereas two with mild aortic valve disease and two asymptomatic men with bilateral iliac artery occlusion (Judkin's femoral approach unsuccessful) were excluded. Of the remaining 105, 69 had pathologic angiograms, of whom 50 were completely asymptomatic. Of 2014 men tested, then, 50/2014 (2.5%) had silent myocardial ischemia, suggesting a major, latent community health problem (2, 3). The clinical course among these 50 middle aged men appeared benign during the first years. Thus, as reported previously, the first event occurred after approximately 3 years (6). Although the number of events increased rapidly during the years immediately preceding the report at 8 years mortality rate at that time was rather low (6). During the further 4.5 years observation, mortality has increased rapidly, and more so in those with baseline 2VD and 3VD than among those with 1VD. Moreover a considerable number of men have also developed angina and/or myocardial infarctions.

These data are somewhat discouraging, since it seems that CAD progresses when only "common" measures are taken to prevent progression. On all annual examinations all were asked to stop smoking (if they had not), the necessity of adhering to the low fat diet was repeated and mild exercise was recommended. This regime has apparently been insufficient in preventing CAD-progression, although the unproven impression is that those who adhered strictly had a more benign course than those who did not (Erikssen: unpublished data). The impact of a strict CAD preventive approach in such patients can only be tested during a randomized clinical trial.

The impact of bypass surgery on the final outcome in our men is uncertain. The CASS study indicates that early surgery cannot be recommeded in mildly symptomatic men if improvement in mortality is the final goal (9). It is, however, noteworthy that all 12 who have had bypass surgery are still alive. All deaths thus took place in non-operated subjects, four of whom died while awaiting a second angiographic examination to see if bypass surgery was possible.

The present data strongly suggests that asymptomatic CAD is a progressive disease. Discussion on the use of lipid lowering drugs etc. is beyond the scope of this presentation, as is the use of PTCA.

The problem of silent myocardial ischemia in patients with known CAD has recently become a field of major interest, since it has been shown that some 75% of all ischemic episodes seem to be asymptomatic (10). Moreover, limited experience indicates that an increase in such episodes may have grave prognostic significance (10). Data on such testing in the asymptomatic population is largely unknown. However, our data suggest that such testing during the asymptomatic stage would have contributed only marginally to the prognostication in our population, since only one man died without having developed symptoms and/or signs of CHD. Death and MI were almost universally preceded by angina. This possibly indicates that 24 hour monitoring should be reserved for symptomatic subjects when resources are limited, although the important aspect of gathering information with this test for epidemiological purposes in the normal population should be kept in mind. After angina has developed, ECG monitoring over 24 hours may be one way of detecting patients prone to develop more serious complications.

Conclusions

Asymptomatic CAD is a serious progressive disease which deserves continuous surveillance.

The optimal way of treating this condition is still to be defined.

References

1. Borer JS, Brensike JF, Redwood DR, Itscoitz SB, Passamani ER, Stone NJ, Richardson JM, Levi RI, Epstein SE (1975) Limitations of the electrocardiographic response to exercise in predicting coronary artery disease. New Engl J Med 293: 367—371
2. Cohn PF (1985) Silent myocardial ischemia: Classification, prevalence and prognosis. Am J Med 79, Suppl 3 A: 2—6

3. Cohn PF (1986) Silent myocardial ischemia: Dimensions of the problem in patients with and without angina. Am J Med 80, Suppl 4 C: 3—8
4. Erikssen J, Enge I, Storstein O, Forfang K (1976) Circulation 53: 371—376
5. Erikssen J, Mundal R (1981) The non-infarct patient with coronary artery disease: Can a high risk group be identified? Ann NY Acad Sci: 438—451
6. Erikssen J, Thaulow E (1984) Follow up of patients with asymptomatic myocardial ischemia. In: Rutishauser W, Roskamm H (eds) Silent myocardial ischemia. Springer Verlag, Berlin, pp 156—164
7. Froelicher VF, Thompson AJ, Longo MR, Triebwasser WJ, Lancaster MC (1976) Progr Cardiovasc Dis 18: 265—276
8. Froelicher VF, Yanowitz FG, Thompson AJ (1973) The correlation of coronary angiography and electrocardiographic response to maximal treadmill testing in 76 asymptomatic men. Circulation 48: 597—604
9. National Blood, Lung and Heart Institute Coronary Artery Surgery Study (CASS) (1981) Principal Investigators and their Associates. Circulation, Suppl I
10. Pepine CJ (1986) Clinical aspects of silent myocardial ischemia in patients with angina and other forms of coronary heart disease. Am J Med 80, Suppl 4 C: 25—34
11. Proudfit WL, Bruschke AV, Sones FM Jr (1978) Natural history of obstructive coronary artery disease: Ten-year study of 601 non-surgical cases. Progr Cardiovasc Dis 22: 53—78

Author‘s adress:
J. Erikssen, M.D., Ph.D.
Medical Department
Central Hospital of Akershus
1474 Nordbyhagen
Norway

Prognostic implications of silent ischemia in patients with stable angina pectoris

K. M. Fox

National Heart Hospital, Westmoreland Street, London, England

Summary

Twenty-four-hour ambulatory monitoring of the ST segments coupled with hemodynamic and radionuclide studies in patients with angina has shown that silent myocardial ischemia is frequent. Hemodynamic studies, nuclear imaging and ambulatory pulmonary artery monitoring has shown that silent ST segment depression is accompanied by alterations in left ventricular filling pressure and alterations in myocardial perfusion very similar to those seen during angina pectoris. Whilst the prognostic implications of silent ischemia are unknown, circumstantial evidence would suggest that silent ischemia is important. Long term follow up studies have shown that silent ischemia in completely asymptomatic subjects is associated with subsequent death and the development of symptoms. Approximately one quater of all myocardial infarctions occur without chest pain and half of these are completely silent; the long term outlook from silent myocardial infarction does not differ form infarction accompanied by chest pain. Finally, recent investigations in unstable angina show that silent myocardial ischemia is an important predictor of future coronary events.

Thus, silent ischemia should not be considered in any way different to angina pectoris in terms of prognosis. The mechanisms responsible for producing silent ischemia do not differ from angina and in any one patient the pathophysiological mechanism may change depending on the stage of the disease. Therapeutic approaches should not be confined to simply alleviating silent ischemia in patients with chronic stable angina, but should be aimed at preventing the subsequent probable outcomes, i.e., sudden death, unstable angina and myocardial infarction.

Twenty-four-hour ambulatory monitoring has been used in the diagnosis of cardiac arrhythmias for many years. More recently, patients with angina pectoris have been undergoing ambulatory monitoring studies and it has been observed that during angina pectoris, ST segment depression occurs; this is to be expected since ST segment depression is known to indicate the presence of myocardial ischemia. However, it has also been found that ST segment depression can occur in patients with angina pectoris in the absence of chest pain (1, 2). At first it was suggested that these ST segment changes did not reflect myocardial ischemia since such changes could be recorded in normal subjects. However, ST segment depression in a normal volunteer has very different characteristic features to those recorded in patients with known coronary artery disease (3). In normal volunteers, they are usually accompanied by a tachycardia and are rarely more severe than 2 mm depressed. In contrast, in patients with coronary artery disese, ST segment changes will often occur at much lower heart rates and very frequently several millimetres of ST segment depression will be observed. Indeed, the ST segment changes accompanied by angina cannot be distinguished morphologically from those that are not accompanied by chest pain.

In patients with coronary artery disease, it has been found that approximately one third of all episodes of ST segment depression are accompanied by chest pain (4). In general, however, the more severe the ST segment depression, the more frequently chest pain is an accompanying feature, such that approximately 15% of episodes of 1 mm ST segment depression are accompanied by chest pain, whilst approximately 35% of episodes of 4 mm ST segment will be accompanied by chest pain. However, even in 4 mm ST segment depression the majority of episodes will be pain-free. Also episodes of ST segment depression accompanied by pain tend to be longer in duration than those not accompanied by pain. In a recent study, the relationship between heart rate and the development of ST segment changes has been analyzed (5). It has been found that in the majority of episodes, the heart rate preceded the onset of ST segment depression which again preceded the onset of chest pain. This occurred in both episodes that were present during the day, as well as those seen at night. However, of particular interest was that the pattern of the relationship between heart rate and ST segment changes was identical between painful episodes and painless episodes, such that they can be distinguished only by the late development of chest pain. It was also found that the circadian distribution of ST segment changes was identical in terms of the number of episodes and duration, whether or not the episodes were accompanied by chest pain (4).

Thus, morphological studies using ambulatory monitoring have shown that both painful and painless ST segment depression are indistinguishable when they occur in patients with coronary artery disease. However, painless ST segment depression in normal volunteers can easily be distinguished from the ST segment changes described in patients with angina pectoris. Of equal importance, particularly in terms of the prognostic and therapeutic implications is that the mechanism responsible for the development of painful ST segment depression appears to be identical to that responsible for painless ST segment depression. In other words, in patients in whom effort and increased myocardial oxygen demand is responsible for the generation of angina, it will also be responsible for the development of silent ST segment changes; likewise in those patients with variant angina ST segment elevation, whether it is accompanied by pain or not, will be generated by a similar mechanism and the circadian distribution of ST segment elevation in these circumstances will be identical, i.e., predominantly in the early hours of the morning. Many patients have multiple mechanisms generating their angina and in such circumstances the mechanisms generating silent ST segment changes will be similar.

The significance of painless ST segment depression

The frequency of painless versus painful ST segment depression is unrelated to the extent of coronary artery disease. Studies using a nuclear stethoscope have shown that in both painful and painless ST segment depression there are increases in left ventricular volume and these increases precede the development of chest pain where it occurs. Furthermore, using positron tomography it has, on occasion, been possible to record positron scans during painless ST segment changes. These scans using Rubidium 82 show that during painless ST segment depression, defects in the regional myocardial uptake of rubidium occur. Invasive investigations following cardiac catheterization, in which catheters have been left in the left ventricle, have shown that during painless ST segment depression, there is an increase in left ventricular filling pressure although this increase is not as great as during episodes of painful ST segment depression (6).

The recent development of ambulatory pulmonary artery monitoring has provided a means of recording ambulatory pulmonary artery diastolic pressure (7). In the absence of obstructive lesions of the mitral valve and in the absence of pulmonary hypertension a pulmonary artery diastolic pressure equates with left ventricular filling pressure. This allows for indirect assessment of left ventricular function to be made while the patient is ambulant and going about his everyday activities. Such recordings in patients have shown that during painless ST segment depression there is an increase in pulmonary artery diastolic pressure (8). Such increases in pulmonary artery diastolic pressure were not seen in normal controls and indeed were equal in magnitude to the increase that occurred during painful ST segment depression. Also, the increases in pulmonary artery diastolic pressure were unrelated to the severity of ST segment depression.

Prognostic Implications

These results show that painless ST segment depression cannot be distinguished either morphologically, or on the basis of their hemodynamic effects, from painful ST segment depression. Further studies are necessary to determine the prognostic significance of myocardial ischemia. Circumstantial evidence, however, would suggest that silent ischemia does have important prognostic implications. In a recent update from the Framingham study, it was noted that of 708 myocardial infarctions occurring amongst 5, 127 participants, more than 25% were discovered only through the apperance of a routine electrocardiogram (9). Of these unrecognised infarctions, almost half were silent while the other half had atypical symptoms. In a recent study of silent ischemia in patients with unstable angina, survival curve analysis demonstrated that silent ischemia is associated with a higher incidence of myocardial infarction, bypass graft surgery or angioplasty (10). A multi-variant analysis showed that myocardial ischemia was the best predictor of these outcomes amongst the 15 variables tested.

Perhaps the most compelling evidence, however, comes from the studies of Eriksson in which follow-up data has been obtained in 50 patients who were completely asymptomatic and screened from a population of over 2,000 office workers (11). Over 8 years, 6% died, 14% developed an acute myocardial infarction, 32% developed angina and 22% underwent coronary artery bypass surgery.

Undoubtedly, silent ST segment depression truly reflects silent myocardial ischemia and this has important implications. Theoretically, it could be argued that patients die because they develop ischemic ventricular arrhythmias or because they develop coronary spasm leading to unstable angina and myocardial infarction. Finally, patients may die because they develop unstable angina or acute myocardial infarction following rupture of their atherosclerotic plaque. Silent ischemia, whether or not angina pectoris is present, indicates that there is underlying atherosclerotic heart disease or, less frequently, coronary spasm in the presence of normal coronary arteries. Thus, the mechanism is present for the development of ischemic ventricular arrhythmias, coronary spasm or plaque rupture. Further research is necessary to determine why stable silent ischemia or angina pectoris become unstable.

References

1. Schang SJ, Pepine CJ (1977) Transient asymptomatic ST segment depression during daily activity. Am J Cardiol 39: 396—402
2. Selwyn AP, Fox K, Eves M, Oakley D, Dargie H, Shillingford J (1978) Myocardial ischemia in patients with frequent angina pectoris. Br Med J 2: 1594—1596
3. Quyyumi AA, Wright C, Fox K (1983) Ambulatory electrocardiographic ST segment changes in healthy volunteers. Br Heart J 50: 460—464
4. Deanfield JE, Maseri A, Selwyn AP et al (1983) Myocardial ischemia during daily life in patients with stable angina: its relation to symptoms and heart rate changes. Lancet ii: 753—758
5. Quyyumi AA, Wright CA, Mockus LJ, Fox KM (1984) Mechanisms of nocturnal angina pectoris: importance of increased myocardial oxygen demand in patients with severe coronary artery disease. Lancet i: 1207—1209
6. Maseri A, Severi S, Denes M et al (1978) "Variant angina": One aspect of a continuous spectrum of vasospastic myocardial ischemia. Am J Cardiol 42: 1019—1035
7. Levy RD, Cunningham AD, Shapiro LM, Wright C, Mockus L, Fox KM (1986) Continuous ambulatory pulmonary artery pressure monitoring: A new method using a transducer tipped catheter and a simple recording system. Br Heart J 55: 336—343
8. Levy RD, Shapiro LM, Wright C, Mockus L, Fox KM (1986) The hemodynamic significance of asymptomatic ST segment depression assessed by ambulatory pulmonary artery pressure monitoring. Br Heart J 56: 526—530
9. Kannel WB, Abbott RD (1984) Incidence and prognosis of unrecognised myocardial infarction. An update on the Framingham Study. N Engl J Med 311: 1144—1147
10. Gottlieb SO, Weisfeldt ML, Ouyang P, Mellits ED, Gerstenblitz G (1986) Silent ischemia as a marker for early unfavorable outcomes in patients with unstable angina. N Engl J Med 314: 1214—1219
11. Erikssen J, Thaulow E (1984) Follow up of patients with asymptomatic myocardial ischemia In: Rutisauser W and Rosham H (eds) Silent Myocardial Ischemia, Springer Verlag, Berlin, pp 156—164

Author's address:
Dr. Kim M. Fox
National Heart Hospital
Westmoreland Street
London W1M 8BA
England

Silent myocardial ischemia in unstable angina: Prognostic considerations

S. O. Gottlieb, M. L. Weisfeldt, G. Gerstenblith

John Hopkins University School of Medicine, Francis Scott Key Medical Center, John Hopkins Medical Institutions, Baltimore, Maryland, U.S.A.

Introduction

Unstable angina is a high risk syndrome which may be defined by the new onset of angina symptoms, a crescendo pattern of angina, and the occurrence of rest angina. The pathophysiology of this condition is complex, and involves a combination of fixed coronary atherosclerosis and superimposed dynamic coronary obstruction, mediated by coronary vasoconstriction, and/or platelet aggregation and thrombosis (1, 2). Although aggressive medical therapy for patients with unstable angina often successfully controls symptoms in the coronary care unit, a significant proportion of patients whose symptoms are initially ameliorated nevertheless experience cardiac death, myocardial infarction, and recurrent angina requiring revascularization (3—6).
Continuous electrocardiographic monitoring has demonstrated a high number of ischemic episodes in patients with coronary artery disease (7—13), and these changes have been shown to represent true ischemic events through correlations with abnormalities of myocardial perfusion and function (14—16). This review will discuss the utility of the technique of continuous electrocardiographic monitoring to detect ischemic episodes, many of which are silent, in patients with unstable angina. The use of this technique will also be correlated with prognosis and therapy.

The detection of ischemic events with continuous electrocardiographic recording

Holter first reported the use of continuous electrocardiographic recording in ambulatory patients for the diagnosis of cardiac rhythm abnormalities in 1961, and in the original paper a continuous electrocardiographic tracing demonstrating ST segment depression was published (17). In 1974, Stern and Tzivoni reported the results of electrocardiographic monitoring to detect ischemic episodes. They found that nearly one half of stable angina patients studied had ischemic episodes on Holter monitoring, which they correlated with the occurrence of cardiac events over 6—12 months of follow-up (7). Shang and Pepine demonstrated the occurrence of ischemic episodes which were often asymptomatic during ordinary daily activities (8). Other investigators including Maseri, Selwyn, Deanfield and others have demonstrated a much higher incidence of silent ischemic events in patients with coronary artery disease than was previously appreciated (9—16), and these episodes have been correlated with abnormalities of myocardial perfusion and function (14—16) as well as elevations of left ventricular filling pressures (18). In contrast to the frequent documentation of ischemic episodes in patients with coronary artery disease, there appears to be a low incidence of transient ST-segment changes in patients who do not have coronary artery disease (19).

Early investigations utilized frequency-modulated recording systems for ST-segment analysis. Certain amplitude-modulated systems have frequency-response characteristics sufficient to detect ST-segment changes, and comparative studies have demonstrated that the diagnostic accuracy of certain amplitude-modulated systems are similar to frequency-modulated systems (20).

Incidence and importance of silent ischemia in unstable angina

A high incidence of silent ichemic episodes has been detected in several studies using the continuous electrocardiographic recording technique in patients with unstable angina (11—13). In the Johns Hopkins study, 70 patients at rest in the coronary care unit with angina who had ischemic electrocardiographic changes accompanying episodes of pain (21) were studied. The patients were treated with a triple combination of anti-ischemic therapy including long-acting nitrates, propranolol, at least 160 mg daily, and nifedipine 80 mg daily. Holter monitoring was performed during the first 48 h in the CCU. The two leads which initially demonstrated the most pronounced ischemic changes on the 12 lead electrocardiogram were chosen for monitoring. The definition of ischemic episodes was: the occurrence of ST-segment elevation or horizontal or downsloping ST-segment depression of at least 1 mm, occurring 80 ms after the J point and lasting for at least 1 min. Of the 70 patients, 37 (53%) experienced a total of 205 ischemic episodes on the Holter, and the median duration per episode was 20 min. Over 90% of all episodes were asymptomatic; only 8 of the 37 patients with ischemic episodes had accompanying angina; 29 had only silent ischemia. The clinical characteristics of the patients with and without silent ischemia demonstrated no significant differences with regard to age, sex, cardiovascular risk factors, or the extent of obstructive coronary artery disease documented at angiography. The mean left ventricular ejection fraction in the group with silent ischemia (56 ± 14%) was lower than the group without silent ischemia (64 ± 13%), possibly related to the repeated ischemic episodes causing stunned myocardium.

The total number of ischemic episodes, both symptomatic and asymptomatic, appear be correlated with the occurrence of unfavorable clinical outcomes in patients with unstable angina (12, 13, 21). In the Johns Hopkins study (21), 20 patients experienced outcomes including myocardial infarction ($n = 7$) or recurrent angina which required revascularization ($n = 13$). Sixteen of the 20 patients who experienced unfavorable outcomes were in the group with silent ischemia. In addition, Kaplan-Meier analysis demonstrated that the patients with silent ischemia had a statistically significant higher cumulative probability of experiencing an unfavorable outcome over one month ($p > 0.002$, Fig. 1). Similar analysis of the 29 patients with only silent ischemia, i.e. who had no angina accompanying the ST-segment changes during the two day period also demonstrated that silent ischemia was associated with a higher risk of outcome.

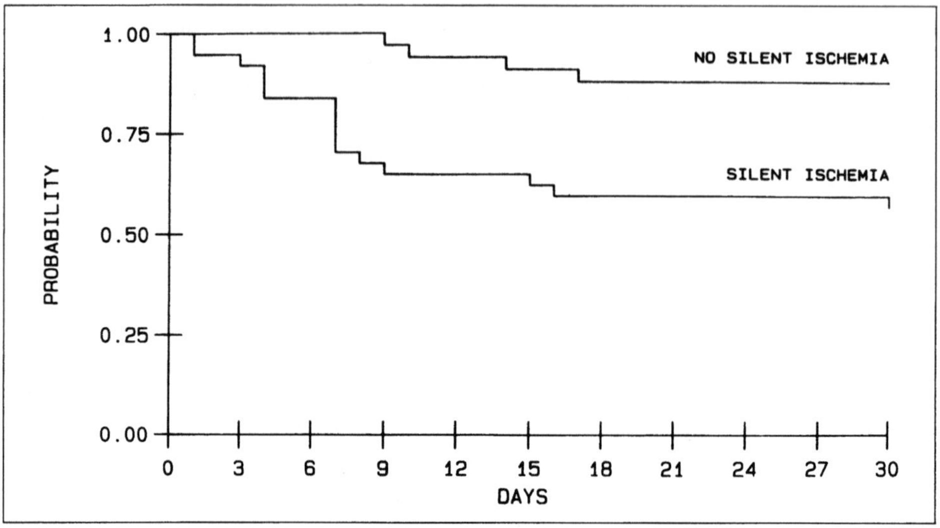

Fig. 1. Kaplan-Meier curves comparing the probability of not experiencing an unfavorable outcome (myocardial infarction of revascularization for symptoms) over 30 days, for 37 unstable angina patients with silent ischemia and 33 patients without silent ischemia detected by continuous electrocardiographic monitoring ($p < 0.002$); (21).

The total cumulative duration of all silent ischemic episodes over the 48 h monitoring period was also associated with the occurrence of clinical outcomes. Those patients who experienced $\geqslant$ 60 min per 24 h of silent ischemia had a worse prognosis than those with less than 60 min per 24 h ($p < 0.04$). Using a multivariate analysis, silent ischemia was also compared to a number of clinical, electrocardiographic and angiographic variables which have previously been considered predictive of outcome in patients with ischemic heart disease. In this multivariate analysis, silent ischemia was found to be the most predictive variable of unfavorable outcomes.
These results demonstrate that the presence and the extent of silent ischemia, as detected by continuous electrocardiographic recording, are significantly correlated with early unfavorable outcomes, providing a measure of the level of dynamic disease activity and abnormal physiology which my be used, together with the anatomic findings at angiography, to provide better risk stratification for unstable angina patients.

Therapeutic considerations

Holter monitoring for the detection of ischemic episodes has provided important insight into the frequent occurrence and severity of asymptomatic ischemia, the extent of which has prognostic significance in unstable angina patients. The finding or persistent ischemia on Holter monitoring with its adverse prognostic implications suggests that further anti-ischemic therapy is warranted.

Medical therapy

Controlled clinical trials have demonstrated the efficacy of combination medical therapy including nitrates, beta blockers and calcium antagonists in unstable angina (4—6). The calcium antagonist nifedipine added to therapy with propranolol and nitrates has been demonstrated to be efficacious in reducing the incidence of recurrent ischemia requiring revascularization, and in reducing the incidence of infarction or cardiac death in patients with post-infarction angina (4, 22). In another trial, the beta blocker propranolol has been shown to be effective in unstable angina when added to coronary vasodilator therapy with nitrates and nifedipine, in reducing both symptomatic and asymptomatic ischemic episodes (6). Initial therapy with nifedipine has been shown to be comparable to the combination of beta blockers and nitrates in another randomized trial (5); however, considerable evidence supporting the combination of beta blockers and calcium antagonists suggests that this is the best initial strategy which provides additional synergistic benefit beyond the effect of either drug alone.
Anticoagulation with heparin has been reported in one study to reduce the incidence of subsequent myocardial infarction in patients with unstable angina (23), and two large multicenter randomized trials have demonstrated the benefit of aspirin in reducing death or reinfarction (24, 25). There is a growing body of angiographic (26, 27) and angioscopic (28) evidence supporting the concept that unstable angina is commonly the result of a complex unstable atherosclerotic lesion involving ruptured plaque and with subsequent thrombosis. In addition, initial studies suggest that thrombolytic therapy may provide clinical benefits in subsets of unstable angina patients (29, 30).

Bypass surgery and angioplasty

Two randomized unstable angina trials have failed to demonstrate a reduction in mortality with early bypass surgery (3, 31); this procedure is effective therapy for patients with continued symptoms despite aggressive medical therapy. Patients with adverse coronary anatomy (i.e. left main disease, triple vessel disease) where a large proportion of the myocardium is threatened, should undergo coronary bypass surgery as well.
Percutaneous transluminal coronary angioplasty (PTCA) is a relatively new and effective therapeutic option for patients with both stable and unstable angina. Several reports have demonstrated excellent results with coronary angioplasty for patients with medically refractory unstable angina (32, 33). The long term follow-up in this group of patients is not known, and restenosis may occur in 30% or more of patients. One study has shown that patients with unstable angina may be more likely to develop restenosis than those with stable angina, suggesting a possible further limitation of this procedure for patients with this syndrome (34). However, coronary angioplasty is an excellent stabilizing intervention which may be applied to selected patients and has a low morbidity and mortality and excellent initial results.

Summary

Holter monitoring for ischemic ST changes in patients with unstable angina has demonstrated that a large proportion of patients have asymptomatic ischemic episodes despite control of symptoms with medical therapy. This assessment of the total ischemic burden (both symptomatic and asymptomatic episodes) provides additional sensitivity for the documentation of ischemic episodes and identifies patients who are more likely to experience unfavorable events. This provides complimentary information which may be used along with knowledge of the coronary anatomy, left ventricular function, and exercise performance. Consideration should be given to attempting to reduce or eliminate all ischemic episodes, since the presence and extent of ischemia appears to be correlated with poor prognosis. Initially, this should be attempted using intensive combination medical therapy. If symptoms recur, or if ischemic changes are persistent despite medical therapy, consideration should be given at an early point to revascularization with either coronary artery bypass surgery or coronary angioplasty.

References

1. Maseri A (1986) Pathogenetic classification of unstable angina as guideline to individual management and prognosis. Am J Med 80 (suppl 4C): 48—55
2. Epstein SE, Palmieri ST (1984) Mechanisms contributing to precipitation of unstable angina and acute myocardial infarction: implications regarding therapy. Am J Cardiol 54: 1245—1252
3. Russell RO, Moraski RE, Kouchoukos N, et al (1978) Unstable angina pectoris: National cooperative study group to compare surgical and medical therapy. II. In-hospital experience and initial follow-up results in patients with one, two and three vessel disease. Am J Cardiol 42: 839—848
4. Gerstenblith G, Ouyang P, Achuff SC et al (1982) Nifedipine in unstable angina. A double-blind, randomized trial. N Engl J Med 306: 885—889
5. Muller JE, Turi ZG, Pearle DL, et al (1984) Nifedipine and conventional therapy for unstable angina pectoris: a randomized, double-blind comparison. Circulation 69: 729—739
6. Gottlieb SO, Weisfeldt ML, Ouyang P, et al (1986) Effect of the addition of propranolol to therapy with nifedipine for unstable angina: a randomized, double-blind, placebo-controlled trial. Circulation 73: 331—337
7. Stern S, Tzivoni D (1974) Early detection of silent ischemic heart disease by 24 hour electrocardiographic monitoring of active subjects. Br Heart J 36: 481—86
8. Schang SJ, Pepine CJ (1977) Transient asymptomatic ST segment depression during daily activity. Am J Cardiol 39: 396—400
9. Deanfield J, Maseri A, Selwyn A, et al (1983) Myocardial ischemia during daily life in patients with stable angina: Its relation to symptoms and heart rate changes. Lancet 1983; 753—8
10. Cecchi AC, Dovellini EV, Marchi F, et al (1983) Silent myocardial ischemia during ambulatory electrocardiographic monitoring in patients with effort angina. J Am Coll Cardiol 1 (3): 934—939
11. Biagini A, Mazzei MG, Carpeggiani C, et al (1982) Vasospastic ischemic mechanism of frequent asymptomatic transient ST-T changes during continuous electrocardiographic monitoring of selected unstable angina patients. Am Heart J 103: 13—19
12. Nademanee K, Intarachot V, Piontek M, et al (1984) Silent myocardial ischemia on Holter: has it clinical significance? (abstr) Circulation: 70 (suppl) II: II-452
13. Johnson SM, Mauritson DR, Winniford MD, et al (1982) Continuous electrocardiographic monitoring in patients with unstable angina pectoris. Idntification of high-risk subgrop with severe coronary disease, variant angina, and/or impaired early prognosis. Am Heart J 103: 4—12
14. Chierchia S, Lazzari M, Freedman B, et al (1983) Impairment of myocardial perfusion and function during painless myocardial ischemia. J Am Coll Cardiol 1 (3): 924—930
15. Cohn PF, Brown EJ, Wynne J, et al (1983) Global and regional left ventricular ejection fraction abnormalities during exercise in patients with silent myocardial ischemia. J Am Coll Cardiol 1 (3): 931—933

16. Deanfield JE, Shea M. , Ribiero P, et al (1984) Transient ST segment depression as a marker of myocardial ischemia during daily life. Am J Cardiol 54: 1195—1200
17. Holter NJ (1961) New method for heart studies: Continuous electrocardiography of active subjects over long periods is now practical. Science 134: 1214
18. Levy RD, Shapiro LM, Wright C, Mockus L, Quyyumi AA, Fox KM (1986) The significance of painless ST segment depression assessed by ambulatory pulmonary artery pressure monitoring. J Am Coll Cardiol 7: 192A
19. Deanfield J, Ribiero P, Oakley K, et al (1984) Critical analysis of ST segment changes in normal subjects: Implications for ambulatory monitoring of myocardial ischemia in patients with angina. Am J Cardiol 54: 1321—1325
20. Shook TL, Balke CW, Kotilainen PW, Selwyn AP, Stone PH. Accuracy of detection of myocardial ischemia by amplitude-modulated and frequency-modulated holter techniques. J Am Coll Cardiol 7: 104A (abstract)
21. Gottlieb SO, Weisfeldt ML, Ouyang P, Mellits ED, Gerstenblith G (1986) Silent ischemia as a marker for early unfavorable outcomes in patients with unstable angina. N Engl J Med 314: 1214—19
22. Ouyang P, Bulkley BH, Mellits ED, et al (1983) A double-blind, randomized trial of nifedipine in post-infarction unstable angina. Pract Cardiol 3: 30—38
23. Telford AM Wilson C (1981) Trial of heparin versus atenolol in prevention of myocardial infarction in intermediate coronary syndrome. Lancet I: 1225—1228
24. Lewis HD Jr, Davis JW, Archibald DG, et al (1983) Protective effects of aspirin against acute myocardial infarction and death in men with unstable angina. Results of a Veterans Administration Cooperative Study. N Engl J Med 309: 396—403
25. Cairns JA, Gent M, Singer J, et al (1985) Aspirin, sulfinpyrazone, or both in unstable angina-results of a Canadian Multicenter Trial. N Engl J Med 313: 1369—1375
26. Ambrose JA, Winters SL, Stern A, et al (1985) Angiographic morphology and the pathogenesis of unstable angina pectoris. J Am Coll Cardiol 5: 609—616
27. Bresnahan DR, Davis JL, Holmes DR Jr, Smith HC (1985) Angiographic occurrence and clinical correlates of intraluminal coronary artery thrombus: role of unstable angina. J Am Coll Cardiol 6: 285—289
28. Sherman CT, Litvack F, Grundfest W, et al (1985) Fiberoptic coronary angioscopy identifies thrombus in all patients with unstable angina (abstr). Circulation 72: 111—112
29. Vetrovec GW, Leinbach RC, Gold HK, Cowley MJ (1982) Intracoronary thrombolysis in syndromes of unstable ischemia: angiographic and clinical results. Am Heart J 104: 946—952
30. Shapiro EP, Brinker JA, Gottlieb SO, Guzman PA, Bulkley BH (1985) Intracoronary thrombolysis 3 to 13 days after acute myocardial infarction for postinfarction angina pectoris. Am J Cardiol 55: 1453—1458
31. Selden R, Neill WA, Ritzmann LW, Okies JE, Anderson RP (1975) Medical versus surgical therapy for acute coronary insufficiency. A randomized study. N Engl J Med 293: 1329—1333
32. DeFeyter PJ, Serruys PW, Van Den Brand M, et al (1985) Emergency coronary angioplasty in refractory unstable angina. N Engl J Med 313: 342—346
33. Gottlieb SO, Brin KP, Walford GD, McGaughey M, Riegel MB, Brinker JA (1986) Percutaneous transluminal coronary angioplasty for eary post-infarction unstable angina; results and follow-up. J Am Cardiol 7: 21A
34. Leimgruber PP, Roubin GS, Hollman J, Cotsonis GA, Meier B, Douglas JS, King SB III, Gruentzig AR (1986) Restenosis after successful coronary angioplasty in patients with single-vessel disease: Circulation 73: 710—717

Author's address:
Sidney O. Gottlieb, M.D.
Director, Cardiac Catheterization Laboratory
Francis Scott Key Medical Center
John Hopkins Medical Institutions
4940 Eastern Avenue
Baltimore, Maryland 21224

Prevalence of ventricular arrhythmias during silent myocardial ischemia

M. Zehender, T. Meinertz, A. Geibel, S. Hohnloser, C. Weiss, U. Koscheck, H. Just

Innere Medizin III (Leitung: Prof. Dr. H. Just), Universitätsklinik Freiburg, F.R.G.

Symptomatic ST depression at rest and during exercise, as well as the occurrence of ventricular arrhythmias, are known to be independent risk factors in patients with coronary artery disease (1—4). However, the interaction of ischemia and ventricular arrhythmias is frequently difficult to analyze. In patients with coronary artery disease an exercise induced ST depression can secondarily induce ventricular arrhythmias originating in the ischemic or peri-ischemic myocardium, as well as persistent ventricular arrhythmias that can cause ischemic changes in the myocardium. Theroux et al. reported on patients after myocardial infarction a 1-year mortality rate of 16% versus 1% whether or not ST-segment depressions were present and of 11% versus 4% whether or not exercise-induced ventricular arrhythmias were present (1). Udall and Ellestad reported that death due to cardiac causes over a 5-year period occurred in 8% of patients with exercise-induced ventricular arrhythmias and a normal ST-segment response, in contrast to 1.4% of patients with no ventricular arrhythmia and a normal ST-segment response. However, in 22% of patients with exercise-induced ventricular arrhythmias and an abnormal ST-segment response, sudden death was present in the 5 year follow-up (2). Ruberman et al. showed that there is a higher probability of dying from a cardiac event when patients are older, have had previous myocardial infarction and exercise induced ST-segment depression or ventricular arrhythmias (3). The risk further increases when the risk factors are present in combination. In a more recent and well controlled study by Califf et al. (4) in 620 patients with the angiographic diagnosis of coronary artery disease, survival rate after 3 years was 90% in patients with no exercise-induced ventricular arrhythmias, 83% in those with only simple ventricular arrhythmias and 75% in patients with complex ventricular arrhythmias during exercise.

Since the first descriptions of silent myocardial ischemia in patients with coronary artery disease, it has been evident that silent myocardial ischemia is of importance for the occurrence of malignant arrhythmias or sudden death in these patients. In 1981 Denes et al. (5) and Selarno et al. (6) demonstrated an increased incidence of silent ischemia in patients with sudden cardiac death; a similar finding is documented in Fig. 1. However, silent myocardial infarction seems to be only one parameter among other interacting factors. Pratt and coworkers demonstrated that in 15 patients who died during Holter monitoring from spontaneous occurrence of ventricular fibrillation, a ventricular tachycardia was the initiating arrhythmia. However, in only one of these patients a change in the ST-segment was observed prior to the beginning of the ventricular tachycardia. In 14/15 of these patients autopsy proved the presence of significant coronary artery disease.

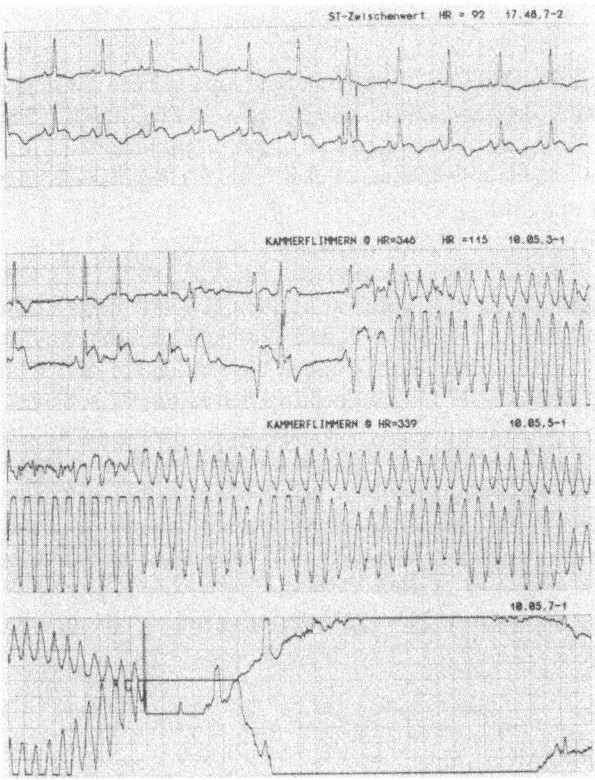

Fig. 1. Spontaneous occurrence of ventricular fibrillation after episodes of silent ST elevation.

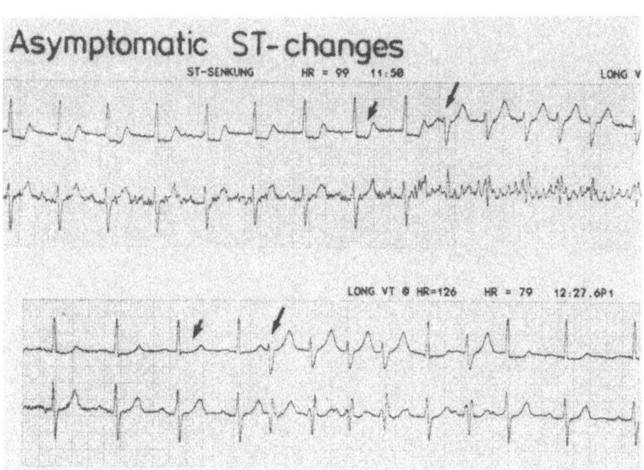

Fig. 2. Occurrence of a short run of tachycardia during an episode of asymptomatic ST depression and of the same tachycardia slightly later without evidence of myocardial ischemia.

Figure 2 shows the combination between episodes of myocardial ischemia and the occurrence of a tachycardia episode; however, the same tachycardia was observed slightly later without evidence of ischemia.

Prevalence and diagnostic evaluation of silent myocardial ischemia

The prevalence of silent myocardial ischemia in a larger population has been estimated by the Framingham study. Of 5127 patients who underwent routine ECG monitoring, 708 patients (14%) had evidence of myocardial infarction without such a history. Fifteen percent of these patients had never had any evidence of chest pain (7). Similar findings have been reported by other authors (8—12).

Deanfield et al. demonstrated the presence of silent myocardial ischemia in 30 patients with coronary artery disease by the intravenous application of Rubidium-82 (9). Other authors have used ventriculography to directly visualize segmental hypokinesia of the myocardium during asymptomatic ST depression (14) and proved a simultaneous increase in enddiastolic pressure (15). More frequently, exercise tests which are known for a high specificity in symptomatic patients (16, 17) have been used to demonstrate asymptomatic ST depression. However, when the patient is asymptomatic during significant ST depression, a "false positive" result is difficult to separate from silent myocardial ischemia. Coronar angiography in such patients results in an incidence of coronary artery disease in 22%—72% of patients (18, 19). Specificity of detection of silent myocardial ischemia improves when an exercise thallium scan is used (20). Altogether, the incidence of silent myocardial ischemia is described as 29%—75% during ventriculography, in 17%—47% of patients during exercise test and 29%—75% during exercise thallium scan,

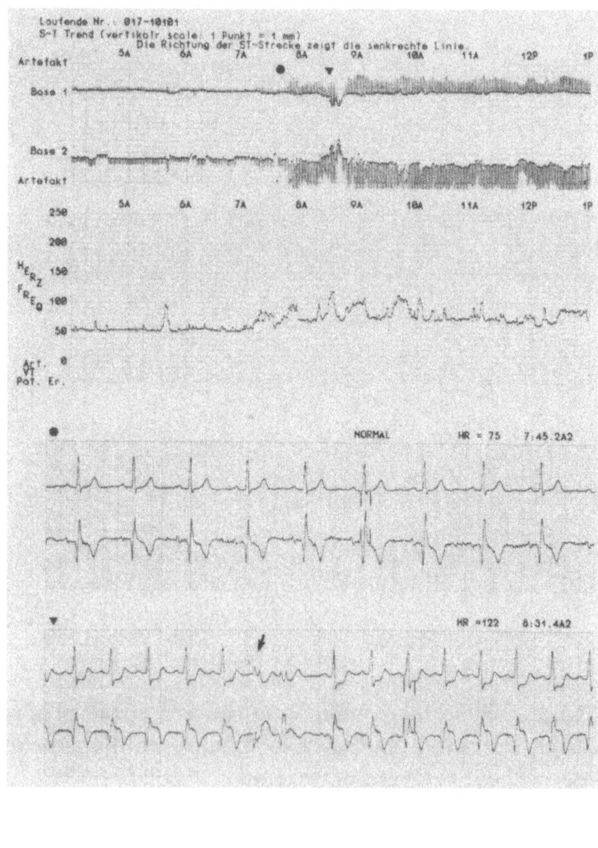

Fig. 3. Occurrence of asymptomatic ST-segment depression and elevation associated with an increasing heart rate and the occurrence of complex ventricular arrhythmias (Base 1 and 2: averaged change in ST-segment as compared to the isoelectrical line in both channels; the vertical line at the trend represents the slope of the ST-segment; patient's events are marked in the middle line).

although some of these studies are handicapped by a lack of proof of the underlying heart disease (16, overview 21).

With an improved technical standard, long term electrocardiography is used increasingly in the evaluation of silent ST-segment depression. Thus, in 197 patients with the angiographic diagnosis of coronary artery disease, the incidence of silent ST-segment was found to be 20%—60% of patients (22—24). The interesting advantage to obtain data on the ST-segment during normal daily activity is in contrast to the smaller amount of information available from such registration, as compared to a 12-lead exercise test. It has been intensively discussed whether ST-segment analysis can be reliably performed from two ECG leads, especially when no angina pectoris is present (25).

From a technical point of view, initial evaluations of the ST-segment changes during long term ECG monitoring were hampered, since Holter systems were designed to evaluate the presence or absence of cardiac arrhythmias (12, 23, 26, 27). Most frequently, a reliable analysis of the ST-segment was limited (1) by an insufficient lower cut-off point which eliminated too much of the lower frequency components of the ST-segment, (2) by a filter mediated phase distortion and (3) by the difficult artefact elimination in the lower frequency range. Based on these considerations there was an initial preference for frequency modulated Holter systems, as compared to amplitude modulated Holter systems (28). However, since the frequency modulated systems are less effective in the arrhythmia evaluation, much effort has been spent in improving ST-segment analysis by amplitude modulated systems (29—32). Thus, Andresen et al. showed similar cut-off points and a better linearity of signal transfer when newer amplitude modulated systems were compared to available frequency modulated systems. Similar findings were reported by Shook et al. who analyzed the accuracy of amplitude and frequency modulated Holter systems to reproduce ST deviation and QRS-morphology in 14 patients with significant coronary artery disease and exercise test (31).

The system which we use for all arrhythmia and ST analysis is an amplitude modulated Cardiodata MK4 system. This system has proven of a high reliability in the evaluation of changes of the ST-segment, especially as the high degree of linearity of signal transfer in the lower frequency range seems to be the main advantage (29—32).

When the ST-segment is analyzed by the Cardiodata system, two operator mediated points define the isoelectrical line and the point of the first measurement 80 ms after the J-point. To determine the ST slope a third point is automatically set 60 ms after the second point of analysis. Analysis concerns only "dominant" QRS complexes (± 10% deviation of the normal QRS shape). A transient window considers continuously four QRS-ST complexes individually, and eliminates abrupt ST deviations of more than 0.2 mV. An ST-segment trend is given for each minute; at least 16 QRS complexes are considered for analysis. Figure 3 shows an ST-segment trend during an episode of asymptomatic myocardial ischemia. Myocardial ischemia is considered from an ST-segment depression of more than 0.1 mV being present for more than 3 min. During myocardial ischemia complex ventricular arrhythmias occurred.

Silent myocardial ischemia and ventricular arrhythmias

Apart from data on the coincidence of silent myocardial ischemia and ventricular fibrillation, there are little data on the relation between silent myocardial ischemia and an increase in the incidence or severity of cardiac arrhythmias. Nademanee et al. described recently a total of 781 episodes of silent myocardial ischemia; 142 episodes were associated with ventricular arrhythmias, which were classified as ventricular couplets in 14 patients and as ventricular tachycardia in 11 patients. No considerations were made of the incidence and type of ventricular arrhythmia during a 24 h period before exercise (33).

We investigated the prevalence of ventricular arrhythmias during episodes of silent myocardia, detected and induced during exercise-testing, percutaneous transluminal angioplasty (PTCA) and Holter monitoring performed during daily activity.

In 1200 patients, exercise-testing revealed episodes of silent myocardial ischemia in 13% of patients. Silent myocardial ischemia was defined as ST-segment depression of more than 0.1 mV in at least two ECG leads. There was a mean exercise tolerance of patients

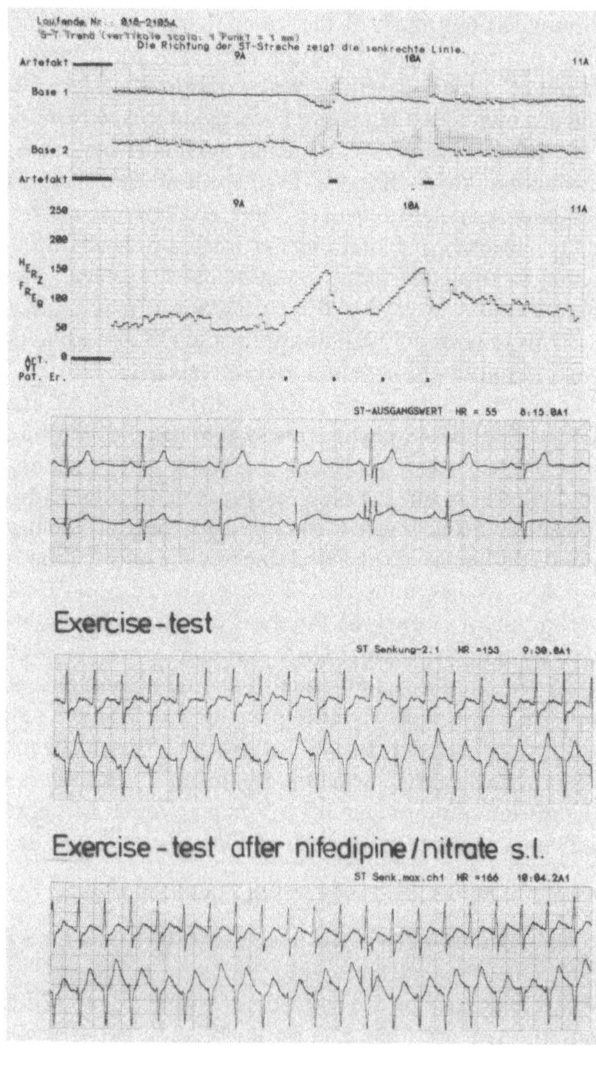

Fig. 4. ST-segment depression during exercise test before and after sublingual nitrate and nifedipine application. The first test was associated with angina pectoris and arrhythmias, but not the second one; ST-segment depression at this time was less as compared to the initial test.

with silent myocardial ischemia of 2 min, 100 W. In these patients a prevalence of ventricular premature beats of 42% was observed. The incidence of frequent ventricular premature beats was 8% and of ventricular pairs and ventricular tachycardia 9% and 1%, respectively. These data did not change when only patients with the angiographic diagnosis of coronary artery disease were considered. We primarily analyzed the total incidence of ventricular arrhythmias over a 24 h period, since a real increase of ventricular arrhythmias during a provocative test such as exercise testing is difficult to verify. Firstly, there is the problem of defining a reference period for the exercise time interval. Secondly, in patients with rare episodes of some types of ventricular arrhythmias, a small period of control or exercise can be influential in registering important temporal episodes. Thirdly, no information is available on the amount of increase of arrhythmias considered as proof of the exercise relation of arrhythmias. Figure 4 demonstrates two

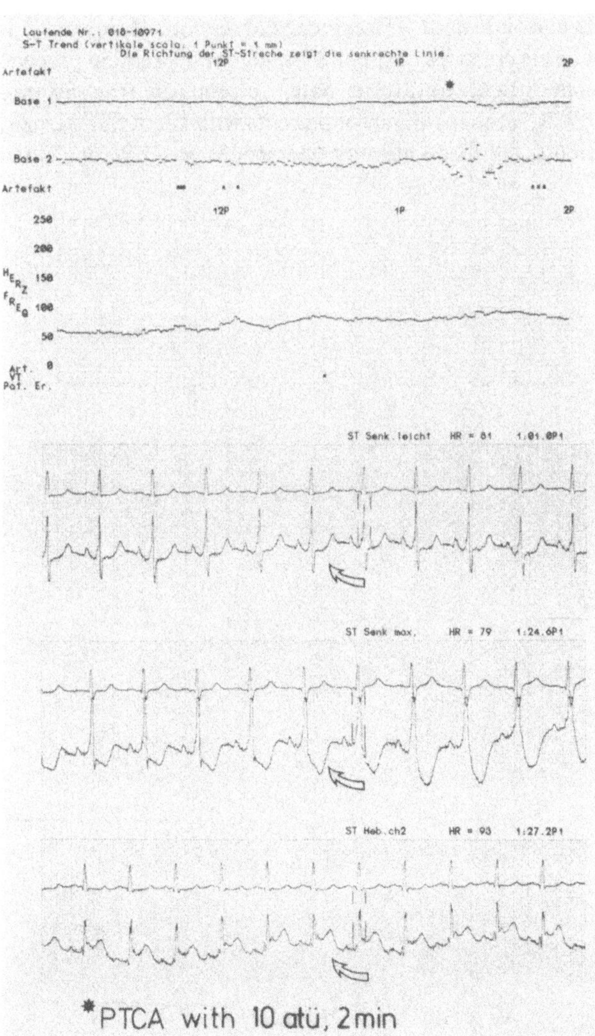

Fig. 5. ST-segment changes during PTCA with 10 atue for 2 min. In the lower part the initial ST-segment depression followed by an increase can be observed.

episodes of exercise test in a 54-year-old patient with coronary artery disease. During the first test, a clear ST-segment depression was observed and frequent supraventricular and single ventricular arrhythmias occurred. After the sublingual application of nitrates and nifedipine the exercise test was repeated and in spite of a higher exercise tolerance and higher heart rate, ST-segment depression was less and nearly no arrhythmias occurred during and after exercise.

PTCA seems to be an excellent situation for better analysis of additional data on the functional, hemodynamic and arrhythmogenic impact of silent myocardial ischemia. Figure 5 demonstrates the changes observed during PTCA in a 53-year-old patient who had been nearly totally asymptomatic (concerning angina pectoris) during marked changes in the ST-segment.

In patients considered for PTCA, we expect a high prevalence of myocardial ischemia during exercise and daily activities. Of 20 patients included in this study we observed in 12 patients a mean of 2.2 episodes of silent ST-segment depression. When these patients underwent PTCA, 17/20 patients showed silent ST-segment depression. However, it is of interest that in most of these patients episodes of silent ST-segment depression precede symptomatic episodes and it seems difficult to discriminate symptomatic from asymptomatic episodes. One week after PTCA the incidence of patients with silent ST-segment depression decreased to 7/20 patients, the mean number of episodes was 1.9/day. When

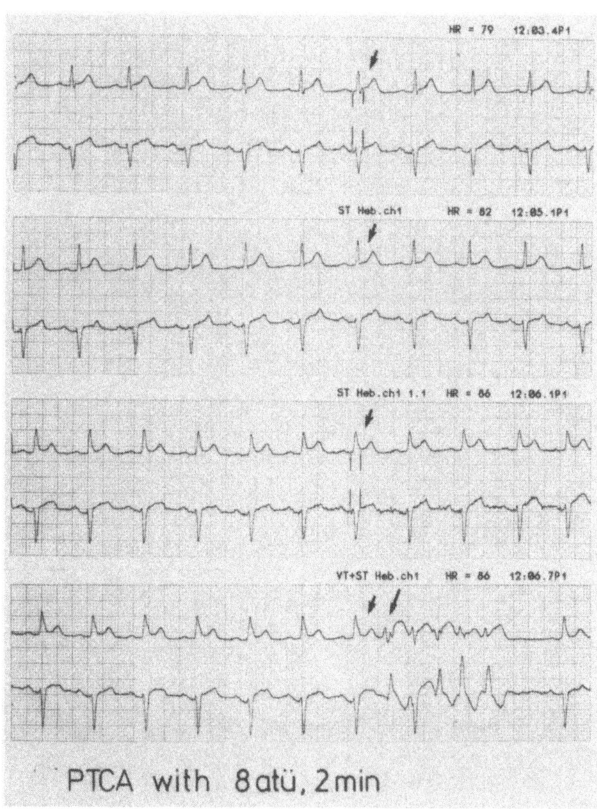

Fig. 6. Induction of ventricular arrhythmias during PTCA.

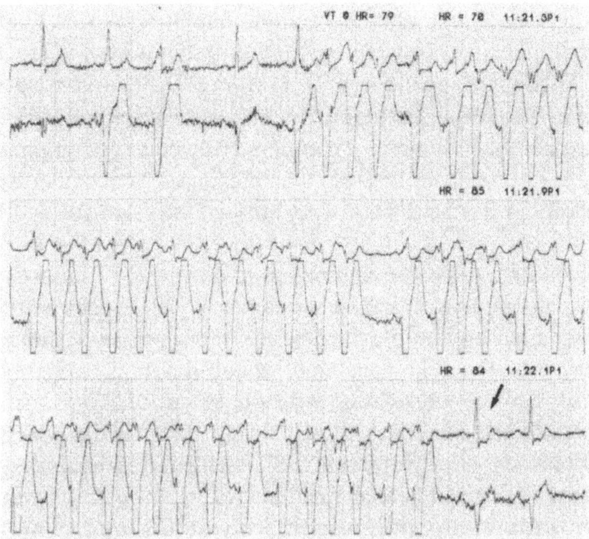

Fig. 7. Occurrence of ventricular arrhythmias after PTCA with and without evidence of myocardial ischemia.

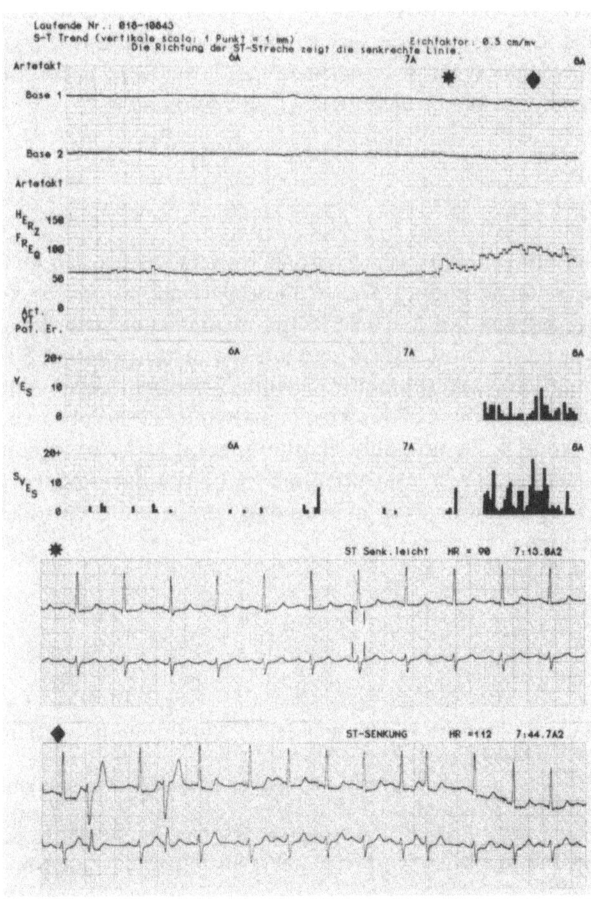

Fig. 8. Increase of ventricular and supraventricular arrhythmias (middle panel) during an asymptomatic episode of ST-segment depression.

an increase in the incidence of ventricular arrhythmias of more than 50%, as well as an increase in severity of such arrhythmias, was considered, 10% of patients showed such an increase during silent ST-segment depression before PTCA. After PTCA the incidence of patients decreased to 5%. During PTCA ventricular arrhythmias increased in 20% of patients. Figures 6 and 7 demonstrate the induction of complex ventricular arrhythmias during and shortly after PTCA. It is of special interest that malignant ventricular arrhythmias were also observed up to 24 h after PTCA with and without significant ST depression in two patients.
From 30 Holter registrations in patients with the angiographic diagnosis of coronary artery disease and with episodes of silent myocardial ischemia per day, we analyzed the influence of silent myocardial ischemia on the prevalence of ventricular arrhythmias during 24 h of normal daily activity. In Fig. 8 an episode of asymptomatic ST-segment depression is demonstrated. As we can see, correlating with the extent of ST-segment depression there is a clear increase in the incidence of ventricular arrhythmias. Of 79 episodes of symptomatic and 39 episodes of asymptomatic ST-segment depression, 9% and 8% of episodes were associated with an increased incidence of ventricular arrhythmias; in no patient sustained ventricular tachycardia was observed at this time. In most patients we observed, before the occurrence of ST-segment depression, an increase in heart rate. This has been discussed and is controversial (25); however, it seems to be of importance, because basic studies determining the occurrence of arrhythmias during acute myocardial ischemia (34) have very recently underlined that lower heart rates during myocardial ischemia decrease the incidence of ventricular arrhythmias.

Clinical implications

In our studies we observed in patients with suspected coronary artery disease, an incidence of silent ST-segment depression of about 13%. In these patients, as well as in patients undergoing normal daily activity, an increase in the incidence or severity of ventricular arrhythmias was observed in about 10% of patients, no matter whether ST-segment depression was symptomatic or asymptomatic. Silent ST-segment depression during PTCA is a common finding. An increase of ventricular arrhythmias was observed in about 20% of patients. There seems to be no doubt about a present arrhythmogenic potential of silent myocardial ischemia; however, at this time we do not have evidence that the prognostic significance is different or even increased as compared to episodes with symptomatic myocardial ischemia.

References

1. Theroux P, Waters DD, Halphen C, Debaisieux JC, Mizgala HF (1979) Prognostic value of exercise testing soon after myocardial infarction. N Engl J Med 301: 341
2. Udall JA, Ellestad MH (1977) Predictive implications of ventricular premature contractions associated with treadmill stress testing. Circulation 56: 985
3. Rubermann W, Weinblatt E, Goldberg JD, Frank CW, Chaudhary BS, Shapiro S (1981) Ventricular premature complexes and sudden death after myocardial infarction. Circulation 64, 2: 297

4. Califf RM, McKinnes RA, McNeer F et al (1983) Prognostic value of ventricular arrhythmias associated with treadmill exercise testing in patients studied with cardiac catheterization for suspected ischemic heart disease. J Am Coll Cardiol 2: 1060
5. Denes P, Gabster A, Huang SK (1981) Clinical electrocardiographic and follow-up observations in patients having ventricular fibrillation during Holter-monitoring. Am J Cardiol 48: 9
6. Selarno D, Hodges M, Graham E, Asinger RW, Mikell FL (1981) Fatal cardiac arrest during continuous ambulatory monitoring. N Engl J Med 305: 700
7. Kannel WB, Abott RD (1984) Incidence and prognosis of unrecognized myocardial infarction: An update on the Framingham study. N Engl J Med 311: 1144–1147
8. Cecchi AC, Dovellinie EV, Marchi F, Pucci P, Santoro GM, Fazzini PF (1983) Silent ischemia during ambulatory electrocardiographic monitoring in patients with effort angina. J Am Coll Cardiol 1: 934–939
9. Cocco G, Braun S, Strozzi C, Leishman B, Chu D, Rochat N (1982) Asymptomatic myocardial ischaemia in patients with stable and typical angina pectoris. Clin Cardiol 5: 403–408
10. Cohn PF (1980) Silent myocardial ischemia in patients with a defective anginal warning system. Am J Cardiol 45: 697–702
11. Resnekov L (1985) Silent myocardial ischemia: Therapeutic implications. Am J Med 79: 3A, 30–34
12. Schang SJ, Pepine CJ (1977) Transient asymptomatic ST-segment depression during daily activity. Am J Cardiol 39: 396–402
13. Deanfield JE, Shea M, Ribeiro P, Landsheere CM de, Wilson RA, Horlock P, Selwyn AP (1984) Transient ST-segment depression as a marker of myocardial ischemia during daily life. Am J Cardiol 54: 1195–1200
14. Hirzel HO, Leutwyler R, Krayenbühl HP (1985) Silent myocardial ischemia: Hemodynamic changes during dynamic exercise in patients with proven coronary artery disease despite absence of angina pectoris. J Am Coll Cardiol 6: 275–284
15. Grossman W (1985) Why is left ventricular diastolic pressure increased during angina pectoris? JACC 5: 607–608
16. Berman JL, Wynne J, Cohn PF (1978) A multivariate approach for interpreting treadmill exercise tests in coronary artery disease. Circulation 52: 619–626
17. Lindsey HE, Cohn PF (1978) Silent myocardial ischemia during and after exercise testing in patients with coronary artery disease. Am Heart J 95: 441–447
18. Froehlicher VF, Thompson AJ, Longo MR Jr, Triebwasser JH, Lancaster MC (1976). Value of exercise testing for screening asymptomatic men for latent coronary artery disease. Prog Cardiovasc Dis 18: 265–276
19. Erikssen J, Enge J, Forfang K, Storstein O (1976) False positive diagnostic tests and coronary angiographic findings in 105 presumably healthy males. Circulation 54: 371–376
20. Caralis DG, Bailey I, Kennedy HL, Pitt B (1979) Thallium-201 myocardial imaging in evaluation of asymptomatic individuals with ischemic ST-segment depression on exercise electrocardiogram. Br Heart J 42: 562–567
21. Silber S, Vogler A (1986) Die stumme Myokardischaemie: Dimensionierung eines Problems. Intensivmed 23, 2: 52–63
22. Chiariello M, Indolfi C, Cotecchia MR, Sifola C, Romano M, Condorelli M (1985). Asymptomatic transient ST changes during ambulatory ECG monitoring in diabetic patients. Am Heart J 110: 529–534
23. Stern S, Tzivoni D (1974) Early detection of silent ischemic heart disease by 24-hour electrocardiographic monitoring of active subjects. Br Heart J 36: 481–486
24. Wolf E, Tzivoni D, Stern S (1974) Comparison of exercise tests and 24-hour ambulatory electrocardiographic monitoring in detection of ST-T-changes. Br Heart J 36: 90–95
25. Singh B (1986) A symposium: Detection, quantification and clinical significance of silent myocardial ischemia in coronary artery disease. Am J Cardiol 58: 3B
26. Bragg-Remschel DA, Anderson CM, Winkle RA (1982) Frequency response characteristics of ambulatory ECG monitoring systems and their implications for ST-segment analysis. Am Heart J 103: 20–31
27. Bethge KP, Gonska BD (1985) ST-Segment-Analyse im Langzeit-Elektrokardiogramm: Ist die Methode ausgereift? Dtsch Med Wochenschr 26: 1023–1024

28. Armin Th (1985) ST-Segment-Analyse im Langzeit-EKG. Dtsch Med Wochenschr 110: 1047–1051
29. Brüggemann T, Andresen D, Erbherr G, Schröder R (1986) Frequenzantwort verschiedener Langzeit-EKG-Systeme im Vergleich zum Standard-EKG. Z Kardiol 75, 4: 37
30. Hubelbank M, Feldman CL, Glasser SP, Clark PI, Polan BA (1984) ST-Analysis of Holter tapes. IEEE Computers in Cardiology, 269–272
31. Shook TL, Balke W, Kotilainen PW, Selwyn AP, Stone PH (1986) Accuracy of detection of myocardial ischemia by amplitude-modulated and frequency-modulated Holter techniques. J Am Coll Cardiol 7, 2: 104A
32. Hubelbank M, Feldman CL, Kotilainen P (1985) The use of computer aided Holter monitoring for detection of ST-changes. IEEE Computers in Cardiology, 515–517
33. Nademanee K, Intarachot V, Singh P, Josephson MA, Singh BN (1986) Clinical significance of silent myocardial ischemia in unstable angina. Am J Cardiol 58: 26B
34. Bolli R, Fisher DJ, Entman ML (1986) Factors that determine the occurrence of arrhythmias during acute myocardial ischemia. 111: 261

Authors' address:
Dr. M. Zehender
Innere Medizin III
Hugstetterstr. 55
7800 Freiburg

Arrhythmogenic potential of silent myocardial ischemia after myocardial infarction

P. Mathes, A. Reinke, D. Michel

Klinik Höhenried, Bernried, West Germany

Summary

In a series of 300 patients who had suffered a transmural infarction and were undergoing coronary angiography because of ischemia in the surviving myocardium, 17 demonstrated an exercise response indicative of myocardial ischemia, in the absence of any signs or symptoms of angina pectoris. The presence of ischemia in the region of the myocardium under scrutiny was proven by:

1. ST-segment depression during bicycle ergometry of at least 2 mm, in leads without any QRS or ST-T changes at rest
2. > 75% stenosis of vessels supplying the area under investigation, in addition to the vessel supplying the region of infarction
3. a reversible Thallium perfusion defect on exercise.

We compared those 17 patients with silent myocardial ischemia with 21 patients having typical angina pectoris on exertion. All patients underwent 24 h Holter monitoring, treadmill testing at target heart rate (previously determined as inducing signs of myocardial ischemia) swimming and callisthenic programs with telemetric ECG recordings. We concluded that there is no close relationship between myocardial ischemia and the occurrence of complex ventricular arrhythmias. In silent ischemia, complex ventricular arrhythmias do not occur at a higher rate than in patients with angina pectoris.

Introduction

Myocardial ischemia is generally regarded as a cause of ventricular arrhythmias, adding to the risk for the post-infarction patient. On the one hand, the clinical severity of angina pectoris characterizes the prognosis for the coronary patient, and is explicable by its close relationship to the number of diseased coronary vessels. On the other hand, silent myocardial ischemia is regarded as a serious danger, because the warning function of the angina pectoris attack is missing, so the patient may develop more severe ischemia with the resulting danger of arrhythmias, because of the very lack of warning symptoms. Therefore the study presented here should answer the following questions:

- is there any relation between exercise dependent myocardial ischemia and an increased incidence of ventricular arrhythmias?
- is there a special danger for patients with silent myocardial ischemia, who miss the warning function of angina pectoris by the frequent occurrence of ventricular extrasystoles?

Methods

We selected patients according to the following criteria:

1. Transmural infarction at least 6 weeks old
2. Ischemic response during exercise-ECG in leads without QRS or ST-T changes at rest
3. Reproducibility of ST changes during different forms of exercise at comparable heart rates
4. Coronary anatomy demonstrating significant narrowing in arteries supplying the region under examination.

We used the following exclusion criteria:

- Drug therapy with digitalis
- Changes of the drug therapy during the investigation period
- ST-segment changes and/or bundle branch block in the resting ECG.

We compared 21 patients with typical angina pectoris (AP) on exertion with another group of 17 patients who showed objective evidence of exercise-induced ischemia in the absence of any symptoms: in other words, with silent myocardial ischemia (SMI). The mean age of the patients was 53 ± 7 years. In both groups, nearly 30% of the patients had three-vessel-disease with stenoses of at least 75% of the major branches. The mean ejection fraction was 61% (AP) and 58% (SMI)

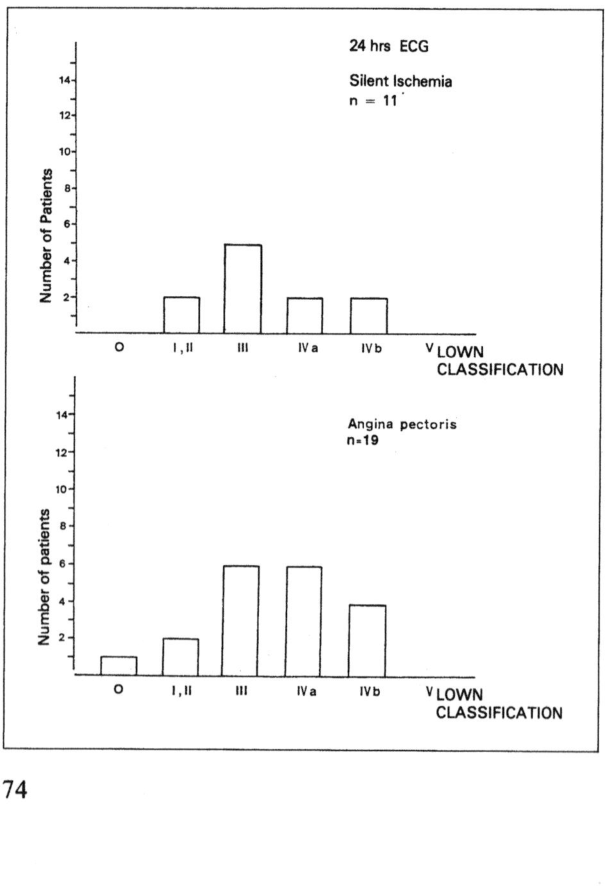

Fig. 1. Lown classification during the 24 h Holter monitoring in patients with silent ischemia (upper panel) and in patients with angina pectoris (lower panel)

All patients were investigated by bicycle ergometry and the following exercise tests: The patients performed a bicycle ergometry in a sitting position with an initial load of 50 W and a stepwise increase of 25 W every 4 min. We continuously registered the ECG by a three channel recorder and measured the blood pressure during the last minute of each step up to maximum.

During the 24 h Holter monitoring the patients were instructed to take part in their usual daily exercise programs, which consisted of gymnastics, callisthenics and endurance training. They kept diaries during this period to note, if necessary, the exact time of onset, duration and severity of chest discomfort and their activity at the time of pain.

The treadmill test was started at a rate of 3 km/h, equivalent to slow walking, and raised every 4 min by about 1 km/h. We also continuously monitored the ECG. A special program was developed for the swimming telemetry. It included gymnastics in the water as an initial adaptation, as well as certain swimming distances. The ECG monitoring by telemetry enabled recording during the entire program.

In the same manner we observed the patients daily during their morning gymnastics. This activity took 40 min and was performed in small groups of patients having a similar exercise capacity.

The exercise tests were stopped when any of the following endpoints were reached: angina pectoris, severe fatigue or dyspnea, appearance of frequent multifocal or paired extrasystoles, or an abnormal blood pressure response. ST-segment depressions of more than 1.5 mm were not taken as an indication to stop exercise.

All the ECGs recorded during these different stress tests were evaluated for changes in heart rate and ST-segment changes, as well as being graded according to the Lown classification.

Results

Only patients with a transmural infarction took part in this study, who demonstrated an unequivocal ischemic response during bicycle ergometry, showing an ST-segment depression of at least 2 mm in leads without any ST-T changes at rest.

During the 24 h Holter monitoring, not only patients with angina pectoris, but also patients with silent myocardial ischemia showed, with one exception, ventricular arrhythmias. We found predominantly multifocal and paired extrasystoles. These arrhythmias appeared at the same time that we registered a rate dependent ST-segment depression in five patients in the angina pectoris group (25%) and in six patients in the silent myocardial ischemia group (30%) (Fig. 1).

Ventricular arrhythmias appeared during the bicycle ergometry at nearly the same rate in both groups. Patients with angina pectoris and patients with silent myocardial ischemia did not show frequently severe extrasystoles. It was generally noticed that all patients with more complex arrhythmias, corresponding to the Lown classification III and IV, showed more prominent ST-segment depressions of between 2.5 and 4 mm during exercise (Fig. 2).

During the treadmill-test, we reached the highest maximum work load, as judged by the heart rate. During this test, we observed results similar to those of the ergometry. All patients were exercised until they had ST-segment depressions of more than 1.5 mm. In nearly 80% of the patients no extrasystoles appeared. A higher graded arrhythmia was

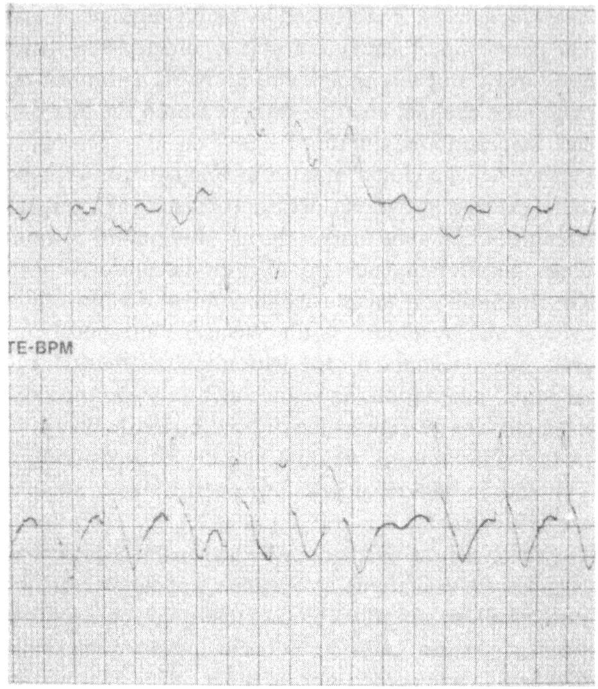

Fig. 2. ST depression during Holter monitoring

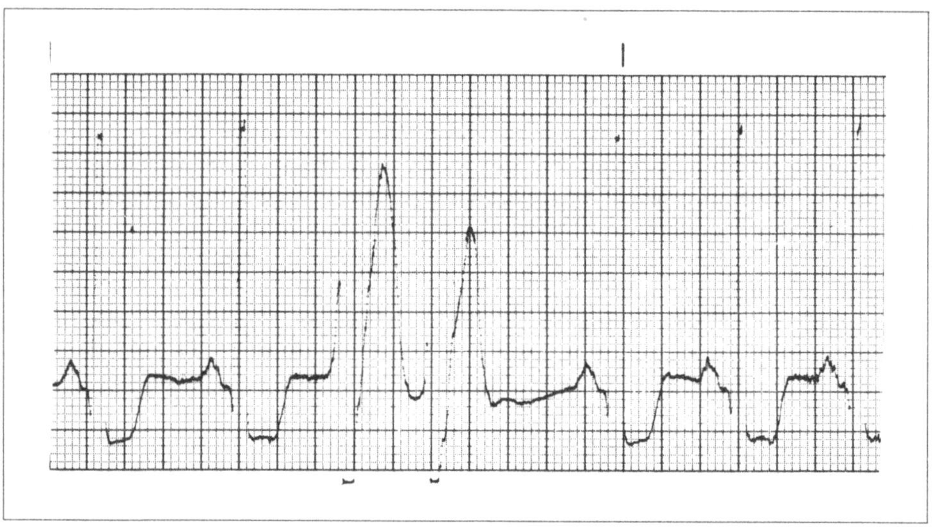

Fig. 3. ST depression during treadmill exercise

found only in one patient with silent myocardial ischemia. He also had a considerable ST-segment depression of 5 mm (Fig. 3).
The exercise with the lowest work load was performed during the morning gymnastics. Only a few patients showed ischemic reactions, none of more than 2 mm ST depression.

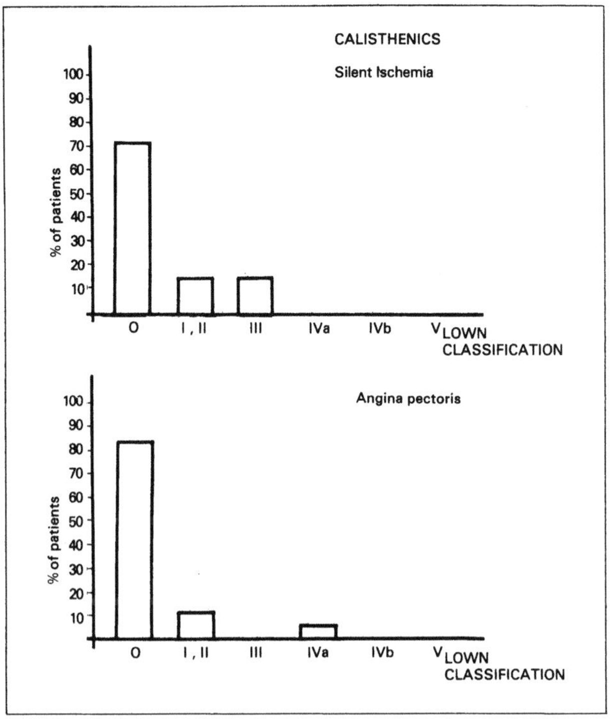

Fig. 4. Lown classification during morning gymnastics in patients with silent ischemia (upper panel) and in patients with angina pectoris (lower panel)

On the other hand, 30% of the patients with silent myocardial ischemia demonstrated arrhythmias of Lown class I and II, nearly twice as much as found in the other exercise tests so far described (Fig. 4).

The results of the swimming telemetry were markedly different: more than half the patients showed arrhythmias during the swimming program, the majority being lower graded arrhythmias. However, in relation to the other exercise forms, a high proportion of coupled and paired ventricular extrasystoles were seen in patients with silent myocardial ischemia. We were unable to detect a relationship between severe ST-segment depression and arrhythmias. However, one must keep in mind that ST-segment depressions of between 1.5 and 5 mm appeared during the swimming program in only 50% of all patients examined.

Discussion and Conclusions

As previously documented by Deanfield and others (1—3) the phenomenon of silent myocardial ischemia is not a rare event in patients with coronary heart disease, as also demonstrated by our study. It was interesting to note that during the 24 h Holter monitoring, the episodes of silent myocardial ischemia were not related to ventricular arrhythmias.

During the different forms of exercise tests, we found a frequent occurrence of substantial ST-segment depressions. No correlation to ventricular arrhythmias could be established.

However, in particular during bicycle ergometry and treadmill testing, we found higher graded arrhythmias in those patients showing marked ST-segment depressions. No statistical relationship, however, could be established either.

The occurrence of ventricular arrhythmias during the usual daily activities within the rehabilitation center and during exercise tests seemed to be nearly the same in patients with angina pectoris as in those with silent myocardial ischemia. For this latter group, the risk in regard to the occurrence of severe ventricular arrhythmias was not higher than in patients with angina pectoris. It appears that exercise forms resulting in high heart rates, e.g., treadmill testing, will lead to an overdrive suppression of ventricular arrhythmias because of the high sinus rate observed. On the contrary, exercise forms such as swimming, with a relatively slower heart rate caused by diving and the cold reflex, will cause more ventricular arrhythmias because of a relative lack of overdrive suppression.

In conclusion, we can say that:

1. this study did not demonstrate a close relationship between myocardial ischemia and the occurrence of complex ventricular arrhythmias
2. in silent ischemia, complex ventricular arrhythmias do not occur at a higher rate than in patients with angina pectoris.

References

1. Cohn, PF (1980) Silent Myocardial Ischemia in Patients With a Defective Anginal Warning System. Am J Cardiol 45: 697
2. Deanfield JE, Maseri A, Selwyn AP (1983) Myocardial ischemia during daily life in patients with stable angina. Lancet II: 753
3. Shang SJ, Pepine CI (1977) Transient asymptomatic ST-segment depression during daily activity. Am J Cardiol 39: 396

Authors' address:
Prof. Dr. P. Mathes
Klinik Höhenried
8139 Bernried
West Germany

Discussion on Prognosis

Chairmen: J. Erikssen and W. Rutishauser

Asked to compare the life expectancy of his patients with silent ischemia to that of the normal population in Norway, Erikssen answered that he had done several repeat examinations, that follow-up was 95% complete and that the presence of silent ischemia at entry doubled the risk in comparison to the normal population.

Resnekov pointed out fatigue as a symptom in patients who, although they do not have angina, show this symptom as evidence of impaired ventricular function. Erikssen assented and mentioned that from the 1832 normals in his initial group, those with a low exercise capacity had the worst prognosis. In these people low exercise capacity and an elevated erythrocyte sedimentation rate were the most important prognostic factors besides age. The statement by Erikssen during his presentation, that only one of his patients died without preceding anginal symptoms was contrasted with published reports of patients with sudden death showing that around 25% of them had asymptomatic coronary artery disease. Erikssen admitted that in several of the patients who died during follow-up, the anginal symptoms preceding death were of very short duration and did not lead to either medical attention or treatment. Berman questioned the apparently high specificity of exercise ECG testing in Erikssen's study. This was explained by a high exclusion rate of patients who might be expected to fall in a falsely positive group. In thus selected patients, similar findings had been reported from the group in Bethesda.

During the long follow-up time in Erikssen's study, no clear-cut prognostic influence of cholesterol values was found (all patients were under repeated counselling on lipid-lowering diet and smoking). Lichtlen mentioned similar experiences, i.e. the lack of a clear correlation between cholesterol level and progression of coronary artery disease.

Another part of the discussion centered around the question of how to compare and correlate the severity of ischemia on the exercise test with the frequency, severity and duration of ischemia on ambulatory Holter monitoring. Tzivoni presented his findings that — judged from the subsequent coronary events — evidence of ischemia on Holter monitoring added prognostic information beyond that of a positive exercise test. Fox pointed out that, generally speaking, patients with severely positive exercise ECG tests are those with frequent symptomatic and asymptomatic episodes on Holter monitoring. Chierchia also quoted experience of his own and of the Boston group showing an association between the results of treadmill exercise testing and ambulatory ECG monitoring.

In his presentation on prognostic implications of silent ischemia in patients with stable angina, Fox had raised the point that it is probably not the repeated ischemic events, which can be shown on Holter recording, but sudden irreversible changes like plaque-rupture which lead to a sudden worsening of the outlook for the patient. He suggested that different mechanisms may be responsible for stable angina, in contrast to unstable angina and myocardial infarction. He questioned whether by simply removing episodes of ST-segment depression with anti-anginal therapy, the prognosis would be influenced in any way. Gottlieb agreed that in his studies silent ischemia was just a marker for a bad prognostic outcome, which would not necessarily imply that it was also the cause for this outcome.

If plaque-rupture and local thrombosis are important in the transition from stable to unstable angina, then improved methods of analyzing coronary angiograms for the structure of atheromatous plaques and the presence of thrombosis are necessary. Gottlieb assented, from his own and the experience of the Montreal group, that healing of a ruptured plaque is an important mechanism of reversal of unstable angina. Inappropriate coronary vasomotion on top of pre-existing plaques was mentioned by Rutishauser as a mechanism which might lead to rupture of endothelial layers followed by local thrombosis.

It seems difficult, even in the face of a sudden structural change precipitating a cardiac event, to draw a clear-cut line between stable and unstable angina in individual patients (V. Arnim). This applies especially to patients with frequent episodes of ischemia at rest in whom it is conceivable that only minor changes are needed to cause irreversible image. Droste raised the question of whether a totally asymptomatic state of unstable angina existed and if this would necessitate a change in the pain-guided definition of instability. Clearly such patients exist but have not been examined by cardiologists but by pathologists (Fox). These are the patients who suffer sudden death without preceding symptoms, who have been shown to have coronary artery thrombosis and plaque-rupture on top of severe underlying coronary arteriosclerosis, in many cases.

The question by Bolte, of whether the treatment of patients with angina pectoris would give them a different prognosis compared to patients who had silent ischemia and were not treated, was left unanswered and declared an important point for future research in silent ischemia. Malliani pointed out that for future prognostic studies, parameters other than pain would have to be taken into account, like ventricular function, sympathetic activation with sudorimotor crisis and ventricular arrhythmias. From their studies, Mathes and Meinertz remarked that arrhythmias were a rather rare event during silent ischemic episodes and that severe ventricular arrhythmias were associated with severely impaired left ventricular function with scarring.

Finally, Deanfield stated that compared to exercise-induced ischemia, episodes of ischemia detected by Holter monitoring might give different prognostic information. They show a different degree of variability which in itself might be a prognostic marker. Deanfield maintained that not before many patients had been studied through phases of exacerbation of their disease, could answers be given on what might be the triggers of sudden prognostic deterioration.

Prevalence of silent ischemia in patients undergoing coronary angiography

Th. v. Arnim, A. Erath, B. Höfling, M. A. Schreiber

Medizinische Klinik I and Institut für Informationsverarbeitung, Statistik und Biomathematik, Klinikum Großhadern der Ludwig-Maximilians-Universität München

Introduction

One problem in the spectrum of silent myocardial ischemia, which is difficult to ascertain, is its prevalence. Yet the prevalence is of great importance if one wants to understand the medical and socio-economic impact of this disease state. Bayesian analysis (8, 22) has shown that prevalence, or "pre-test-likelihood", has a decisive influence on the usefulness of a diagnostic test in a given patient population. This poses a special problem for the physician dealing with silent ischemia in asymptomatic patients, as there is no prevalence of symptoms to start with, but the disease state needs objective testing for its definition. Information on prevalence of asymptomatic coronary artery disease can be obtained either from post mortem studies or coronary angiography. Results from the study by Diamond and Forrester (8), an example of this type of study, suggested that the prevalence of asymptomatic coronary artery disease in adults is around 5%. This figure increased with age and sex, e.g. to 12% for over 60-year-old males.
The only systematic studies investigating the occurrence of silent ischemia in asymptomatic people were done with exercise testing (9, 11, 17). In these studies, a prevalence of positive exercise tests was found between 2.5% (9) and 9% (17) for middle aged males, screened on the basis of their employment status. For patients in the post-infarction period, studies have shown the diagnostic and prognostic value of exercise testing, which is positive in about 30% of the patients with around 50% of the positive findings occurring without symptoms (4, 6, 19, 26).
While exercise testing is the most widely applied technique to detect silent ischemia, it cannot detect silent ischemic episodes that have been shown to occur frequently in patients with coronary heart disease, during normal daily life (7). In recent years studies with Holter technology have documented silent ischemic episodes under variable circumstances (24). No studies exist to date in which asymptomatic people were screened with Holter monitoring for silent ischemic episodes. In patients with unstable angina under medical treatment, the prevalence of silent ischemic episodes has been found to be between 40% and 60% (2, 14). Recently, in post-infarct patients, a prevalence of 30% was found for occurrence of ischemic episodes (15).
The majority of coronary heart disease patients have more or less stable symptoms, which are more or less effort-dependent, so called "stable angina pectoris". Studies using Holter monitoring to detect ischemic episodes have been done in only highly selected subsets of these patients. Thus, high prevalences of between 50% and 100% were found for the

occurrence of transient ischemia (5, 7, 12). These data are probably not representative of the patient population that most cardiologists will see on an out-patient basis or even in hospital. Therefore we conducted a study to find the prevalence of transient ischemic episodes on Holter monitoring by consecutively screening a larger patient population. The 296 patients investigated were referred to us for coronary angiography for suspected or manifest coronary heart disease.

Methods

Patient population

We consecutively included 296 patients who underwent coronary angiography at our institution. Patients were excluded for atrial fibrillation, left or right bundle branch block (both interfering with Holter analysis of ST segments), valvular heart disease, cardiomyopathy. There were 241 male patients (81% of the total; age: mean 52.9 years, range 21—73 years) and 55 female patients (19%; age: mean 54.9 years, range 33—69 years).

ST Segment monitoring

24-hour electrocardiographic monitoring was carried out as previously described (2, 3) with the frequency-modulated, calibrated recording system Medilog II (Oxford Electronics). The patients were in hospital, but in an ambulatory state. From the day before the recording, the patients were taken off calcium channel blockers and long-acting nitrate medications. Short acting nitrates were allowed as necessary to alleviate angina, and beta-adrenergic blocking agents were continued with the previously given dosage. 65% of the patients were on beta blockers at the time of study.

Episodes of ST segment deviation were identified visually and documented with analog recordings at the beginning of an episode, one minute before the episode, at the maximum of ST segment deviation and at the end of the episode. Episodes were counted if there was ST segment deviation of at least 1 mm (0.1 mV) for at least 1 min. An increase of the heart rate preceding the episode was defined as a rate increase of 10% or more, from 1 min before to the beginning of the episode.

Patients were asked to mark painful events either by pressing the event button of the electrocardiographic recorder or by writing a note in a purpose-made diary.

Patients questionnaire / routine ECG

From every patient anamnestic data were asked directly and collected on a questionnaire for computerized evaluation. Blood pressure and cholesterol values were taken from the charts. A routine 12-lead ECG was recorded before the procedure and evaluated for evidence of previous Q-wave or non-Q-wave infarction (10). Exercise ECGs were evaluated following standard criteria (25).

Coronary angiography

Coronary angiography was carried out following the Judkins procedure. All major coronary vessels were opacified in at least three different projections. All coronary films were reviewed and stenoses graded according to the consent of two experienced examiners. For quantification, the Gensini-score was used, which combines the degree of narrowing an the position of a stenosis for grading (13). The indications for coronary angiography were recorded for all patients and were as follows:
Angina pectoris despite medical therapy: 131/196 (44%)
Previous acute myocardial infarction with angina: 93/296 (31.4%)
Previous acute myocardial infarction, no angina: 24/296 ((8.1%)
Undefined chest pain: 19/296 (6.4%).

Data analysis and statistics

All results were analysed by computer, using a data bank system developed at the Institut für Informationsverarbeitung, Statistik und Biomathematik, in our institution (23). For evaluation of group differences the Chi-square test was used.

Results

Prevalence and patient characteristics

Table 1 shows the prevalence of symptomatic and asymptomatic ischemic episodes, a) for the patients studied and b) among the ischemic episodes detected. 70 patients, or just under a quarter of our patient population, did show transient episodic ECG changes. One half of these patients did not note the occurrence of anginal pain together with the episodes. Of the total number of episodes, however, 65% were asymptomatic. The number of episodes per patient ranged from 1 to 8 episodes in patients with ST depression (median 2 episodes) and from 1 to 13 with ST elevation (median 5 episodes). As we recorded the occurrence of pain by the patients diary and event markers on the tape, we also have occurrences of pain where the ECG did not show concordant ischemic changes. This was the case in 77 patients.
When patients with and without ischemic episodes were compared for their prevalence of risk factors and concomitant diseases, the data-base analysis did not show any significant group differences. Thus, an anamnestic or diagnostic marker for patients with transient ischemic episodes could not be found: Neither the incidence of ECG signs of previous myocardial infarctions (44% vs 46%) nor the proportion of positive ECG exercise tests (72% vs 71%) were different between patients with or without transient ischemic episodes. As the results of coronary angiography from all patients were also part of the data base, we were also able to compare patients with and without transient ischemic episodes for the severity of fixed coronary disease. This was done by comparing the frequency of 1-, 2-, 3-vessel disease and by comparing the Gensini scores in absolute numbers and qualified groups. This type of analysis also did not show significant differ-

Table 1. Prevalence of symptomatic and asymptomatic ischemic episodes.

a) *Patients studied*	*n*	%
	296	100
Patients with one or more ischemic episodes	70	23.6
Patients with one or more ischemic episodes, symptomatic*	35	11.8
Patients with ST depression	60	20.2
Patients with ST depression, symptomatic*	27	9.1
Patients with ST depression and elevation, symptomatic*	1	0.3
Patients with ST elevation	9	3,0
Patients with ST elevation, symptomatic* ·	7	2.4
Patients with ST depression, not tachycardia**	15	5.0
Patients with ST depression, no tachycardia, symptomatic*	8	2.7
b) *Ischemic episodes detected*	*n*	%
all episodes	221	100
all episodes with pain***	77	34.8
episodes of ST elevation	56	25.3
episodes of ST elevation with pain***	19	(33.9% of ST elevation)
episodes of ST depression	165	74.7
episodes of ST depression with pain***	58	(35.2% of ST depression)

* at least one painful episode/24 h.

** increase by more than 10% or HR > 100 min, 1 min before ST depression.

*** noted either by pressing an event button on the recorder or by making a note in the diary.

ences between the patient groups with and without transient ischemic episodes. For patients with ST elevation and/or ST depression without tachycardia, however, we found a significantly increased prevalence of 2- and 3-vessel disease: of the 25 patients with ST elevation or ST depression without tachycardia, 21 (84%) had 2- or 3-vessel disease, while of the other 271 patients, 153 (56.5%) had 2- and 3-vessel disease ($p < 0.05$).

Characteristics of silent and symptomatic episodes

Degree of ST depression

Of the total number of 221 episodes 77 were recorded as painful. The fraction of painless or silent episodes was similar for ST elevation and ST depression. In episodes of ST depression the degree of change did not correlate with the occurrence of pain. Of 118 episodes with ST depression of 0.1 and 0.15 mV, 39 (33.1%) were painful, and of 47 episodes with ST depression of 0.2 mV or more, 19 (40.4%) were painful (p = N.S.).

Duration of episodes

Figure 1 shows the duration of episodes, separated for silent and symptomatic episodes and separated for episodes of ST elevation or ST depression. It is apparent that there are

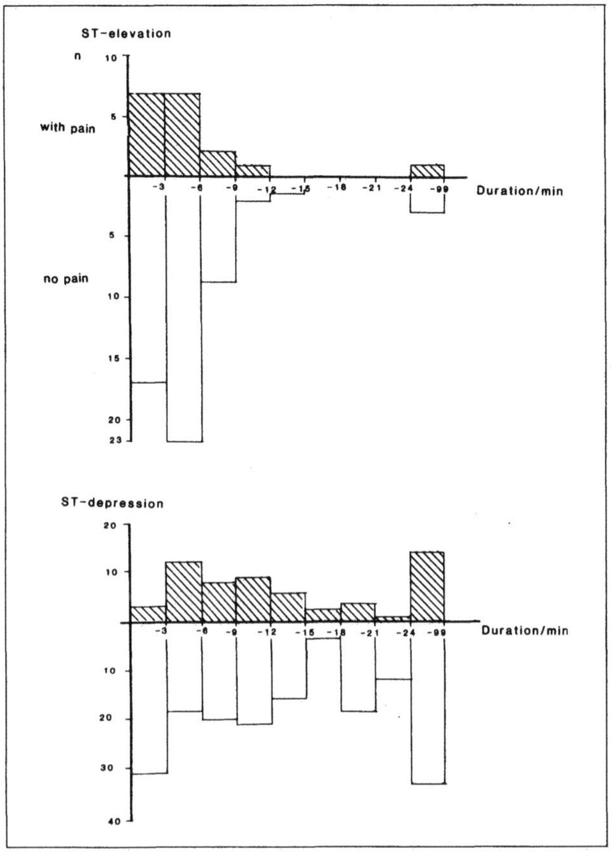

Fig. 1. Number of episodes of ST elevation and ST depression against duration of the episode. There were more short episodes with ST elevation ($p < 0.001$). The proportion of painful episodes is not significantly greater with longer episodes (> 10 minutes).

more short duration episodes of ST elevation and more longer duration episodes of ST depression. This difference is significant ($p > 0.05$) with Chi-square testing, if the decision line is taken at 10 min duration.

Whether an episode is silent or not does not depend on the episode duration, because there are many short duration episodes with pain and long lasting episodes without pain.

Heart rate increases by more than 10 beats/min occurred more often with episodes of more than 10 min duration ($p < 0.05$).

We compared the duration of anginal attacks as described by the patients when they were asked in the questionnaire, to the duration of their transient ischemic episodes: there was a clear difference. 71.6% of the patients reported a duration of 1—5 min for their angina, yet in this large group of patients the majority of episodes lasted for 7 min or longer (92 of 140 episodes, 65.7%). Thus, there is not only a great number of transient ST changes that go unnoticed, but also the duration of ischemia is misjudged when estimated from the duration of anginal attacks.

Heart rate changes

Figure 2 shows the episodes of ST elevation and ST depression divided according to the heart rate at which the ischemic changes started. ST elevation starts predominantly at heart rates of 90/min or lower and this difference is significant if compared to ST depression ($p < 0.001$). An increase of the heart rate by 10 beats or more, 1 min before the beginning of ST changes was found in 110 of 165 episodes of ST depression (66.7%) and in only 6 of 56 episodes of ST elevation (10.7%, $p < 0.001$). The occurrence of silent episodes does not show a strong dependence on the heart rate. However for episodes with ST elevation, a tendency to more painful episodes can be seen in the small fraction of episodes with ST elevation occurring at higher heart rates: for ST elevation at heart rates over 90/min the percentage of silent episodes was only 47%. Thus with ST elevation and tachycardia, more patients feel anginal pain compared to episodes at lower heart rates (Chi-square $p < 0.05$).

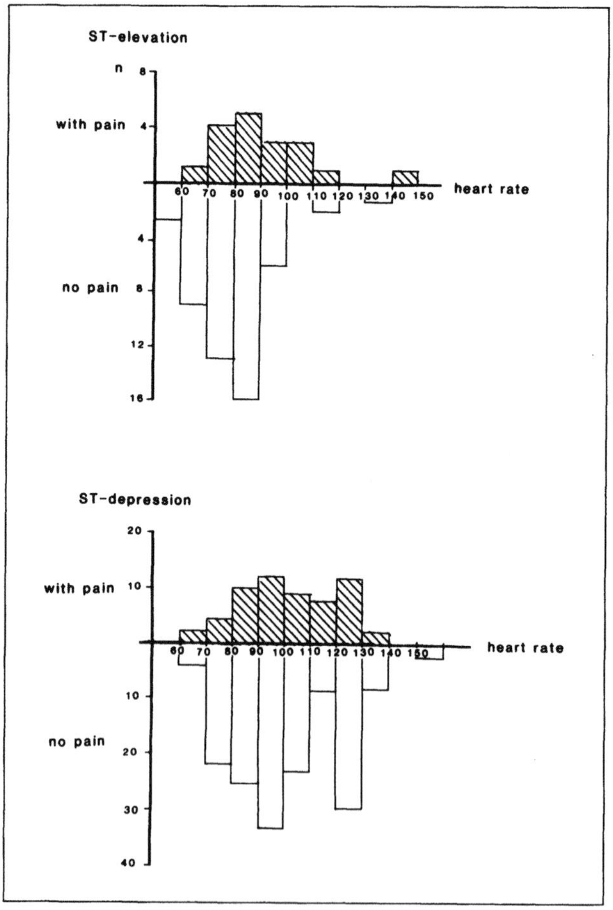

Fig. 2. Number of episodes of ST elevation and ST depression against heart rate at which ischemia became apparent. Most episodes with ST elevation occurred at heart rates below 90 beats/min.

Circadian variation

Figure 3 shows the time of day at which episodes of ST elevation and ST depression occurred. This diurnal distribution of episodes is somewhat different for ST elevation and ST depression, with ST elevation showing a peak in the early morning hours and no decrease during the night-time, while episodes of ST depression have a more broad day-time peak with the highest number of episodes occurring between 8 and 12 o'clock a.m. The percentage of silent episodes remained stable throughout the day; the appearance of silent ischemia is not dependent on the time of day.

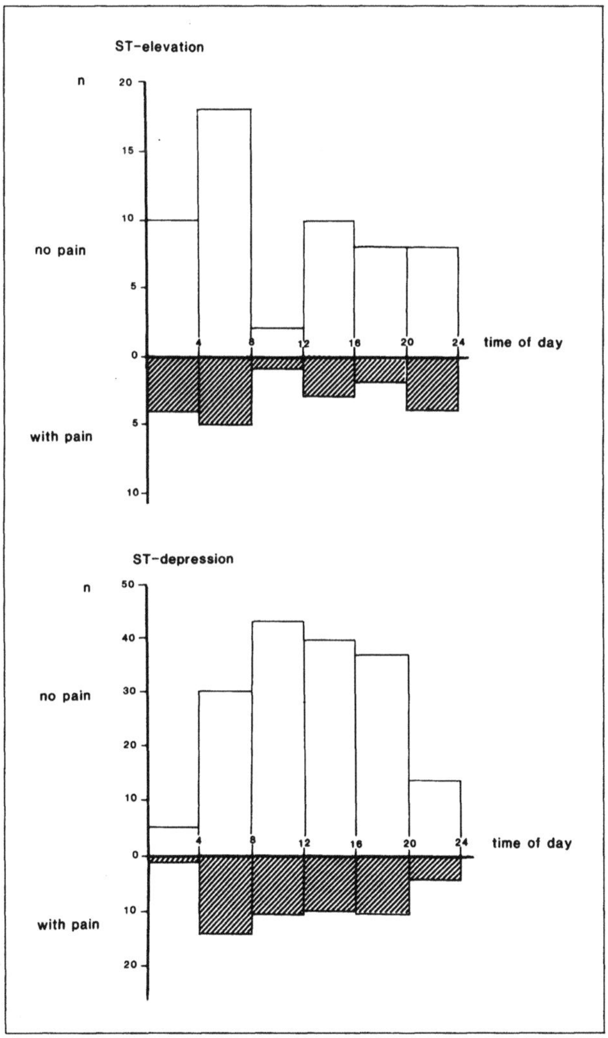

Fig. 3. The time of day at which episodes of ST elevation and ST depression occurred. ST elevation was most common during the early morning and there was broad daytime peak for ST depression. The occurrence of pain was not related to the time of day.

Discussion

In a population of consecutive patients who were referred for coronary angiography, we found ischemic episodes in just under a quarter of all patients. This is markedly less then other authors have found in more selected subgroups of patients (7, 12), but our population may be more representative of common clinical practice. If patients are preselected for ambulatory monitoring on the basis of strongly positive exercise tests (7, 12) or otherwise known severe coronary disease (21) then the percentage of positive results for ischemic episodes may be higher, but the added diagnostic value may be less. Higher percentages of patients positive for transient ischemic episodes are found in unstable angina (1, 14). The separation of unstable angina from stable angina pectoris has become more difficult with the information gained from ambulatory monitoring. In many patients with so-called stable angina, frequent episodes of ischemia at rest are documented with ECG changes, and represent important parts of the definition of unstable angina (20).

Although the ischemic origin of transient ST deviations in patients with coronary heart disease is well validated (7, 24), in patients without severe coronary stenoses who may or may not have dynamic obstructions, false-positive results may be a problem. Therefore in all patients with silent ischemia, the documentation of ischemia by two independent methods is crucial, especially in the decision for invasive treatment.

Another problem are patients who in our study had symptoms but no changes on the ambulatory ECG. Clearly a dual-channel recorder will not pick up all ischemic events reliably and therefore, in these patients, atypical or non-cardiac pain cannot easily be separated from true angina pectoris.

In our study, the occurrence of transient ischemic episodes was not clearly correlated with the severity of fixed coronary stenoses. Only in the sub-group of patients with ST elevation, or ST depression at lower heart rates, was an increased incidence of 2- and 3-vessel disease found. These types of episodes, in which increased oxygen demand of the heart does not seem to be the trigger of ischemia, are more frequent in patients with underlying severe obstructions. This fits very well with the concept of dynamic coronary stenoses but does not make ambulatory monitoring a useful test for predicting severity of fixed coronary disease. The purpose of the method, however, is to show objective signs of ischemia independent of activity through the day. As there is no "gold standard" for the transient ischemic events that are documented by Holter monitoring, calculations of sensitivity and specificity are not possible on the basis of our data. The prognostic relevance, however, that has been shown for transient ischemic episodes in patients with unstable angina (1, 14) may give the results of Holter monitoring a predictive value also for other groups of patients. Quantification of this predictive value must await further prognostic studies.

In our study, as in others, the degree of ST depression, duration, heart rate and circadian variation did not differ between silent and symptomatic ischemic episodes. Therefore, we think that silent ischemic episodes, in general, represent ischemia of a similar degree as that accompanied by angina pectoris.

In conclusion, the prevalence of silent ischemic episodes is high and has prognostic significance in patients with unstable angina pectoris. This prevalence is lower in post-infarct patients or in a coronary heart disease population like the one we have studied. The prevalence of silent ischemic episodes in totally asymptomatic people is still unknown and will be problematic to investigate as this prevalence will be low. However, in this large group of potential patients there are hidden those for whom sudden death or acute myocardial infarction will be the first manifestation of their disease (16, 18).

References

1. v. Arnim Th, Gerbig HW, Krawietz W, Höfling B (1986) Prognostic implications of transient spontaneous — predominantly silent — ischemia in patients with stable and unstable angina. Circulation 74. Suppl II: 359
2. v. Arnim Th (1985) ST-Segment-Analyse im Langzeit-EKG. Deutsch Med Wschr 26: 1047—1051
3. v Arnim Th, Höfling B, Schreiber M (1985) Characteristics of episodes of ST elevation or ST depression during ambulatory monitoring in patients subsequently undergoing coronary angiography. Brit Heart J 54: 484—488
4. Benjamin ST, MacDonald PS, Horowitz JD, Goble AJ, Doyle AE (1986) Usefulness of early exercise testing after non-Q-wave myocardial infarction in predicting prognosis. Am J Cardiol 57: 738—744
5. Campbell S, Barry J, Rebecca GS, Rocco MB, Nabel EG, Wayne RR, Selwyn AP (1986) Active transient myocardial ischemia during daily life in asymptomatic patients with positive exercise tests and coronary artery disease. Am J Cardiol 57: 1010—1016
6. Davidson DM, DeBusk RF (1980) Prognostic value of a single exercise test 3 weeks after uncomplicated myocardial infarction. Circulation 61: 236—242
7. Deanfield JF, Maseri A, Selwyn AP, Ribeiro P, Chierchia S, Krikler S, Morgan M (1983) Myocardial ischemia during daily life in patients with stable angina: its relation to symptoms and heart rate changes. Lancet II: 753—758
8. Diamond GA, Forrester JS (1979) Analysis of probability as an aid in the clinical diagnosis of coronary artery disease. New Engl J Med 300: 1350—1358
9. Erikssen J, Thaulow E (1984) Follow-up of patients with asymptomatic myocardial ischemia. In: Rutishauser W, Roskamm H (eds) Silent Myocardial Ischemia, Springer Verlag Berlin Heidelberg New York Tokyo, pp 156—164
10. Fisch C (1984) Electrocardiography and vectorcardiography. In: Braunwald E (ed) Heart Disease. W. B. Saunders, pp 195—257
11. Froelicher VF, Thompson AJ, Longo MR Jr, Triebwasser JH, Lancaster MC (1976) Value of exercise testing for screening asymptomatic men for latent coronary artery disease. Prog Cardiovas Dis 16: 265—276
12. Fazzini PF, Marchi F, Pucci P, Zambaldi G, Santoro GM (1984) Asymptomatic myocardial ischemia in patients with effort angina. In: Rutishauser W, Roskamm H (eds) Silent Myocardial Ischemia, Springer Verlag Berlin Heidelberg New York Tokyo, pp 112—116
13. Gensini GG (1975) Coronary arteriography. Mount Kisco, Futura Publishing Co., New York
14. Gottlieb SO, Weisfeldt ML, Ouyang P, Mellits ED, Gerstenblith G (1986) Silent ischemia as a marker for early unfavorable outcomes in patients with unstable angina. New Engl J Med 314: 1214—1219
15. Gottlieb SH, Gerstenblith G, Achuff SC, Mellits FD, Gottlieb SO (1986) Ischemic ST segment changes by ambulatory Holter predict one year mortality in high risk post-infarct patients. Circulation 74, Suppl II: 231
16. Harper RW, Kennedy G, DeSanctis RW, Hutter AM (1979) The incidence and pattern of angina prior to acute myocardial infarction: A study of 577 cases. Am Heart J 97: 178
17. Langou RA, Huang EK, Kelley MJ, Cohen LS (1980) Predictive accuracy of coronary artery calcification and abnormal exercise test for coronary artery disease in asymptomatic men. Circulation 62: 1196—1203
18. Lown B (1979) Sudden cardiac death: The major challenge confronting contemporary cardiology. Am J Cardiol 43: 313
19. Miller DH, Borer JS (1982) Exercise testing early after myocardial infarction: risks and benefits. Am J Med 72: 427—435

20. Muller JE, Turi ZG, Pearle DL, Schneider JF, Serfas DH, Morrison J, Stone PH, Rude RE, Rosner B, Sobel BE, Tate C, Scheiner E, Roberts R, Hennelens CH, Braunwald E (1984) Nifedipine and conventional therapy for unstable angina pectoris: a randomized, double-blind comparison. Circulation 69: 728—739
21. Quyyumi AA, Wright C, Fox K (1983) Ambulatory electrocardiographic ST segment changes in healthy volunteers. Brit Heart J 50: 460—464
22. Rifkin RD, Hood WB Jr (1977) Bayesian analysis of electrocardiographic exercise stress testing. New Engl J Med 297: 681—686
23. Selbmann HK, Raab A (1980) SAVOD-Q: Sammel- und Auswertungssystem volldynamischer Datenbestände. Technische Berichte d. Inst. f. Med. Informationsverarbeitung, Statistik und Biomathematik, Universität München, Nr. 3
24. Selwyn AP, Shea MJ, Deanfield JE, Wilson RA, deLandsheere C, Jones T (1985) Clinical problems in coronary disease are caused by a wide variety of ischemic episodes that affect patients out of hospital. Am J Med 79, Suppl 3A: 12—17
25. Sheffield LT (1984) Exercise stress testing. In: Braunwald E (ed) Heart Disease, WB Saunders, 258—276
26. Theroux P, Waters DD, Halphen C, Debaisoeux JC, Mizgala HF (1979) Prognostic value of exercise testing soon after myocardial infarction. New Engl J Med 301: 341

Authors' address:
Dr. Th. v. Arnim
Medizinische Klinik I
Klinikum Großhadern
Marchioninistraße 15
8000 München 70

Identification of patients with silent myocardial ischemia by metabolic, scintigraphic and angiographic findings

C. W. Hamm, W. Kupper, A. Hinrichs, and W. Bleifeld

Dept. of Cardiology, Medical Clinic, University Hospital Eppendorf, Hamburg, West Germany

Introduction

Episodes of painless myocardial ischemia occur frequently in patients with chronic stable angina (2, 6) and unstable angina (9, 14). Silent myocardial ischemia has also been observed in patients with documented coronary heart disease who are completely asymptomatic (4, 8). Defective pain perception (5, 7, 10), as well as less severe ischemia (3), has been proposed to underly painless ischemia. Its diagnosis is most frequently based on ST-segment analysis during Holter monitoring (1, 17) or stress testing (12). In the present study we investigated how these electrocardiographic findings relate to scintigraphic, angiographic, hemodynamic and metabolic parameters of coronary heart disease and myocardial perfusion.

Patients and methods

The study included 13 patients (3 females, 10 males; 43—60 years old). In 9 patients no angina or angina like – symptoms were found, while 4 patients reported dyspnea or atypical precordial pains on effort. During treadmill exercise, according to the Bruce protocol, asymptomatic ST depression of more than 0.15 mV in at least 2 precordial leads was documented in all patients. In addition, biphasic thallium-201 scintigrams and ambulatory 24 h Holter ECG's (Medilog MR 14, Oxford Instruments) were obtained. All patients underwent routine coronary and left ventricular angiography, followed by coronary sinus blood flow measurements with the thermodilution technique as previously described (13). In arterial and coronary venous blood samples the oxygen and lactate content were determined, to calculate myocardial oxygen uptake and the lactate extraction rate. Arterial, pulmonary artery and pulmonary wedge pressures were continuously recorded via fluid filled catheters. Cardiac output was calculated by means of Fick's principle. Throughout the study the ECG was registered by 6 standard precordial Wilson leads. After all baseline values were obtained, the patients were paced atrially until ST-segment depression or AV-block occurred, and measurements were repeated.

Results

Based on the coronary angiograms the patients were subdivided in two groups (Table 1). Patients in group A (3 females, 1 male) showed only mild to moderate vessel wall irregularities. The angiographic result was confirmed by a normal thallium scintigraphy and the lack of lactate production during atrial pacing. The ST-segment depression was therefore interpreted as a false-positive result.

The other 9 patients had two- (n = 1) or three- (n = 8) vessel disease (group B) including an 80% or more cross-sectional area stenosis of the left anterior descending coronary artery. In all cases the ejection fraction was within the normal range of our laboratory. According to the transcardiac lactate gradient during atrial pacing, group B was further subdivided in group B_1 (n = 3) with normal lactate metabolism (lactate extraction rate: 17%) and group B_2 (n = 6) with lactate production (22%) indicating myocardial ischemia. In group B_2, 4/6 patients exhibited regional perfusion defects by means of thallium scintigraphy (Fig. 1), while all patients of group B_1 showed normal tracer distribution during

Table 1. Patient groups with asymptomatic ST depression.

	Group A (n = 4)	Group B_1 (n = 3)	Group B_2 (n = 6)
Coronary Angiography	no relevant stenoses	2- or 3-vessel disease	
Thallium-201	normal	normal	normal n = 2 defects n =4
Lactate metabolism	normal	normal	production
Holter	normal	normal	ST ↓

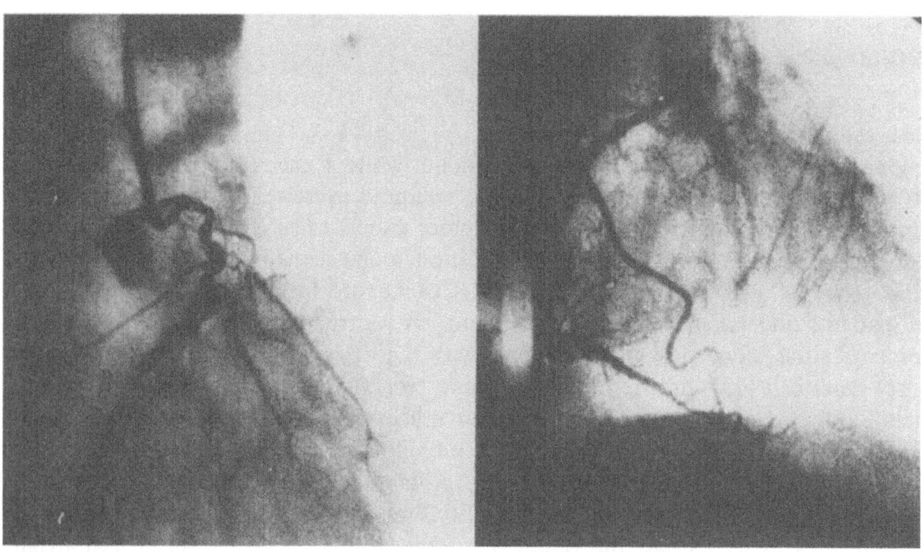

Fig. 1a

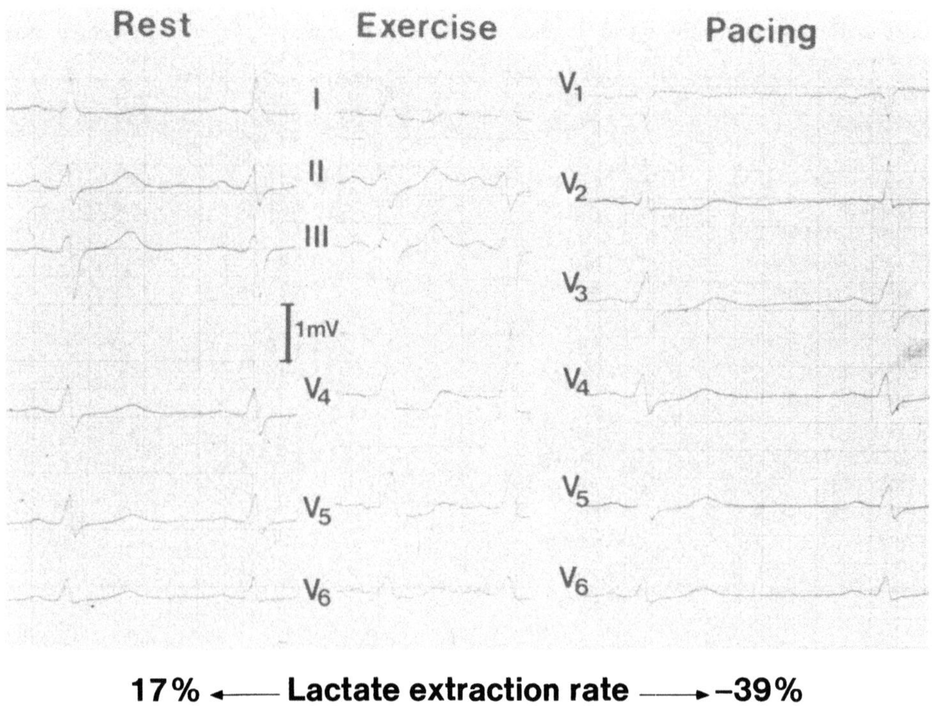

Fig. 1b

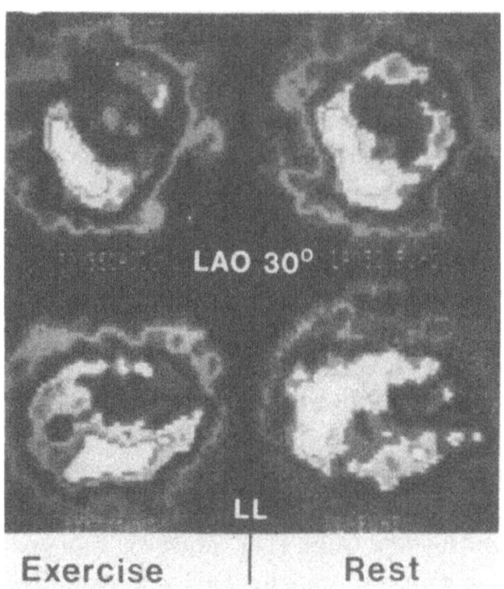

Fig. 1c

Fig. 1. Example of data from an asymptomatic patient (57-year-old male)
a) Subtotal occlusion on the left anterior descending coronary artery, with collaterals from the right coronary artery in the coronary angiogram.
b) ST-segment depression during rest, exercise and atrial pacing accompanied by lactate production.
c) Perfusion defect during exercise, revealed by thallium scintigraphy.

rest and exercise. Holter monitoring revealed ST-segment depression in all patients of group B_2, but not in group B_1. There was a trend to higher pulmonary pressures in group B_2 which was accompanied by lower coronary sinus blood flow and oxygen consumption (Table 2).

Table 2. Hemodynamic and metabolic data in patients with angiographically documented heart disease.

ST-segment	exercise	0.30±0.14	0.36±0.10
depression	pacing	0.17±0.08	0.16±0.05
[mV]			
Pressure-rate	exercise	209±41	218±33
product	pacing	216±21	166±37
[mm Hg/min × 10^2]			
Mean pulmonary	rest	12±2	17±2
artery pressure	pacing	9±2	18±2
[mm Hg]			
Coronary sinus	rest	74± 9	60±23
blood flow	pacing	125±44	100±48
[ml/min]			
Myocardial O_2	rest	7.1±3.1	6.0±2.3
consumption	pacing	13.8±3.4	9.8±4.5
[ml/min]			
Lactate extraction	rest	35±28	6±10
rate	pacing	17±20	–22±17
[%]			

Discussion

There is growing evidence that patients with coronary artery disease frequently sustain episodes of painless ischemia. Asymptomatic ECG changes compatible with myocardial ischemia have been found in patients with chronic stable angina as well as totally symptom-free patients (4, 6, 8, 10, 14, 16). Asymptomatic patients may easily miss adequate treatment and suffer an adverse prognosis (9). Consequently, elaborate diagnostic techniques should supplement ECG findings in order to prove or rule out major coronary heart disease.

The results of our study confirm that severe coronary heart disease may be present in completely asymptomatic patients. False-positive stress tests, however, need to be considered, as our study demonstrates.

In patients with angiographically documented high grade coronary obstructions we found evidence for two different subgroups. In the first group (B_1) we could not detect ischemia by conventional scintigraphy or by coronary sinus lactate measurements. These findings may suggest less severe ischemia or a lesser amount of myocardium in jeopardy. This hypothesis is consistent with hemodynamic data reported by Chierchia et al. (3), but conflicting with the angiographic findings of Lindsey and Cohn (14). However, any possible controversy may be resolved by the second group of patients (B_2) who exhibited clear metabolic evidence of myocardial ischemia. In this group, defective pain perception (5, 7, 10) possibly represents the underlying mechanism for the lack of angina.

Thus, in patients with angiographically documented coronary heart disease and evidence of silent ischemia, two distinct, independent mechanisms – less ischemia and defective pain perception – need evaluation. With respect to therapeutic consequences, refined diagnostic tools, such as cardiac metabolic studies, may be warranted in certain patients.

References

1. v Arnim T, Höfling B (1985) Characteristics of episodes of ST elevation or ST depression during ambulatory monitoring in patients subsequently undergoing coronary angiography. Brit Heart J 54: 484—488
2. Cecchi AC, Dovellini LV, Marchi F, Pucci P, Santoro GM, Fazzini PF (1983) Silent myocardial ischemia during ambulatory electrocardiographic monitoring in patients with effort angina. J Am Coll Cardiol 1: 934—939
3. Chierchia S, Lazzari M, Freedman B, Brunelli C, Maseri A (1983) Impairment of myocardial perfusion and function during painless myocardial ischemia. J Am Coll Cardiol 1: 924—930
4. Cohn PF (1977) Severe asymptomatic coronary artery disease. A diagnostic, prognostic, and therapeutic puzzle. Am J Med 62: 565—568
5. Cohn PF (1980) Silent myocardial ischemia in patients with a defective anginal warning system. Am J Cardiol 45: 697—702
6. Deanfield JE, Selwyn AP, Chierchia S, Maseri A, Ribeiro P, Krikier S, Morgan M (1983) Myocardial ischemia during daily life in patients with stable angina: its relation to symptoms and heart rate changes. Lancet 2: 753—758
7. Droste E, Roskamm H (1983) Experimental pain measurements in patients with asymptomatic myocardial ischemia. J Am Coll Cardial 1: 940—945
8. Erikssen J, Thaulow E, Myhre E (1982) Coronary artery disease with and without angina — two different entities? Acta Med Scan 211: 243—248
9. Eriksen J, Thaulow E (1984) Follow-up of patients with asymptomatic myocardial ischemia. In: Rutishauser W, Roskamm H (eds) Silent myocardial ischemia. Springer Verlag, Berlin Heidelberg New York Tokyo, pp 156—164
10. Glazier JJ, Chierchia S, Brown MJ, Maseri A (1986) Importance of generalized defective perception of painful stimuli as a cause of silent myocardial ischemia in chronic stable angina pectoris. Am J Cardiol 58: 667—672
11. Gottlieb SO, Weisfeldt ML, Ouyang P, Mellits ED, Gerstenblith G (1986) Silent ischemia as a marker for early unfavorable outcomes in patients with unstable angina. N Eng J Med
12. Kattus AA, Jorgensen CR, Worden RE, Alvaro AB (1971) ST-segment depression with near-maximal exercise in detection of preclinical coronary heart disease. Circulation 44: 585—595
13. Kupper W, Bleifeld W (1981) Regionale and globale Koronarsinusflußmessungen mit dem kontinuierlichen Thermodilutionsverfahren. II. Klinische Untersuchungen bei Koronarkranken. Z Kardiol 70: 116—123
14. Lindsey HE, Cohn PF (1978) Silent myocardial ischemia during and after exercise testing in patients with coronary artery disease. Am Heart J 95: 441—447
15. Nademanee K, Intarachot V, Singh PN, Josphson MA, Singh BN (1986) Characteristics and clinical significance of silent myocardial ischemia in unstable angina. Am J Cardiol 58: 26B—33B
16. Schang SJ Jr, Pepine C (1977) Transient asymptomatic ST segment depression during daily activity. Am J Cardiol 39: 395—402
17. Stern S, Tzivoni D (1974) Early detection of silent ischemic heart disease by 24 hour electrocardiographic monitoring of active subjects. Br Heart J 36: 481—486

Authors' address:
Dr. C. W. Hamm
Dept. of Cardiology
Medical Clinic
University Hospital Eppendorf
Martinistraße 52
2000 Hamburg 20
West Germany

The frequency, pathophysiology, and prognosis of exercise-induced silent ischemia

A. Rozanski, D. Berman

Division of Cardiology, Department of Medicine, and the Department of Nuclear Medicine, Cedars-Sinai Medical Center, and the Department of Medicine, UCLA School of Medicine, Los Angeles, California

Introduction

Silent myocardial ischemia in now recognized to be a frequent occurrence in patients with coronary artery disease. Many of the recent observations regarding the occurrence of silent myocardial ischemia have been made using ambulatory electrocardiography, but silent ischemia can also be detected using exercise tests. These two forms of testing offer potentially complementary information. Exercise testing may be used to assess the extent and severity of "potentially inducible" silent myocardial ischemia, whereas ambulatory electrocardiography may be used to assess the frequency and duration of "spontaneously occurring" silent ischemia. In this article, we specifically focus on the frequency and prognostic implications of exercise-induced silent ischemia.

Methods of assessing exercise-induced silent ischemia

When myocardial ischemia is induced during exercise, a constellation of physiologic and metabolic abnormalities occurs. Myocardial hypoperfusion results in anaerobic metabolism, diminution in myocardial contractile function, and electrophysiologic changes characteristic of myocardial ischemia. Each of these alterations can be detected during exercise testing, using either electrocardiography or radionuclide imaging (Table 1). As-

Table 1: Objective measurements of myocardial ischemia during exercise testing.

Physiologic abnormality	Exercise test
myocardial hypoperfusion	thallium-201 scintigraphy rubidium-82 scintigraphy*
anaerobic metabolism	18-F-Fluoro-deoxy glucose* C-11 palmitate*
diminished contractile function	radionuclide ventriculography.
electrophysiologic changes	electrocardiography

* assessed using positron emission tomography

sessment of anaerobic metabolism, however, is currently impractical, except for research purposes, since it requires the use of positron emission tomography, a very costly imaging procedure. Thus, we have focused on the assessment of silent myocardial ischemia using exercise electrocardiography and conventional radionuclide stress tests: stress-redistribution thallium scintigraphy (used to assess myocardial perfusion) and exercise radionuclide ventriculography (used to assess regional wall motion and ejection fraction).

Working definition of exercise-induced silent myocardial ischemia

There is presently no noninvasive "gold standard" for determining the presence of myocardial ischemia. However, the presence of myocardial ischemia may be identified with *high probability* in patients in whom multiple tests indicate the presence of myocardial ischemia (e.g., an abnormal electrocardiographic test response combined with a reversible thallium perfusion defect or exercise-induced regional wall motion abnormality). In patients who have a high pre-test probability of coronary artery disease, such as male patients with typical angina, or patients who have a history of prior myocardial infarction, even a single abnormal test response may be sufficient to establish a high probability of silent myocardial ischemia. This is because the frequency of false-positive test responses for myocardial ischemia and coronary artery disease is low in such patients, given the high prevalence of coronary artery disease (1). In patients who are asymptomatic, however, or who have only nonanginal chest pain, a single abnormal test response is *not* sufficient to establish a diagnosis of myocardial ischemia. This is because such patients have a low prevalence of coronary artery disease. Thus, as predicted by Bayes theorem, the majority of abnormal test responses in such patients will be falsely positive for coronary artery disease or myocardial ischemia. For instance, an asymptomatic 50-year-old male (pre-test CAD probability = 5%) with a positive exercise electrocardiogram still has less than a 20% post-test probability of coronary artery disease (1). In other words, the odds are greater than 4 : 1 that a positive exercise electrocardiographic response in asymptomatic individuals is falsely positive. The probability of coronary disease and myocardial ischemia, however, increases significantly if such asymptomatic individuals also have an abnormal response during radionuclide stress testing (1), particularly if either the electrocardiographic or radionuclide response is markedly abnormal.

Exercise-induced silent ischemia is simply the development (of evidence) of myocardial ischemia during exercise in the *absence* of exercise-induced chest pain. In patients with a low pre-test probability of coronary artery disease, this determination should not be made unless there are *at least* two tests indicating evidence of myocardial ischemia.

On a practical basis, this means that exercise electrocardiography may be used to diagnose the presence of (a high probability of) silent myocardial ischemia in patients with typical angina (unless young or female) or prior myocardial infarction. However, radionuclide stress testing is also needed to establish the presence of a high probability of myocardial ischemia in those asymptomatic or nonanginal chest pain patients having an abnormal exercise electrocardiogram. If the radionuclide stress test response is abnormal in such patients, then the probability of silent ischemia increases to a high level, especially if the thallium response is strongly positive. If the radionuclide test response is normal, however, then the probability that the abnormal exercise electrocardiographic response represents silent ischemia is low.

Frequency of exercise-induced silent ischemia

In patients with evidence of significant coronary artery disease by coronary angiography who have positive exercise electrocardiograms, the frequency of exercise-induced ST segment depression which occurs painlessly is approximately 33% (2—12). Approximately one-third of catheterized patients with evidence of exercise-induced hypoperfusion by thallium scintigraphy or wall motion abnormalities during radionuclide ventriculography have also been reported to have no chest pain during stress (13—14). In uncatheterized patients with chest pain syndromes but as yet unproven CAD, the frequency of exercise-induced painless ST segment depression has been reported to be higher. For instance, in the follow-up of 1402 patients with chest pain syndromes and positive exercise electrocardiograms. Cole and Ellestad found that the frequency of painless ST depression was 75%, more than twice as high as in the patients who were not catheterized (15). But since there was no radionuclide confirmation of ischemia or angiographic confirmation of disease, the frequency of ST depression which represented true silent ischemia in their uncatheterized population cannot be determined. Since there is generally a preferential selection of patients who are more sick to angiography (16), the frequency of exercise-induced silent ischemia in the total population of CAD patients with exercise ST depression is probably higher than the 33% observed in catheterized patients, but lower than the 75% observed in uncatheterized patients.

Exercise tests as predictors of patient prognosis

Various studies indicate that the magnitude of exercise-induced myocardial ischemia is an important predictor of patient prognosis (17—19). Important individual predictors of cardiac risk for exercise electrocardiography, thallium scintigraphy, and radionuclide ventriculography are listed in Table 2 (20—40). In general, those parameters which indicate ischemia of great magnitude (e.g., multiple [19] or severe exercise-induced thallium defects [27]) or ischemia which is easily provocable at a low level of stress (e.g., marked ST depression in Stage I of the Bruce protocol) [17] are the most powerful predictors of high risk. Each of the exercise tests has been shown to add incremental information to the results of angiography and clinical history (41—43). The radionuclide stress tests are more powerful predictors of prognosis than is exercise electrocardiography (28, 41—43, 45) and they add incremental prognostic information to the exercise electrocardiography results (28, 41—43). This is due to the greater inherent sensitivity of radionuclide tests for detecting the presence of myocardial ischemia and their ability to characterize both the global extent of myocardial ischemia (predictive of the proportion of the myocardium subtended by stenosed vessels) and the regional severity of ischemia (predictive of the severity of stenosis subtending a given myocardial region). The abnormalities noted on exercise electrocardiography do not have such localizing ability.

Prognosis of exercise-induced silent ischemia

Although exercise testing is an effective means of inducing silent myocardial ischemia, the prognostic implications of this finding are not yet as well defined. Recently, however,

Table 2: Exercise parameters used to assess prognosis in patients with coronary artery disease.

Exercise ECG	Thallium scintigraphy	Radionuclide ventriculography
Proven predictors		
Magnitude of ST ↓ (20–21)	Extent of perfusion defects (19)	LVEF response (33–36)
Duration of ST ↓ (22)	Severity of perfusion defects (27)	Segmental wall motion abnormalities (36)
Timing of ST ↓ (23)	Lung uptake (28)	
Exercise duration (24)	Washout abnormalities (29)	
Chest pain (25)		
Hypotension (26)		
Potential but unproven predictors		
	Rate of defect reversibility (30)	RVEF response (37–38)
	Transient ischemia dilatation (31)	Timing of WMA (39)
	Basal myocardial uptake (32)	Postexercise persistence of exercise WMA
		Magnitude of WMA
		Postexercise reversal of resting WMA (40)

↓ = depression; RVEF = right ventricular ejection fraction; WMA = wall motion abnormalities.

information regarding the prognostic importance of exercise-induced silent ischemia has begun to emerge.

Assessment by exercise electrocardiography

Exercise electrocardiography has been used to evaluate potentially inducible silent ischemia in three groups of patients: (1) totally asymptomatic individuals in whom testing is being performed for screening purposes (2) asymptomatic individuals following myocardial infarction and (3) patients with chest pain syndromes, in whom there may be no elicitable ischemia, painless ischemia, or symptomatic ischemia during exercise.

With respect to totally asymptomatic individuals, many investigators have now demonstrated that the elicitation of exercise-induced ST segment depression signifies an increased risk of cardiac events (46–57). The average increase in risk is nearly five-fold (46–57), but the overall frequency of cardiac events in totally asymptomatic individuals in still relatively small, given both the very low pre-test probability of cardiac events in these patients, and the fact that, as previously mentioned, most positive ECG results in such individuals are falsely positive, not indicative of silent ischemia (1).

The same problem is not true for asymptomatic individuals following myocardial infarction. In such patients, the prevalence of coronary artery disease is nearly 100%, so that the frequency of false-positive responses for myocardial ischemia is very low. Not surprisingly, therefore, the predictive accuracy of exercise-induced ST segment depression for subsequent cardiac events is much higher in these patients. For instance, Theroux et al. performed submaximal exercise electrocardiography prior to hospital discharge in

210 patients recovering from acute myocardial infarction (58). Each patient had been asymptomatic for at least four days prior to testing. The frequency of unstable angina, myocardial infarction, or death during the ensuring year was 32% in the subgroup of 37 patients with silent ST segment depression during exercise, and 30% in the 27 patients who had both chest pain and ST segment depression during exercise. Thus, the prognosis of silent and symptomatic ischemia was similar in this important subgroup of patients. Among the 146 patients without ST segment depression, the frequency of these cardiac events was still 13%, a not insubstantial event rate. The frequency of myocardial infarction, or death, alone was 10%. Other investigators have also recently reported that the cardiac event rate is not inconsequential following a negative predischarge test response in asymptomatic post-MI patients (42, 45). This may represent a relative insensitivity of the exercise electrocardiogram for detecting silent ischemia, especially when using only submaximal stress. The predictive accuracy of pre-discharge submaximal exercise thallium scintigraphy and exercise electrocardiography in asymptomatic post-infarction patients has now been compared, with the former found to be more accurate (42, 45). Specifically, whereas a positive response during exercise electrocardiography or thallium scintigraphy are both highly predictive of subsequent cardiac events, a negative thallium response was found to be significantly more predictive of *no* subsequent events than was exercise electrocardiography (42).

With respect to patients with chronic chest pain syndromes, a number of investigators have demonstrated a similar frequency of cardiac events in patients having silent or symptomatic ST depression during exercise testing (59—60). For instance, Weiner et al. followed 1583 patients with documented CAD for seven years. They observed a similar frequency of cardiac events in the patients with silent and symptomatic ischemia during stress testing (59). In contrast, Ellestad et al., found a higher frequency of cardiac events in patients having symptomatic rather than silent ST depression among the 1402 patients they followed for five years after exercise testing (15). Seventy-one percent of the patients with symptomatic ST segment depression developed a myocardial infarction or angina or had a cardiac death, compared to 52% of the patients with silent ST segment depression during the period of follow-up. Even so, the frequency of cardiac events in their subgroup with silent ST segment depression was high, further indicating that the identification of potentially inducible silent ischemia is prognostically important.

Assessment by radionuclide stress tests

The reported assessment of silent ischemia using radionuclide stress tests has so far been more sparse, related to the relative newness of these tests, thus providing less time for follow-up, and the relative newness of focus on the prognosis of silent ischemia. Nevertheless, some follow-up studies have now been performed after radionuclide stress testing for each of the three types of patient populations referred to above:

1. Totally asymptomatic individuals

Fleg and colleagues performed a 30-month follow-up in a large group of 245 volunteers who underwent stress-redistribution thallium scintigraphy (61). They assessed the subsequent frequency of new anginal syndromes, myocardial infarction, or subsequent cardiac events. These cardiac events occurred in only 2% of the volunteers who had a normal study during stress-redistribution scintigraphy, but occurred in 14% having an abnormal response — a seven-fold increase. Similarly, we assessed the one-year frequency of myocardial infarction, cardiac death, or late coronary bypass surgery (> 60 days post-testing) in 599 asymptomatic patients undergoing stress redistribution thallium scintigraphy (44). The frequency was five-fold higher in the patients with an abnormal thallium response. To assess the prognostic significance of silent myocardial ischemia in asymptomatic individuals, we further compared the prognosis of a reversible exercise-induced thallium defect in 83 asymptomatic patients and 77 patients with typical angina (62). The one-year incidence of the aforementioned cardiac events was approximately twice as high in the patients with typical angina (18%), but the frequency in the patients who were asymptomatic was not insubstantial (8%). Furthermore, the one-year cardiac event rate was essentially the same (19% vs 16%) in the typical angina and asymptomatic subgroups who manifested a reversible thallium defect at a low level of stress (< 85% of maximal predicted heart rate) (62). Thus, as with exercise electrocardiography, studies using radionuclide imaging also indicate that the elicitation of potentially inducible silent ischemia is prognostically important.

2. Predischarge evaluation of asymptomatic post-MI patients

Two investigative groups have employed radionuclide testing for pre-hospital discharge evaluation in asymptomatic post-MI patients (42, 45). Gibson et al. followed 140 patients for 15 months following submaximal exercise thallium scintigraphy (42). The frequency of subsequent cardiac death, re-infarction or progressive angina was 59% in the patients demonstrating evidence of a reversible thallium defect, compared to only 6% in the patients without a reversible defect. Twenty-two (16%) of the 140 patients had chest pain during exercise, so abnormal thallium responses in this small subgroup (cross-correlative results not reported) would not represent true silent ischemia. It is evident from their data, however, that the vast majority of thallium responses in their event group must have occurred silently (in at least 34/47 = 72%). Leppo et al. employed dipyridamole infusion rather than stress testing in 51 asymptomatic post-MI patients followed for a mean of 16 months (45). The subsequent rate of cardiac events during a mean follow-up of 19 months was 33% in the patients with inducible hypoperfusion, versus a rate of only 6% in the patients with no reversible hypoperfusion.

3. Patients with chest pain syndromes

Bonow et al. recently followed 131 patients with coronary artery disease who underwent exercise radionuclide ventriculography (63), divided into patients having silent and symptomatic evidence of myocardial ischemia (i.e., inducible wall motion abnormalities with exercise). The frequency of subsequent cardiac events was similar in both groups. Similarly, Walters et al. followed a group of 55 patients with coronary artery disease who performed stress-redistribution thallium scintigraphy, divided evenly into 27 patients with silent exercise-induced ischemia (i.e. having transient perfusion defects without chest pain) and 28 patients in whom both ischemia and chest pain were induced (64). Again, the frequency of cardiac events was similar in both groups. Thus, these studies further illustrate the importance of potentially inducible silent myocardial ischemia.

Comparison to ambulatory electrocardiography

Recent studies indicate that ambulatory electrocardiography may also be used to identify high risk patient subgroups, by identifying those patients having evidence of spontaneously occurring silent myocardial ischemia (65—67). The relative efficacy of stress testing and ambulatory electrocardiography for identifying silent myocardial ischemia is not known. Relatively little direct comparison of these two forms of testing has been reported so far. In a recent study, Campbell et al. were able to make some initial comparisons (68). Among their findings, they noted no evidence of spontaneously occurring silent ischemia (as assessed by ambulatory monitoring) among the patients who did not have potentially inducible myocardial ischemia (as assessed by exercise electrocardiography). Further study is needed to confirm this observation, which, if valid, could provide a means for determining which patients might be candidates for ambulatory monitoring. From a practical point of view, the frequency of cardiac events is already very low (one year rate of 1% or less) in patients having a normal response with radionuclide stress testing (69—71). The added usefulness of ambulatory monitoring in patients with such a low probability of an event would appear to be dubious.

Pathophysiology

The reason(s) as to why exercise-induced myocardial ischemia is sometimes silent and sometimes not is not well understood. Speculation has most commonly centered around two explanations: (1) that silent ischemia, in general, is a less severe ischemia than that occurring with chest pain (72—73) and (2) that silent ischemia occurs due to a "defective (73) anginal warning system", the result of either a heightened threshold for pain or defective transmission of painful stimuli (74—76). Other explanations have also been proposed (77), but at this time there is no definitive answer as to this question. A reasonable speculation is that symptomatic ischemia represents a greater magnitude of ischemia than silent ischemia, but in recent studies of spontaneously occurring ischemia using ambulatory electrocardiography, a wide overlap in the measured magnitude of silent and symptomatic ischemic responses has been noted (78—79). This issue requires further study in broader spectrums of patients. Regardless of the comparative magnitude of silent and symptomatic ischemia, it is evident from the prognostic data cited above that silent ischemia is "bad enough" to warrant clinical attention.

Conclusion

An increasing accumulation of data now suggests that the identification of potentially inducible silent ischemia has strong prognostic significance. In many studies, silent ischemia detected during stress testing has had the same prognostic significance as symptomatic ischemia. Radionuclide stress tests are the most potent means of assessing the magnitude of potentially inducible myocardial ischemia during exercise. Their prognostic effectiveness, relative to that of ambulatory electrocardiography, remains to be determined by future study.

Acknowledgements

We would like to thank Lisa Hestrin, M.P.H., for her technical assistance, and Dwana Williams for her word processing assistance. Funded is part by a grant from the MacArthur Foundation and National Institute of Health SCOR grant # 17651.

References

1. Berman DS, Rozanski A, Knoebel S (1987) The detection of silent ischemia: cautions and precautions. Circulation 75
2. Allen RD, Gettes LS, Phalan C, Avington ND (1976) Painless ST segment depression in patients with angina pectoris: correlation with daily activities and cigarette smoking. Chest 69: 467—473
3. Rios JC, Hurwitz LE (1974) Electrocardiographic responses to atrial pacing and multistage treadmill exercise testing: correlation with coronary arteriography. Am J Cardiol 34: 661—666
4. Piessens J, Van Meighem WV, Kesteloot H, DeGeest H (1974) Diagnostic value of clinical history, exercise testing and atrial pacing in patients with chest pain. Am J Cardiol 33: 351—356
5. Allen RD, Gettes LS, Phalan C, Avington ND (1976) Painless ST segment depression in patients with angina pectoris; Correlation with daily activities and cigarette smoking. Chest 69: 467—473
6. Jelinek VM, Herman MV, Schweitzer P, Gorlin R (1976) The significance of chest pain occurring with the master two step test. Aust NZ J Med 6 : 22—25
7. Tompkin MJ, Miller RR, DeMaria AN, Vismara LA, Amsterdam EZ, Mason DT (1977) Multifactor evaluation of the determinants of ischemic electrocardiographic response to maximal treadmill testing in coronary disease. Am J Med 62: 339—346
8. Berman JL, Wynne J, Cohn PF (1978) A multivariate approach for interpreting treadmill exercise tests in coronary artery disease. Circulation 58: 505
9. Cole JP, Ellestad MH (1978) Significance of chest pain during treadmill exercise: Correlation with coronary events. Am J Cardiol 41: 227—232
10. Lindsey HE Jr, Cohn PF (1978) „Silent" myocardial ischemia during and after exercise testing in patients with coronary artery disease. Am J Heart J 95: 441—47
11. Selwyn AP, Fox K, Eves M, Oakley D, Dargie H, Shilingford J (1978) Myocardial ischemia in patients with frequent angina pectoris. Br Med J 2: 1594—1596
12. Weiner DA, McCabe C, Heuter DC, Ryan TJ, Hood WB Jr (1978) The predictive value of anginal chest pain as an indicator of coronary disease during exercise testing. Am Heart J 458—462
13. Bailey IK, Griffith LSC, Rouleu J, Strauss HW, Pitt B (1977) Thallium-201 myocardial perfusion imaging at rest and during exercise: comparative sensitivity to electrocardiography in coronary artery disease. Circulation 55: 79—87
14. Borer JS, Kent KM, Bacharach SL, Green MV, Rosing DR, Seides SF, Epstein SE, Johnston GS (1979) Sensitivity, specificity and predictive accuracy of radionuclide cineangiography during exercise in patients with coronary artery disease: comparison with exercise electrocardiography. Circulation 60: 572—580
15. Cole J, Ellestad MH (1978) Significance of chest pain during treadmill exercise. Am J Cardiol 41: 227—235
16. Rozanski A, Diamond G, Berman DS, Forrester JS, Morris D, Swan HJC (1983) The declining specificity of exercise radionuclide ventriculography. NEJM 309: 518—522

17. McNeer JF, Margolis JR; Lee KL et al (1978) The role of the exercise test on the evaluation of patients for ischemic heart disease. Circulation 57: 64—70
18. Bonow RO, Kent KM, Rosing DR, Gordon KK, Lakatos E, Borer JS, Bacharach SL, Green MV, Epstein SE (1985) Exercise-induced ischemia in mildly symptomatic patients with coronary-artery disease and preserved left ventricular function. N Eng J Med 312: 389—394
19. Ladenheim ML, Pollack H, Rozanski A, Berman DS, Stanilff HM, Forrester JS, Diamond GA (1986) Extent and severity of myocardial hypoperfusion as orthogonal indices of prognosis in patients with suspected coronary artery disease. JACC 7: 464—471
20. Dagenais GR, Rouleau JR; Christen A, Fabia J (1982) Survival of patients with a strongly positive exercise electrogram. Circulation 65: 452—6
21. Staniloff H, Diamond G, Forrester J, Berman D, Swan HJC (1982) Prediction of death, infarction and worsening chest pain with exercise electrocardiography and thallium scintigraphy. Am J Cardiol 49: 967
22. Reisman S, Rozanski A, Maddahi J, Berman D (1985) Prolonged post exercise ST segment depression in an indicator of hemodynamically severe and extensive coronary artery disease (CAD). JACC 7: 163A (abstr)
23. Schneider RM, Seaworth JF; Dohman ML, et al (1982) Anatomic and prognostic implications of an early positive treadmill exercise test. Am J Cardiol 50: 682—8
24. Weiner DA, McCabe CH, Ryan TJ (1983) Prognostic assessment of patients with coronary artery disease by exercise testing. Am Heart J 105: 749—755
25. Ellestad MH, Wan MKC (1975) Predictive implications of stress testing. Follow up of 2,7000 subjects after maximum treadmill stress testing. Circulation 51: 363—369
26. Hammermeister KE, DeRoven TA, Dodge HT; Zia M (1983) Prognostic and predictive valve of exertional hypotension in suspected coronary heart disease. Am J Cardiol 51: 1261—1266
27. Reisman S, Berman D, Maddahi J, Swan HJC (1985) The severe stress thallium defect: An indicator of critical coronary stenosis. Am Heart J 110: 128—134
28. Gill JB, Ruddy TD, Newell JB, Sexton J, Strauss HW, Boucher CA (1986) Long-term prognostication with exercise thallium imaging. Circulation 74: II-505
29. Maddahi J, Gurewitz T, Bateman T, Staniloff H, Cohen I, Berman D (1986): Prognosis in coronary artery disease: Assessment by quantitative stress-redistribution thallium-201 myocardial scintigraphy. J Am Coll Cardiol 7: 4A (abstr).
30. Gutman J, Berman DS, Freeman M, Rozanski A, Maddahi J, Waxman A, Swan HJC (1983) Time to completed redistribution of thallium-201 in exercise myocardial scintigraphy: Relationship to the degree of coronary artery stenosis. Am Heart J 106: 989—995
31. Weiss T, Berman D, Garcia E, Swan HJC; Waxman A, Maddahi J (1987) Transient ischemic dilatation of the left ventricle on stress-redistribution T1-201 scintigrams: A marker of severe and extensive coronary artery disease. J Am Coll Cardiol (in press)
32. Canhasi B, Dae M, Botrinick E, Lanzer P, Schecthmann N, Faulkner D, O'Connell W, Schiller N (1985) Interaction of „supplementary“ scintigraphic indicators of ischemia and stress electrocardiography in the diagnosis of multivessel coronary disease. JACC 6: 581—588
33. Pryor DB, Harrell FE, Lee KL, Rosati RA, Coleman RE, Cobb FR, Califf RM, Jones RH (1984) Prognostic indicators from radionuclide angiography in medically treated patients with coronary artery disease. Am J Cardiol 53: 22
34. Dewhurst NG, Muir AL (1983) Comparative prognostic value of radionuclide ventriculography at rest and during exercise in 100 patients after first myocardial infarction. Br Heart J 49: 111—121
35. Hung J, Goris ML, Nash E, Kraemer HC, DeBusk RF, Berger WE, Lew H (1984) Comparative value of maximal treadmill testing, exercise thallium myocardial infarction. Am J Cardiol 53: 1221—1227
36. Kottler TS, Work JW, Rozanski A, Berman DS, Diamond GA (1986) Integrated prognostic interpretation of exercise radionuclide angiographic ejection fraction and wall motion. J Nucl Med: 934 (abstr)
37. Maddahi J, Berman DS, Matsuoka DT, Waxman AD, Forrester JS, Swan HJC (1980) Right ventricular ejection fraction during exercise in normal subjects and in coronary artery disease patients: Assessment by multiplegated equilibrium scintigraphy. Circulation 62: 133—140
38. Berger HJ, Johnstone ED, Sands JM, Gottschalk A, Zaret BL (1979) Response of right ventricular ejection fraction of upright bicycle exercise in coronary artery disease. Circulation 60: 1292—300

39. Kimchi A, Rozanski A, Fletcher C, Maddahi J, Swan HJC; Berman D (1982) The time of onset of exercise wall motion abnormalities aids in the prediction of the presence and severity of coronary artery disease. Circulation 66: II-340 (abstr)
40. Rozanski A, Berman DS, Gray R, Diamond G, Raymond M, Prause J, Maddahi J, Swan HJC, Matloff J (1982) Preoperative prediction of reversible myocardial asynergy by postexercise radionuclide ventriculography. New Eng J Med 307: 212—216
41. Brown KIA, Boucher CA, Okada RD, Guiney TE, Newell JB, Strauss HW, Pohost G (1983) Prognostic value of exercise thallium-201 imaging in patients presenting for evaluation of chest pain. JACC 1: 994—1001
42. Gibson RS, Watson DD, Craddock GB, Crampton RS, Kaiser DL, Denny MJ, Beller GA (1983) Prediction of cardiac events after uncomplicated myocardial infarction: a prospective study comparing predischarge exercise thallium-201 scintigraphy and coronary angiography. Circulation 68: 321—336
43. Hakki AH, Iskandrian A, Kane SA (1984) The use of exercise thallium-201 imaging in risk stratification in patients with suspected coronary heart disease. Circulation 70 (Suppl II): 286 (abstr)
44. Rozanski A, Maddahi J, O'Byrne G, Staniloff H, Said N, Berman D (1986) Comparison of the prognostic usefulness of thallium scintigraphy according to the population referred for testing. Clin Nucl Med 11: P17 (abstr)
45. Leppo JA, O'Brien J, Rothendler JA, Getchell JD, Lee VW (1984) Dipyridamole-thallium-201 scintigraphy in the prediction of future cardiac events after acute myocardial infarction. N Eng J Med 310: 1014-8
46. Brody AJ (1959) Master two-step exercise test in clinically unselected patients. J Am Med Assoc 171: 1193—1198
47. Robb GP, Marks HH (1967) Postexercise electrocardiogram in arteriosclerotic heart disease: Its value in diagnosis and prognosis. J Am Med Assoc 200: 110—118
48. Kattus AA (1977) Prevention of heart disease in the normal subject with a positive exercise test. Prim Care 4: 225—28
49. Froelicher VF, Thompson AJ, Longo MR Jr, Triebwasser JH, Lancaster MC (1976) Value of exercise testing for screening asymptomatic men for latent coronary artery disease. Progr Cardiovasc Dis 18: 265—276
50. Aronow WS, Cassidy J (1975) Five year follow up of double master's test, maximal treadmill stress test, and resting and postexercise apexcardiogram in asymptomatic persons. Circulation 52: 616—618
51. Cummings GR, Samm J, Borysyk LK (1975) Electrocardiographic changes during exercise in asymptomatic men: 3 year follow-up. Canad Med J 112: 578—581
52. Allen WH, Aronow WS, Goodman P, Stinson P (1980) Five-year follow-up of maximal treadmill stress test in asymptomatic men and women. Circulation 62: 522-27
53. Bruce RA, DeRouen TA, Hossack KF (1980) Value of maximal exercise tests in risk assessment of primary coronary heart disease events in healthy men: Five years' experience of the Seattle Heart Watch Study. Am J Cardiol 46: 371—378
54. Langou RA, Huang EK, Kelley MJ, Cohen LS (1980) Predictive accuracy of coronary artery calcification and abnormal exercise test for coronary artery disease in asymptomatic men. Circulation 62: 1196—1203
55. MacIntyre NR, Kunkler JR, Mitchell RE, Oberman A, Graybiel A (1981) Eight-year follow-up of exercise electrocardiograms in healthy, middleaged aviators. Aviation, Space and Environmental Med 256—259
56. McHenry PL, O'Donnell J, Morris SN, Jordan JJ (1984) The abnormal exercise electrocardiogram in apparently healthy men: A predictor of angina pectoris as an initial coronary event during long-term follow-up. Circulation 70: 547—551
57. Giagnoni E, Secchi MB, Wu SC, Morabito A, Oltrona L, Mancarella S, Volpin N, Fossa L, Bettazi L, Arangio G, Sachero A, Folli G (1983) Prognostic value of exercise EKG testing in asymptomatic normotensive subjects: A prospective matched study. N Engl J Med 309: 1085—1089
58. Theroux P, Waters DD, Halphen C, DeBaisieux JC, Mizgala HF (1979) Prognostic value of exercise testing soon after myocardial infarction. N Eng J Med 301: 341—345
59. Weiner DA, Ryan TJ, McCabe CH, Luk S, Chaitman BR, Sheffield LH, Tristani FE (1986) The significance of silent myocardial ischemia during exercise testing. Circulation 74: II-502 (abstr)

60. Falcone C, de Servis, Ardiosino A, Foglia MG, Scire A, Specchia G (1986) Significance of exercise-induced silent myocardial ischemia in patients with coronary artery disease. Circulation 74: II-503 (abstr)
61. Fleg JL, Gerstenblith G, Becker LC, Lakatta EG, Weisfeldt ML (1983) Prognostic value of exercise electrocardiography and thallium scintigraphy in asymptomatic subjects. Circulation 68: III-503 (abstr)
62. Reisman S, Ladenhein M, Staniloff H, Rozanski A, Berman DS (1985) Asymptomatic patients with exercise T1-201 hypoperfusion: Identification of a high risk subset. Circulation 72: III-45 (abstr).
63. Bonow RO, Bacharach SL, Green MV, LaFreniere RL, Epstein SE (1986) Prognostic implications of "silent" vs symptomatic ischemia induced by exercise testing in mildly symptomatic patients with coronary artery disease. Circulation 74: II-59 (abstr)
64. Walter GL, Assey AE, Hendrix GH, Usher BW, Carabello BA, Spann JF (1986) Increased incidence of myocardial infarction in patients with exercise-induced silent myocardial ischemia. Circulation 74: II-58 (abstr)
65. Stern S, Tzivoni D (1974) Early detection of silent ischemic heart disease by 24-hour electrocardiographic monitoring of active subjects. Br Heart J 36: 481—486
66. Gottlieb SO, Weisfeldt ML, Duyang P, Mellits ED, Gersternblith G (1986) Silent ischemia as a marker for early unfavorable outcomes in patients with unstable angina. N Eng J Med 314 (19): 1214—9
67. Gottlieb SH, Gerstenblith G, Achuff SC, Mellits ED, Gottlieb SO (1986) Ischemic ST segment changes by ambulatory holter predict one year mortality in high risk post-infarct patients. Circulation 74: II-58 (abstr)
68. Campbell S, Barry J, Rocco MB, Nabel EG, Mead-Walters K, Rebecca GS, Selwyn AP (1986) Features of the exercise test that reflect the activity of ischemic heart disease out of hospital. Circulation 74: 72—80
69. Wackers FJT, Russo D, Clements JP (1985) Prognostic significance of normal quantitative planar thallium-201 stress scintigraphy in patients with chest pain. JACC 6: 27—30
70. Wahl JM, Hakki A, Iskandrian AS (1985) Prognostic implications of normal exercise thallium-201 images. Arch Intern Med 145: 253—256
71. Pamelia FX, Gibson RS, Watson DD, Craddock GB, Sirowatka J, Beller G (1985) Prognosis with chest pain and normal thallium-201 exercise scintigrams. Am J Cardiol 55: 920—926
72. Cecchi AC, Dovellini EV, Marchi F, Pucci P, Santoro GM, Fazzini PF (1983) Silent myocardial ischemia during ambulatory electrocardiographic monitoring in patients with effort angina. J Am Coll Cardiol 1: 934—9
73. Chierichia S, Lazzari M, Freedman B, Brunelli C, Maseri A (1983) Impairment of myocardial perfusion and function during painless myocardial ischemia. J Am Coll Cardiol 1 (3): 924—30
74. Cohn PF (1980) Silent myocardial ischemia in patients with a defective anginal warning system. Am J Cardiol 45: 697—702
75. Droste C, Roskamm H (1983) Experimental pain measurement in patients with asymptomatic myocardial ischemia. J Am Coll Cardio 1(3): 940—5
76. Glazier JJ, Chierchia S, Brown MJU, Maseri A (1986) Importance of generalized defective perception of painful stimuli as a cause of silent myocardial ischemia in chronic stable angina pectoris. Am J Cardiol 58: 667—672
77. Selwyn AP, Deanfield J, Shea M, Jones T (1986) Different pathophysiology of painful and silent myocardial ischemia Circulation 74: II-57 (abstr)
78. Deanfield JE, Selwyn AP, Chierchia S, Maseri A, Ribeiro P, Krikler S, Morgan MM (1983) Myocardial ischemia during daily life in patients with stable angina: Its relation to symptoms and heart rate changes. Lancet II: 753—758
79. Stern S, Gavish A, Weisz G, Benjorin J, Tzivoni D, Holim B (1986) Characteristics of silent and symptomatic myocardial ischemia during every day activity. Circulation 74: II-57 (abstr)

Authors' address:
Alan Rozanski, M.D.
Division of Cardiology
Cedars-Sinai Medical Center
8700 Beverly Boulevard
Los Angeles, California 90048

Regional wall motion disorders during exercise with and without angina

D. Faßbender, J. Vogt, H. Mannebach, U. Gleichmann

Herzzentrum Nordrhein-Westfalen, Kardiologische Klinik, Bad Oeynhausen, FRG

Introduction

Angina is the most frequent subjective symptom of myocardial ischemia in patients with coronary heart disease. During recent years, several studies have revealed that only a part of the ischemic periods are accompanied by angina. Some patients are completely asymptomatic. Others experience numerous asymptomatic episodes with otherwise symptomatic coronary heart disease (2—4).
Since Cohn (3, 4) defined silent myocardial ischemia and established a clinical classification, this clinical variation of coronary heart disease was evaluated using different diagnostic procedures. Previous studies in asymptomatic patients have shown that before the occurrence of angina there is firstly an impairment of diastolic and systolic ventricular function with a drop in dp/dt_{min} and dp/dt_{max} and with prolongation of the isovolumic relaxation time. Secondly there is an increase in left ventricular enddiastolic pressure (LVEDP) which is followed by anginal symptoms (2, 23). However, there are patients who are completely asymptomatic even during severe ischemia (11, 13, 16).
It was the aim of our study to investigate the incidence and extent of exercise-induced wall motion disorders by left ventricular angiography and to correlate it with the occurrence of angina.

Methods

During routine heart catheterization 158 patients with coronary heart disease underwent left ventricular angiography at rest and during supine bicycle exercise. The control group consisted of 17 patients with atypical thoracic complaints and/or slight ECG changes, in whom any significant organic heart disease was excluded by noninvasive and invasive data (11, 13, 14, 16, 20, 22, 25).
Biplane left ventricular angiography (Judkins technique/50 frames/s) was done at rest and — mostly before coronary angiography — during supine bicycle exercise. Work load was 40—140 W over a period of 3 min and depended on previous findings of the severity of angina and exercise capacity in various noninvasive exercise tests.
Angiography and measurement of hemodynamic parameters (heart rate, systolic and enddiastolic left ventricular pressure, cardiac output) during exercise were performed

either at the occurrence of subjective complaints or at the occurrence of one or more of the following parameters: increase of ST segment depression ≥ 0.3 mV, of LVEDP ≥ 40 mm Hg, or of heart rate to more than 110—120 beats/min. Methodological details have been described previously (13, 14, 22, 25). Analysis of left ventricular volumes and assessment of ejection fraction was done according to Dodge and Sandler (7). In a first study of 141 patients wall motion disorders were evaluated by visual criteria and independent assessment of two experienced cardiologists.

In a second study, 17 patients with a proximal isolated stenosis of the left anterior descending artery (LAD) of more than 75% were examined in the same way. In this group wall motion disorders were quantified by a modified radial axes system (Fig. 1) (15, 19, 21). Analysis was done by means of a computerized system (AVD — Siemens Corp.) (18). Excluding the aortic valve region the shortening of 90 radial axes with an angle distance of 4 ° was measured. Every 14% of the radial axes were combined into one region (in the apex area 16% of the axes) resulting in 7 regions in RAO- and LAO-projection (Table 1).

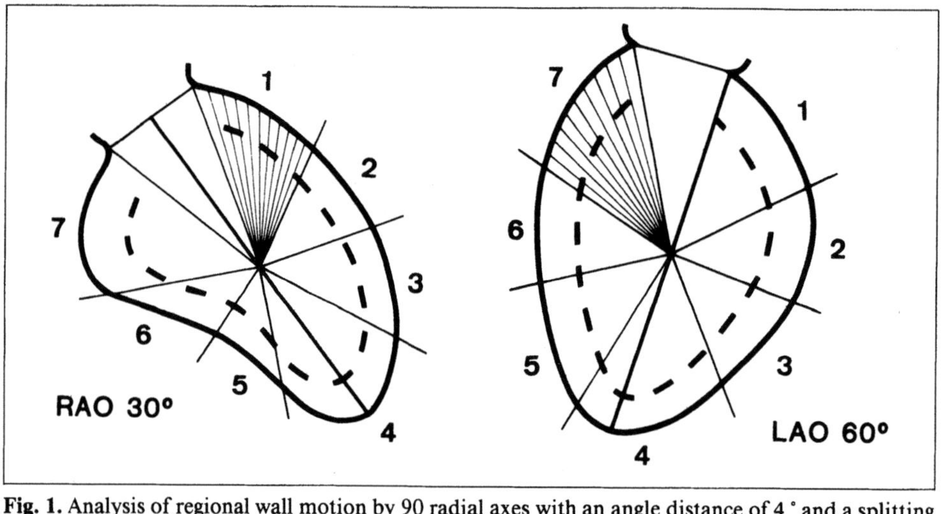

Fig. 1. Analysis of regional wall motion by 90 radial axes with an angle distance of 4 ° and a splitting up of the axes into 7 regions.

Table 1. Anatomical definition of regions in RAO- and LAO-projection.

Region	RAO-Projection	LAO-Projection
1	Anterobasal wall	High posterolat. wall
2	High anterolat. wall	Mid posterolat. wall
3	Low anterolat. wall	Low posterolat. wall
4	Apex	Apex
5	Apical diaphragmatic wall	Apical septum
6	Mid diaphragmatic wall	Mid septum
7	Posterobasal wall	Subvalvular septum

Because of an overprojection of the mitral valve with parts of the posterobasal region (RAO-projection) and the high posterolateral wall (LAO-projection) these regions were excluded from further analysis.
Hypokinetic or akinetic wall motion disorder was defined as mean radial axes shortening of a region, which corresponded to less than the double standard deviation of the normal collective. Patients with scar were investigated with regard to extent of wall motion disorders.

Results

Study 1

During exercise, 35 (25%) of the total group of 141 patients had angina as well as wall motion disorders; 31 (22%) had wall motion disorders without angina: 23 (16%) reported angina without wall motion disorders and 52 (37%) showed neither angina nor wall motion disorders (Table 2).
Out of 141 patients, 66 had already suffered myocardial infarction and accordingly showed a scar in resting angiogram; 75 patients without previous infarction had normal left ventricular function at rest. In both subgroups we investigated the occurrence of angina and wall motion disorders with regard to the extent of coronary heart disease.
Those 75 patients without a scar showed the following results: 14 out of 22 patients with one-vessel-disease had wall motion disorders, but only 3 of them complained of angina. This means that the majority of patients with one-vessel-disease were asymptomatic, although exercise-induced ischemic wall motion disorders had already been observed.

Table 2. Left ventricular angiography during exercise. Incidence of wall motion disorders (WMD +) and angina pectoris (AP +) in 141 patients with coronary heart disease. WMD — = no wall motion disorders; AP — = no angina pectoris.

	all pts $n = 141$	pts without scar $n = 75$	pts with scar $n = 66$
WMD + / AP +	35	17	18
WMD + / AP —	31	22	9
WMD — / AP +	23	16	7
WMD — / AM —	52	20	32

Table 3. Left ventricular angiography during exercise. Incidence of WMD and AP in 75 patients without infarction with 1-, 2-, and 3-vessel-disease (VD). Abbreviations as in Table 2.

	50% st. $n = 23$	1-VD $n = 22$	2-VD $n = 18$	3-VD $n = 12$
WMD + / AP +	1	3	7	6
WMD + / AP —	2	11	6	3
WMD — / AP +	6	5	4	1
WMD — / AP —	14	3	1	2

Out of 18 patients with two-vessel-disease 13 developed wall motion disorders, seven of them being symptomatic. In the group of 12 patients with three-vessel-disease, however, the situation was different. The majority (six out of nine patients) had wall motion disorders accompanied by anginal symptoms, only three showed no complaints (Table 3). In the group of 66 patients with scar a similar correlation between incidence of angina and extent of coronary heart disease could be observed (Table 4). The majority, 16 of 25 patients with one-vessel-disease were asymptomatic and without additional wall motion disorders, as expected. Half of the 22 patients with two-vessel-disease were asymptomatic and without additional wall motion disorders. Out of eight patients with wall motions disorders, five were symptomatic. Out of 17 patients with three-vessel-disease, 14 developed wall motion disorders, only two of them asymptomatic (Table 4).

Table 4. Left ventricular angiography during exercise. Incidence of WMD and AP in 66 patients with scar and 1-, 2-, and 3-vessel-disease. Abbreviations as in Table 2.

	50% st. $n = 2$	1-VD $n = 25$	2-VD $n = 22$	3-VD $n = 17$
WMD + / AP +	–	3	3	12
WMD + / AP –	–	2	5	2
WMD – / AP +	–	4	3	–
WMD – / AP –	2	16	11	3

Table 5. Hemodynamic data of 17 patients without coronary heart disease with normal ventricular function (normals) and of 11 out of 17 patients with significant LAD-stenosis and exercise-induced WMD (5 patients with AP, 6 patients without AP). Abbreviations as in Table 2; EF = ejection fraction.

		17 normals	5 pts with AP	6 pts without AP
exercise (Watt)		64±26	58±8	83±34
rate-pressure-product		15860	16395	18596
LVEDP	rest	10± 3	10±2	8± 4
mm Hg	exercise	19± 6	28±6	27± 9
EF %	rest	76± 6	71±7	70± 5
	exercise	83± 6	64±8	64± 8

Study 2

The investigation of 17 patients without a scar with isolated LAD-stenosis showed 11 patients with wall motion disorders, five of them with and six without angina; four patients had complaints without a significant drop in radial axes shortening. Two patients with a small and relatively short LAD had neither angina nor wall motion disorders. Hemodynamic evaluation showed no significant differences between the symptomatic and asymptomatic group regarding enddiastolic pressure, volumes and ejection fraction (Table 5). In comparison to normals, all patients showed a highly significant drop in radial axes shortening of the LAD-corresponding regions (Table 6). Of five patients with angina 22 regions showed a significant drop in radial axes shortening as did 25 regions of six patients without angina. There was no significant difference in the extent of wall motion disorders during exercise between both subgroups of patients with LAD-stenosis (Table 7).

Figures 2 and 3 give an example of wall motion disorders in a 55-year-old male patient with severe proximal LAD-stenosis during ergometric exercise with 140 W without angina. At rest, contraction is normal; during exercise akinesia of the anterior wall can be

Table 6. Mean regional radial axes shortening during exercise in 17 normals and 11 patients with proximal LAD-stenosis (5 patients with AP and 6 patients without AP with exercise-induced WMD). Abbreviations as in Table 2.

Region		17 normals	5 pts with AP	6 pts without AP
RAO				
Ant. Wall	1	49±17	41±16	28±16*
	2	56±16	39±14*	29±22*
	3	51±15	27±14**	25±21**
Apex	4	39± 6	18± 7**	19± 7*
Inf. Wall	5	49±15	38±11	43± 9
	6	43±11	46±11	44+11
LAO				
Post.-lat. Wall	2	39± 8	29± 8	37± 9
	3	41±11	34±12	44±11
Apex	4	44±11	29±13*	40±15
Septum	5	36± 8	10± 5**	22±13*
	6	56±14	15±17**	17±21**
	7	52±19	19±17*	14±21**

* $p < 0.05$; ** $p < 0.001$ (Comparison to normals)

Table 7. Regional wall motion disorders in 11 patients with proximal LAD-stenosis. Abbreviations as in Table 2.

	5 pts with AP	6 pts without AP	
total amount of regions with WMD	22	25	N.S.
hypokonesia	17	20	N.S.
akinesia	4	4	N.S.
dyskinesia	1	1	N.S.
regions/patient	4.4±1.5	4.2±1.6	N.S.

observed. Ejection fraction decreases from 71% to 57%. LVEDP rises from 6 mm Hg to 22 mm Hg. Mean radial axes shortening decreases from 48% to 6% in RAO-region 2, from 40% to 6% an RAO-region 3, and from 22% to 13% in RAO-region 4; from 37% to 19% in LAO-region 5, from 55% to 25% in LAO-region 6, and from 44% to 24% in LAO-region 7.

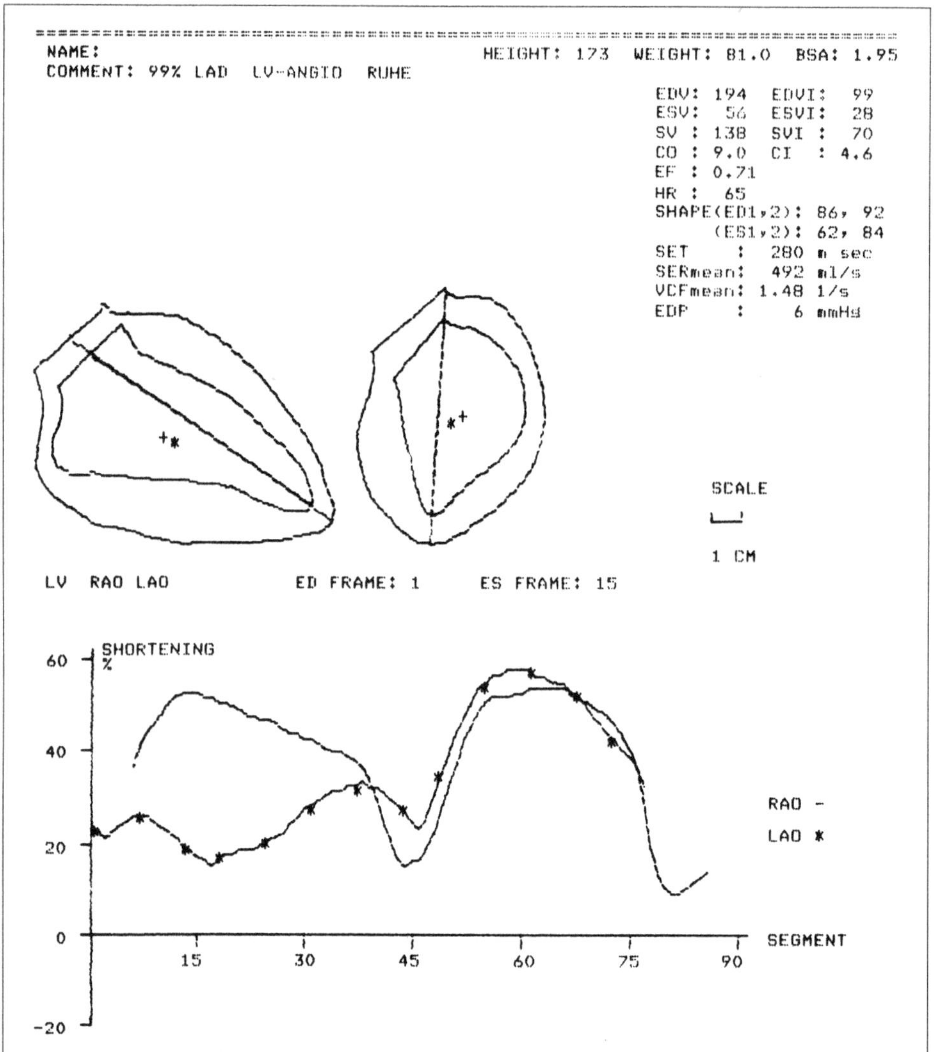

Fig. 2. Computerized analysis of left ventricular wall motion at rest in a 55-year-old male patient with proximal LAD-stenosis.

Discussion

These results show that increasing extent of coronary heart disease (from one- to multiple-vessel-disease) increases the proportion of patients in whom wall motion disorders during exercise are accompanied by angina pectoris. However, about 50% of the patients with

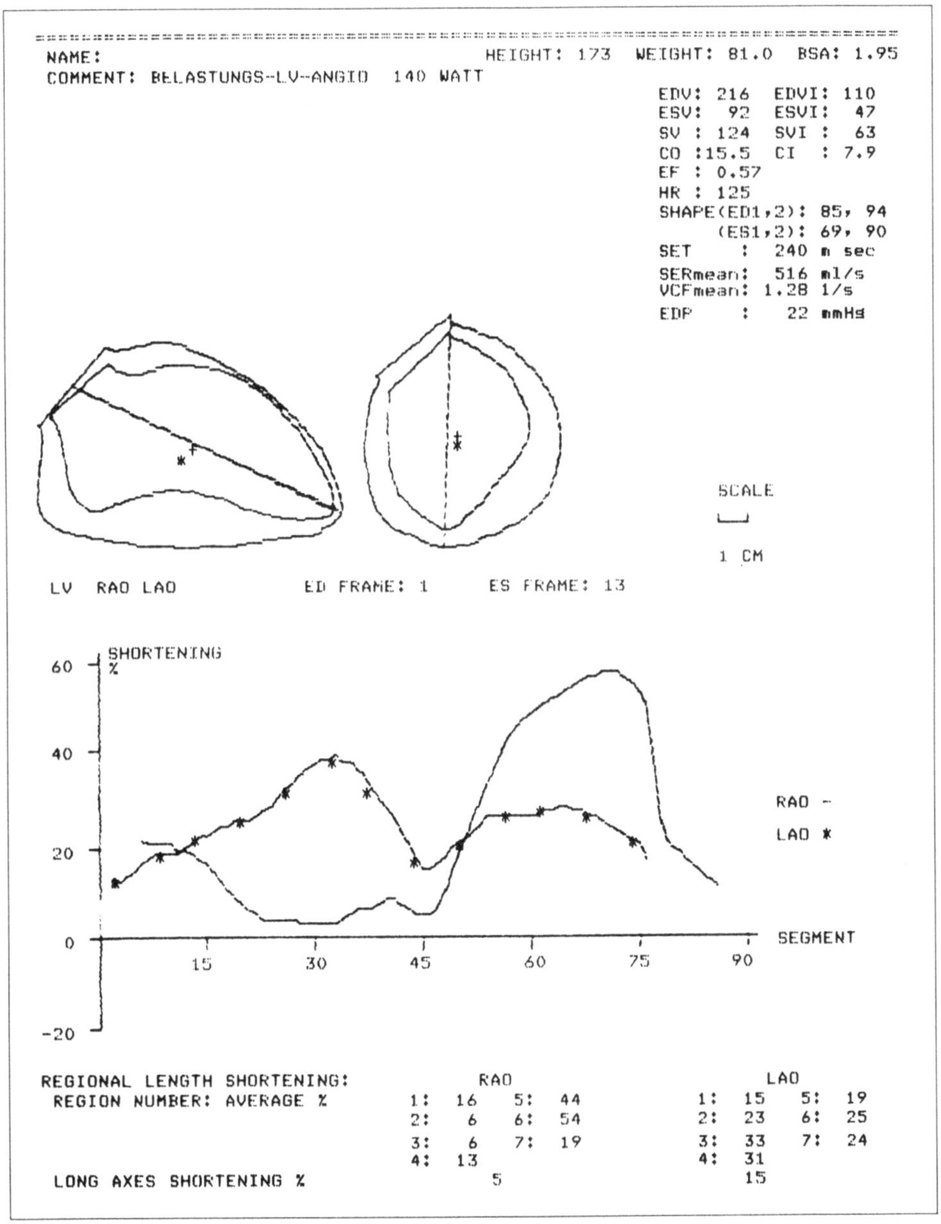

Fig. 3. Computerized analysis of left ventricular wall motion during exercise (140 W).

one-vessel-disease developed wall motion disorders without angina, compared to less than 25% of the patients with three-vessel-disease. A comparison of the hemodynamic data, however, showed no significant difference in heart rate, blood pressure, rate-pressure-product, enddiastolic pressure and drop in ejection fraction during exercise between patients with and without angina.

The group of patients with one-vessel-disease was analyzed with regard to a possible correlation of the occurrence of angina and the extent of ischemic myocardium. In this group, too, which is relatively small but exactly defined as to severity of disease, quantitative analysis of wall motion disorders, by means of radial axes shortening, showed no significant difference in the extent of wall motion disorders between the five patients with wall motion disorders and angina, on the one hand, and six patients with silent myocardial ischemia on the other.

From these results, three questions could not be answered: First: what is the cause of angina in those patients who do not have any corresponding wall motion disorders? Second: what is the reason for silent exercise-induced myocardial ischemia? Third: how should patients with silent myocardial ischemia be treated?

In those patients with angina without corresponding wall motion disorders, the complaints have to be assumed to be a sign of ischemia. This group, too, shows a pathologic increase in enddiastolic pressure, although a localized or general change in contraction cannot be observed. The symptoms are possibly caused by small localized ischemias, which lead to subjective complaints and changes of diastolic function, but do not result in any significant wall motion disorders.

Obviously, the anginal phenomenon does not only depend on hemodynamic changes and the degree of wall motion disorders. It seems to be caused by other mechanisms as well, such as peripheral pain reception, central pain perception, endorphine level and possibly local adenosine concentration (5, 8, 9, 10, 12, 24).

Only 30% to 50% of the patients with first infarction are symptomatic before infarction. Numerous patients with sudden cardiac death never before had cardiac complaints (17, 26). For patients with minor anginal symptoms, randomized studies have not so far shown any superiority of surgical myocardial revascularization with regard to survival rate (1, 6). As it is not yet clear which specific stimuli or special mediators are the originators, both patient groups are treated according to the same principles. This means that asymptomatic patients with significant coronary heart disease, and identification of objective parameters, should be treated the same way as patients with symptomatic ischemia.

References

1. CASS Principal Investigators and their Associates (1983) Coronary artery surgery study (CASS): a randomized trial of coronary artery bypass surgery survival data. Circulation 68: 939—950
2. Chierchia S, Lazzari M, Freedman B, Brunelli C, Maseri A (1983) Impairment of myocardial perfusion and function during painless myocardial ischemia. J Am Coll Cardiol 1: 924—930
3. Cohn PF (1977) Severe asymptomatic coronary artery disease: A diagnostic, prognostic and therapeutic puzzle. Am J Med 62: 565—568
4. Cohn PF (1980) Silent myocardial ischemia in patients with a defective anginal warning system. Am J Cardiol 45: 697—702

5. Cohn PF; Patcha R, Singh S, Vlay SC, Mallis G, Lawson W (1985) Effect of naloxone on exercise tests in patients with symptomatic and silent myocardial ischemia. Clin Res 33: 177 A
6. Detre KM, Takaro T, Hultgren H, Peduzzi P (1985) Long-term mortality and morbidity results of the Veterans Administration randomized trial of coronary artery bypass surgery. Circulation 72 (Suppl V): V—84—89
7. Dodge HT; Sandler H, Ballew DW, Lord JD Jr (1960) The use of biplane angiocardiography for the measurement of left ventricular volume in man. Am Heart J 60: 762—776
8. Droste C, Roskamm H (1983) Experimental pain measurement in patients with asymptomatic myocardial ischemia. J Am Coll Cardiol 1: 940—945
9. Droste C, Roskamm H (1984) Pain measurement and pain modification by naloxone in patients with asymptomatic myocardial ischemia. In: Rutishauser W, Roskamm H (eds) Silent Myocardial Ischemia. Springer, Berlin Heidelberg New York Tokyo, pp 14—23
10. Ellestad MH, Kuan P (1984) Naloxone and asymptomatic ischemia. Failure to induce angina during exercise testing. Am J Cardiol 54: 982—984
11. Faßbender D, Gleichmann U, Mannebach H, Vogt J, Trieb G (1983) Kontrastventrikulographie: Wandbewegungsstörungen ohne Angina pectoris während belastungsinduzierter Ischämie. Z Kardiol 72 (Suppl 2): 73
12. Glazier JJ, Chierchia S, Brown MJ, Maseri A (1986) Importance of generalized defective perception of painful stimuli as a cause of silent myocardial ischemia in chronic stable angina pectoris. Am J Cardiol 58: 667—672
13. Gleichmann U, Trieb G, Sigwart U, Mannebach H, Faßbender D (1982) Methodology of coronary angiography and ventriculography with special reference to exercise. In: Loogen F, Seipel L (eds) Detection of ischemic myocardium with exercise. Springer, Berlin Heidelberg New York, pp 87—97
14. Gleichmann U, Faßbender D, Mannebach H, Vogt J, Trieb G (1984) Contrast ventriculography: Wall motion disorder without angina pectoris during exercise-induced ischemia. In: Rutishauser W, Roskamm H (eds) Silent Myocardial Ischemia. Springer, Berlin Heidelberg New York Tokyo, pp 71—77
15. Heckenberger E, Sigel H, Lippert R (1986) Application of quantitative methods in left ventricular cineangiography: a comparison of 9 models to quantify regional wall motion in patients with coronary artery disease. Z Kardiol 75: 247—255
16. Hirzel HO (1983) Ergometrische Belastung in der invasiven Diagnostik der koronaren Herzkrankheit. Thieme, Stuttgart New York
17. Kannel WB, Abbott R (1984) Incidence and prognosis of unrecognized myocardial infarction: Based on 26 years follow-up in the Framingham Study. In: Rutishauser W, Roskamm H (eds) Silent Myocardial Ischemia. Springer, Berlin Heidelberg New York Tokyo, pp 131—137
18. Mannebach H, Faßbender D, Trieb G, Gleichmann U (1982) AVD: ein neues System zur rechnergestützten Analyse von Wandbewegungsstörungen; erste Erfahrungen. Electromedica 50: 85—89
19. Mathes P, Baxley WA, Neiß A, Kreuz D, Sebening H, Delius W, Blömer H (1979) Ventrikelfunktion nach abgelaufenem Herzinfarkt in Abhängigkeit vom Kontraktionsverhalten des überlebenden Herzmuskels. DMW 104: 175—181
20. Sharma B, Goodwin JF, Raphael MJ, Steiner RE, Rainbow RG, Taylor SH (1976) Left ventricular angiography on exercise: A new method of assessing left ventricular function in ischemic heart disease. Br Heart J 38: 59—70
21. Sigel H, Nechwatal W, Bitter F, Stauch M (1981) Quantitative left ventriculography: comparative investigations in normal patients. Z Kardiol 70: 221—230
22. Sigwart U, Schmidt H, Bonzel T, Mertens HM, Gleichmann U (1975) Biplane cineangiographic evaluation of left ventricular concentration in ischemic heart disease at rest and during bicycle exercise. Circulation 51 (Suppl 11): 11—37
23. Sigwart U, Grbic M, Payot M, Goy JJ, Essinger A, Fischer A (1984) Ischemic events during coronary artery balloon occlusion. In: Rutishauser W, Roskamm H (eds) Silent Myocardial Ischemia. Springer, Berlin Heidelberg New York Tokyo, pp 29—36
24. Sylven C, Beermann B, Jonzon B, Brandt R (1986) Angina pectoris-like pain provoked by intravenous adenosin in healthy volunteers. Br Med J 293: 227—230

25. Trieb G, Sigwart U, Mannebach H, Mertens HM, Gleichmann U (1979) Evaluation of left ventricular dysfunction in coronary heart disease by pressure flow and volume parameter during stress. Z Kardiol 68: 260
26. Weiß B, Donat K, Ziegler WJ (1983) Langzeitbeobachtung nach Herzinfarkt. II. Risikofaktoren, Vorerkrankungen und akut klinischer Verlauf bei Patienten mit überlebtem erstem Herzinfarkt. Herz/Kreislauf 15: 216–221

Authors' address:
Dr. D. Faßbender
Herzzentrum Nordrhein-Westfalen
Kardiologische Klinik
Georgstraße 11
4970 Bad Oeynhausen

Non invasive detection of silent myocardial ischemia with echocardiography

A. Distante

C.N.R., Clinical Physiology Institute, University of Pisa, Pisa, Italy

Limits of traditional markers of myocardial ischemia

In the great majority of cases, the diagnosis of myocardial ischemia can be performed on the basis of clinical and electrocardiographic criteria (11). However, even the most accurate case history, with ECG during the attack, aiming to find out the classical markers of ischemia (i.e., pain and typical ST-segment changes) cannot always reach such a goal. Although ischemia is a difficult task for whatever diagnostic tool, the use of alternative techniques for diagnosing myocardial ischemia serve the purpose of documenting the presence and features of ischemic changes independently of the ECG.
Echocardiography (ECHO) discloses the transient dysfunction typical of myocardial ischemia by means of mechanical markers. Other techniques, providing perfusion, metabolic and hemodynamic parameters, can explore particular aspects of myocardial ischemia but their use, although as ECG independent as ECHO, is highly limited by various factors, such as invasiveness, cost or radiation exposure.

The importance of temporal and spatial resolution

Analogous to ECG, the majority of imaging techniques provide useful information only during the ischemic attack, as the the intercritical period yields few clues, unless a new or old infarction is present or an ischemic attack has left a "stunned myocardium" (1). The transient feature of ischemia therefore requires a "dynamic use" of diagostic techniques since ischemic attacks are characterized both temporally and spatially (they can last only a few seconds and can involve only a very few centimeters). When pathophysiologic answers are required, it is desirable to define the sequence of various parameters altered by the attack: under these circumstances the temporal resolution (of the order of a few ms for ultrasounds) becomes a quality factor of extreme importance as well as spatial resolution (of the order of a few mm for ultrasounds).

Ultrasounds and silent myocardial ischemia

The concept of silent myocardial ischemia is strictly linked to the concept of monitoring techniques. Indeed, when dealing with episodes which are not only transient but also spontaneous, a continuous measurement of appropriate parameters is desirable. In the clinical setting, there are two main ways of documenting mechanical changes induced by ischemia: a) continuous (or semicontinuous) monitoring at the patient's bedside; b) use of stress tests which are to be selective for the mechanism to be studied. In the first instance, the probability can be explored that patients have ischemic attacks in a certain time span, pre-selected according to either historical or ECG (Holter) recordings. In the second instance, clinicians have to use provocative tests which, in the case of primary ischemia, are mainly represented by ergonovine (5), while in secondary ischemia they are mainly represented by dipyridamole (16) and exercise stress testing (2).

Coronary blood flow and regional myocardial function

The relationship between coronary blood flow and systolic wall thickening has been studied both experimentally and in man during cardiac surgery (9). In the anesthetized animal, it has been observed that, at rest, a 20% reduction in subendocardial flow causes a modest reduction in systolic thickening, whereas a clear asynergy occurs if subendocardial flow is reduced up to 80%. In the anesthetized man, the complete occlusion of a coronary branch for 30 s is followed by hypokinesia whereas akinesia seldom occurs. To obtain a kinesia and dyskinesia in man it would probably be necessary to have a more prolonged coronary occlusion, definitely longer than 30 s. Therefore, in resting man, starting from a reduction in coronary flow of at least 80% and reaching the complete coronary occlusion, a continuous spectrum of changes can exist, from hypokinesia to akinesia up to dyskinesia.

The clinical model of Prinzmetal's angina

The first systematic observations of mechanical transient changes induced by myocardial ischemia were obtained in Prinzmetal's angina (3, 4, 7, 17) which represents a particular clinical model of transient coronary occlusion and primary reduction in coronary blood flow (11). More than 100 attacks of Prinzmetal's angina were investigated to explore the relationship between electrocardiographic, mechanical and clinical markers of myocardial ischemia. Studies were performed in one or more of the standard ECHO views during the ischemic attacks, in one or more of the following circumstances: (a) at the appearance of spontaneous ST changes or at the onset of pain in patients under continuous ECG monitoring, with the instrument ready at the bedside, (b) during the ergonovine test with stepwise increments from 0.1 to 0.2 mg i.v. (doubling the dosage every 10 min until ischemia appeared) (5); (c) during ad-hoc bedside monitoring in patients with very frequent ischemic attacks at rest; (d) during hemodynamic monitoring, in a subset of 6 patients (7).
Abnormalities of left ventricular (LV) wall motion both in M-Mode and in 2D were identified according to classically accepted criteria.

M-Mode echocardiographic findings (3)

Ischemic changes occur according to a precise sequence which is quite reproducible in different patients (Table 1). Following the basal condition, there is a phase in which clear-cut reduction in systolic motion and in percentage wall thickening is not accompanied by modifications of ST-segment: this "pre-ECG phase" is almost invariably painless. Mechanical changes occur from 20—140 s before onset of ST changes and before anginal pain. Simultaneous monitoring of ECHO and hemodynamic parameters (7) has shown that the decrease in regional contractility is as early as the decrease in dp/dt, which is considered an early — though global — marker of ischemia. In the next phase both mechanical and ECG changes coexist: this "ECG phase" may or may not be accompanied by pain. At peak ST elevation the LV ischemic wall, when compared to basal state, is found to have a significant reduction in motion (—76 ± 9%) (mean ± SEM), in diastolic thickness (—12 ± 2.5%) and in percentage systolic thickening (—88 ± 6%). An increase in LV end-diastolic diameter (+13 ± 2%) and a decrease in percentage fractional shortening (—38 ± 4%) were also detected at the peak phase of ischemia. The resolution of ischemia ("recovery phase") is characterized, in order, by the disappearance of pain, the return to basal state of mechanical function and of ECG. In a sizeable number of patients with primary ischemia, namely those in whom vasospasm occurs in a coronary artery with a hemodynamically insignificant stenosis, the phenomenon of post-ischemic overshoot has been observed: such a contractile rebound has been proved to be nitrate- and pain-independent and is likely to be due to reactive hyperemia (6) (Figs. 1 and 2).

Two-dimensional echocardiography (4)

This technique is a useful clinical tool and a source of valuable information from diagnostic and pathophysiologic viewpoints. It permits us not only to observe the changes in the involved and contralateral regions, but also the geometric modifications occurring in the heart as a whole, particularly in the LV. At least two of the following transient alter-

Table 1. Time sequence of echocardiographic signs during acute ischemia with ST-segment elevation in man (Prinzmetal's patients).

	Pre ECG phase	ECG phase	Post ECG phase
Electrocardiogram	ST =	ST ↑	ST =
Echocardiogram (M-Mode)			
Wall signs:			
Motion	↓	↓ ↓	↑
End-diastolic thickness	↓	↓	=
End-systolic thickness	↓	↓ ↓	↑
% systolic thickening	↓	↓ ↓	↑
Cavity signs			
End-diastolic diameter	=/ ↑	↑	=/ ↓
End-systolic diameter	↑	↑ ↑	↓
% fractional shortening	↓	↓ ↓	↑
Anginal pain	No	Yes/No	No

Abbreviations: ST = no change; ST ↑ ; ST-segment elevation; ↓ , reduction; ↓ ↓ , marked reduction; ↑ , increase; ↑ ↑ , marked increase; =, no change; No, absent; Yes, present.

From reference 3: reprinted with kind permission of Am Heart Yournal, Mosby Co.

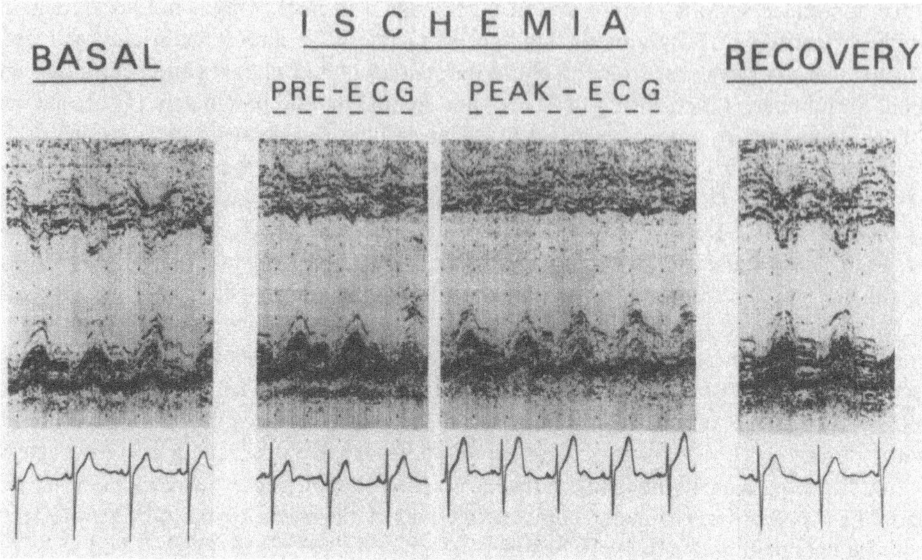

Fig. 1. Selected frames of an original M-Mode tracing documenting the most relevant phases of an ischemic attack induced by ergonovine maleate. The two central "spots" represent, respectively, the pre-ECG and the ECG phase of myocardial ischemia, where it is shown that mechanical markers of ventricular dysfunction precede the clear-cut ECG changes. The sequence of mechanical impairment of septal wall is characterized by a progressive decrease, both in systolic thickening and in wall motion, followed by a contractile overshoot in the recovery phase. (From reference 3; reprinted with kind permission from Am Heart Journal, Mosby Co.)

ations could be observed during ST elevation: (a) a regional asynergy, i.e. hypokinesia, akinesia or dyskinesia; (b) the "step sign" — a sharp demarcation between akinetic/dyskinetic areas and adjacent normal or hypercontractile region; (c) a deformed geometry of the LV, appearing globular in diastole and hour-glass shaped in systole. As with M-Mode, the 2D findings were detected before the onset of pain and clear-cut ST changes. The occurrence of a contractile overshoot after ischemia was also confirmed.

Interpretation of transient minimal T wave changes (17)

In five of Prinzmetal's patients, monitored for a total of 13 h and 20 min, 54 episodes of reversible LV asynergies were detected in association with transient ST elevation (30 episodes) and with transient T wave abnormalities (14 episodes). The latter consisted of peaking (10 episodes), flattening (2 episodes) or diphasic T wave (2 episodes). In each patient, the LV wall showing reversible asynergies was the same both during ST elevation and during T wave changes. The incidence of asymptomatic episodes was higher during T wave abnormalities (9/14 episodes) than during ST elevation (10/30 episodes) ($p < 0.05$). Such abortive attacks of variant angina, very likely linked to an incomplete or short-lasting spasm, might have been easily overlooked if mechanical markers of isch-

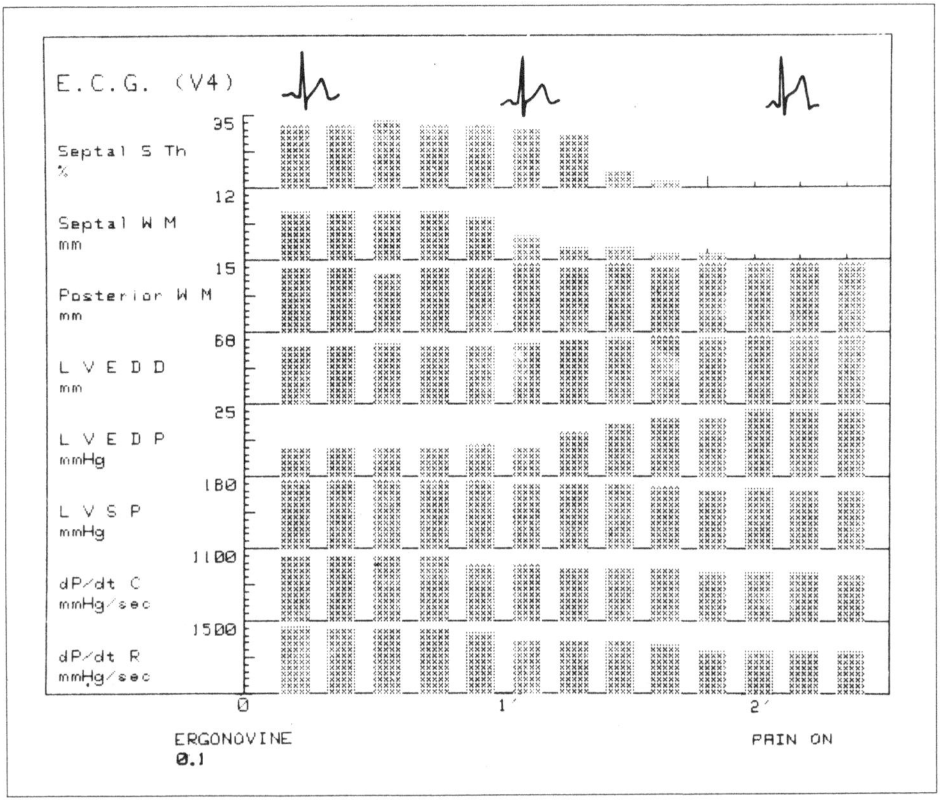

Fig. 2. Computer print-out of an ischemic attack induced by ergonovine maleate during ECHO and hemodynamic monitoring. From top to bottom: ECG, Systolic septal thickening, Septal wall motion, Posterior wall motion, LV end-diastolic pressure, LV systolic pressure, dp/dt of contraction and dp/dt of relaxation. Data have been plotted only up to clear-cut ECG changes (ST elevation) and onset of pain which appeared almost simultaneously. On the contrary, septal wall motion, systolic thickening, dp/dt of contraction and relaxation did change much before, i. e. about 1 min before onset of pain and clear-cut ECG changes.

emia had not been available. The incidence of hypokinesia and akinesia in the two types of ECG changes was statistically different ($p < 0.01$), hypokinesia being present in 1/30 episodes of ST elevation and in 12/14 episodes of T wave changes; on the contrary, akinesia was observed in 25/30 episodes of ST and in 2/14 episodes of T changes. Dyskinesia was detected only with ST elevation (4 episodes). The duration of asynergies accompanying ST elevation (169 ± 83 s) was longer than that accompanying T wave changes (107 ± 76 s) ($p < 0.05$).

Doppler technique

Transient myocardial ischemia with ST elevation has also been studied with Doppler techniques, which permit the measuring of flow velocity in the cardiac cavities and great vessels. The potential for diagnosing ischemia is based on the fact that alterations in diastolic phase (reduced compliance and increased stiffness) can be reflected by changes in transmitral flow. The main changes in flow pattern affect the relationship between the rapid passive phase (E wave) and the late active filling (A wave). Preliminary data in patients with Prinzmetal's angina (12) and in coronary occlusion (obtained by PTCA) (10), have documented that the atrial contribution to ventricular filling increases significantly during ischemia, reverting to basal value in the post-ischemic phase. It is not yet possible to determine whether Doppler parameters of transmitral flow are a real improvement when compared to systolic parameters, such as motion and thickening obtained by classical ECHO: there is, however, agreement on the fact that both modifications precede the ECG changes and, of course, the anginal pain.

The model of subendocardial ischemia (ST depression on ECG)

In subendocardial ischemia ultrasounds may increase specificity and sensitivity of ECG and, more importantly, may localize the site involved. With ST depression, unlike ST elevation, the ECG site of ischemia does not correlate with the anatomical site. The mechanical markers of subendocardial ischemia (hypokinesia, akinesia and dyskinesia, as well as a reduction in systolic percentage thickening) are the same as those for transmural ischemia, which is characterized by ST elevation. It is not possible, however, to directly extend the results obtained in transmural ischemia to subendocardial ischemia: these two models have different behaviours in myocardial perfusion, since in subendocardial ischemia the defect, as shown by radioisotopic techniques, is limited to inner layers. On the other hand, the anecdotal evidence of "proven ischemic changes on ECG" (ST depression) accompanied by hyperkinetic contraction on ECHO has to be further evaluated: in these cases, the mechanical information, although puzzling, is very important. On-going studies with ECHO-stress testing (2) and dipyridamole-ECHO (13—16) testing will clarify the mechanical phenomenon of subendocardial ischemia, and, particularly its relationship to ECG changes, onset of pain and coronary blood flow, thus throwing light on its possibly different pathophysiologic mechanisms.

Discussion and conclusions

The capability of ECHO to detect mechanical signs of myocardial ischemia, independently from ECG and pain and with high spatial and temporal resolution has been well demonstrated. ECHO can help to better evaluate the clinical models of myocardial ischemia and is feasible for a number of reasons: (1) tachycardia or hyperventilation are rarely present, so that both performance and interpretation of findings become possible (this is not always the case with exercise ECHO); (2) the patient is kept quietly in an appropriate position to be monitored from an optimal acoustic window; (3) each patient acts as his own control; (4) the ischemic wall contractility can be simultaneously compared to other, non-ischemic walls.

The proven existence of a pre-ECG phase of ischemia, usually silent, bears some important implications: (a) ECHO-monitoring, when combined with ECG monitoring during the pharmacological tests (ergonovine and dipyridamole for example) permits an early detection of ischemia, thus increasing the safety of the test. In fact, this can be interrupted as soon as the mechanical signs appear, without waiting for ECG changes or even for anginal pain. In addition, mechanical impairment can be detected in the absence of diagnostic ECG changes, increasing the sensitivity of the test (5). (b) In patients with variant angina, minor or atypical T wave changes, although painless, have been shown to be of ischemic nature, on the basis of mechanical changes. The degree of functional impairment, however, appears less severe and chest pain is much less frequent than during episodes of ST elevation (17).

If Holter techniques help to focus on the entity of silent ischemia, ECHO will permit us to demonstrate the phenomenon of "supersilent myocardial ischemia" (i.e., ischemia without electrical or clinical events). In 1980, Maseri (11) stated that "new practical objective criteria (other than ECG changes and pain) for the diagnosis of transient myocardial ischemia are needed. The low sensitivity of the traditional hallmarks of acute transient myocardial ischemia — namely, pain and ST changes — suggests a reconsideration of our set of equations: Pain plus ST changes = ischemia. Pain plus atypical ECG changes or ST changes minus angina = uncertain. Atypical ST changes minus pain = no ischemia".

ECHO criteria, assessing myocardial ischemia on the basis of specific functional changes, introduce another variable in this set of equations, i.e. the mechanical behaviour of LV. The following equations can be, therefore, proposed: Atypical ST changes plus asynergy = ischemia. Pain plus asynergy = ischemia. Atypical ST changes minus pain plus asynergy = ischemia. Being absolutely specific for ischemia, the mechanical marker is the only "stand-alone" criterion, also justifying the equation: Asynergy minus ST changes minus pain = ischemia (the so-called "supersilent ischemia").

However, such statements, although sound from a conceptual viewpoint, should be applied with great caution to the everyday clinical practice since, at present, reliable quantitative criteria for the detection of hypokinesis are missing (B). The risk of overdiagnosis does not exist as to the finding of akinesia and diskinesia. We cannot ignore, anyway, the fact that segmental contraction abnormalities secondary to ischemia can be demonstrated by ECHO, even in the absence of ECG changes and pain; that such a demonstration is clinically useful is beyond question, as Falsetti et al. have pointed out (8).

It is not hard, therefore, to foresee an increasing role of ECHO in the clinical work-up and pathophysiologic characterization of patients with myocardial ischemia, especially considering the great potentiality of ultrasounds to detect silent attacks.

References

1. Braunwald E, Kloner RA (1982) The stunned myocardium: Prolonged, postischemic ventricular dysfunction. Circulation 66: 1146
2. Crawford MH, Amon KW, Vance WS (1983) Exercise 2-dimensional echocardiography. Quantitation of left ventricular performance in patients with sever angina pectoris. Am J Cardiol 51: 1
3. Distante A, Rovai D, Picano E, Moscarelli E, Palombo C, Morales MA, Michelassi C, L'Abbate A (1984) Transient changes in left ventricular mechanics during attacks of Prinzmetal's angina: an M-Mode echocardiographic study. Am Heart J 107: 465—474

4. Distante A, Rovai D, Picano E, Moscarelli E, Morales MA, Palombo C, L'Abbate A (1984) Transient changes in left ventricular mechanics during attacks of Prinzmetal angina: a two-dimensional echocardiographic study. Am Heart J 108: 440—446
5. Distante A, Rovai D, Moscarelli E, Picano E, Morales MA, Palombo C, Sabino F, L'Abbate A (1983) Two-dimensional echocardiography monitoring during ergonovine test: echo-ergo test. Circulation 68: 335
6. Distante A, Picano E, Rovai D, Moscarelli E, Morales MA, Palombo C, L'Abbate A (1983) Post-ischemic contractility overshoot and degree of basal stenosis in coronary artery undergoing spasm: an echocardiographic and angiographic study in Prinzmetal angina. Circulation 68: 256
7. Distante A, Picano E, Moscarelli E, Palombo C, Benassi A, L'Abbate A (1985) Echocardiographic versus hemodynamic monitoring during attacks of variant angina pectoris. Am J Cardiol 55: 1319—1322
8. Falsetti HL, Marcus ML, Kerber RE, Skorton DJ (1981) Quantification of myocardial ischemia and infarction by left ventricular imaging (editorial). Circulation 63: 747
9. Kerber RE, Taylor AL, Hiratzka LR; McPherson DD, Kieso AK (1986) Transient myocardial ischemia: Experimental echocardiographic demonstration and evaluation of myocardial contraction abnormalities. Can J Cardiol (Suppl. A): 136A—141A
10. Labovitz AJ, Lewen M, Kern M, Vandormael M, Habermehl K (1986) Temporal relation of left ventricular systolic and diastolic dysfunction during PTCA. Circulation 74 (Suppl II): 358
11. Maseri A (1980) Pathogenetic mechanisms of angina pectoris: Expanding views. Thomas Lewis Lectures. Br Heart J 43: 648
12. Moscarelli E, Distante A, Rovai D, Lombardi M, Morales MA (1986) Changes in mitral flow induced by transient myocardial ischemia. Circulation 74 (Suppl II): 230
13. Picano E, Distante A, Masini M, Morales MA, Lattanzi F, L'Abbate A (1985) Dipyridamole-Echocardiography test in effort angina pectoris. Am J Cardiol 56: 452—456
14. Picano E, Simonetti I, Masini M, Marzilli M, Lattanzi F, Distante A, De Nes M, L'Abbate A (1986) Transient myocardial dysfunction during pharmacologic vasodilation as an index of reduced coronary reserve: a coronary hemodynamic and echocardiographic study. J Am Coll Cardiol 8: 84—90
15. Picano E, Morales MA, Distante A, Lattanzi F, Moscarelli E, Masini M, L'Abbate A (1986) Dipyridamole-Echocardiography test in angina at rest: non invasive detection of coronary stenosis underlying spasm. Am Heart J 111: 688—692
16. Picano E, Lattanzi F, Masini M, Distante A, L'Abbate A (1986) High dose dipyridamole-echocardiography test in effort angina pectoris. J Am Coll Cardiol 8: 846—854
17. Rovai D, Distante A, Moscarelli E, Picano E, Morales MA, L'Abbate A (1985) Transient myocardial ischemia with minimal electrocardiographic changes: an echocardiographic study in patients with Prinzmetal's angina. Am Heart J 109: 78—82

Author's address:
A. Distante, M.D.
Istituto di Fisiologia Clinica CNR
Universita' di Pisa
Via Savi, 8
56100 Pisa
Italy

Symptomatic versus asymptomatic ischemic episodes during Holter monitoring: patterns of high resolution trend recordings of ST segment and heart rate

E. Hoberg

Medizinische Universitätsklinik III, Universität Heidelberg, West Germany

Introduction

Knowledge about the high incidence of asymptomatic ischemic episodes in patients with coronary artery disease is based on ST segment analysis of Holter recordings (1–4, 10, 11). Most investigators define ST segment elevations and downsloping or horizontal ST segment depressions $\geqslant$ 0.1 mV persisting for at least 30 s (9) or 60 s (4) as ischemic episodes. The detection of such episodes is generally based on visual analysis. But even for experienced operators, visual analysis of the ST segment at 60 or more times normal speed is a potential source of error, especially if the resting ECG is altered. In addition, the determination of onset and offset of the ischemic episodes remains problematic. Gallino et al. (6) reported a computer system which was based on trend recordings of heart rate and QRST parameters with high temporal resolution. This system, however, is not generally available, and its use seems to be time consuming.

By a commercially available trend system it is possible to simultaneously plot heart rate and relative ST segment displacement with high temporal resolution. In this way, the detection and characterization of episodes with ST segment deviations is facilitated. Even short duration episodes of ST segment deviation, such as during coronary angioplasty, can be detected very sensitively (7). Additionally, different patterns of ST segment changes can be defined which may reflect different pathophysiological mechanisms of myocardial ischemia:

1. Episodes with preceding heart rate increase
2. Episodes with a heart increase parallel to the onset of ST segment deviation
3. Episodes without heart rate changes.

The purpose of this study was to use high resolution ST segment/heart rate trend recordings for the determination of the relative frequency of these patterns of ST segment deviation during symptomatic and asymptomatic ischemic episodes in patients with unstable and stable angina pectoris.

Patient population

The study was conducted in 20 consecutive patients with chronic stable angina and in 13 consecutive patients with unstable angina (history of angina pectoris at rest with recent episodes of anginal pain persisting for 15 min or more). All patients had angiographically proven coronary artery disease, i.e. at least one coronary artery obstruction ⩾ 70% (diameter reduction), as assessed by experienced cardiologists. The two study groups did not differ significantly with respect to gender (3 female and 17 males vs 3 females and 10 males), age (56 ± 5 years vs 58 ± 8 years, mean ± 1 SD), or number of coronary vessels obstructed (2.1 ± 0.8 vs 1.9 ± 0.8, mean ± 1 SD).

Holter monitoring

Frequency modulated 24 h Holter monitoring (Oxford Medilog 2-FM) was performed using leads CM5 and CC5. Patients with stable angina were studied out of hospital. Antianginal therapy was limited to sublingual nitrates on demand. Patients with unstable angina were treated with bed-rest, sedatives, and acetyl salicylic acid or heparin. Additional antianginal therapy consisted of a combination of nitrates, calcium channel blockers, and betablockers, if not contraindicated. Patients were asked to keep a detailed diary of their activities and symptoms. Moreover, they were instructed to press the button of the Holter recorder event marker at the onset of anginal pain.

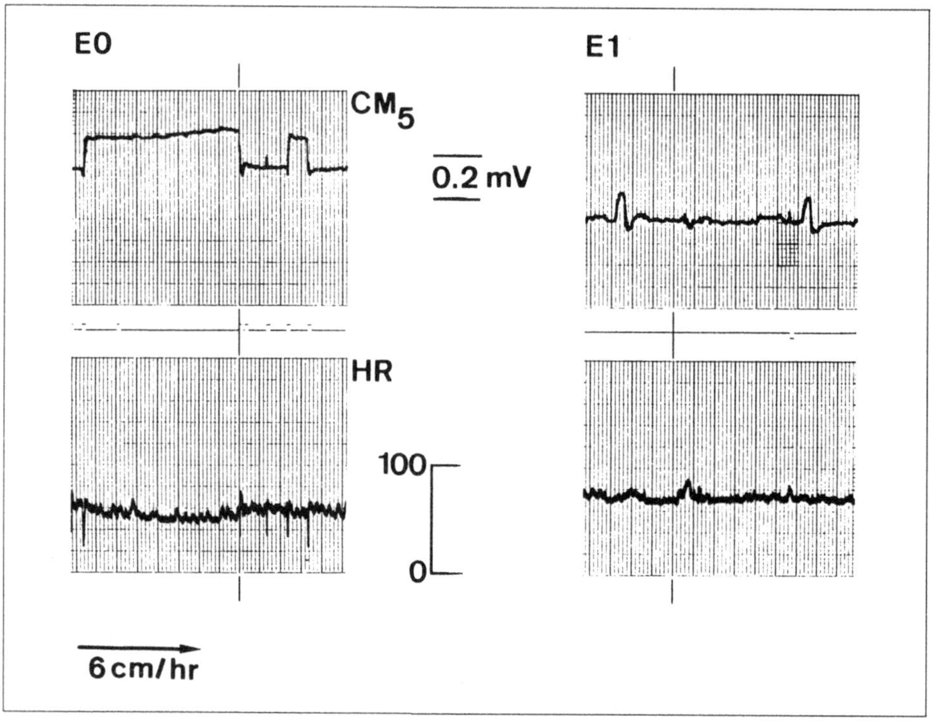

Fig. 1. Patterns of ST segment elevation. EO = abrupt ST segment elevations (⩾ 0.1 mV/15 s), which could be related to postural changes; E1 = episodic ST segment elevations without significant heart rate changes. In the example selected, due to ST depression at baseline, the ST segment crossed the isoelectric line during the 2 episodes of relative ST elevation of 0.14 mV and 0.12 mV, respectively. Episodic ST segment elevations with preceding or concomitant heart rate increases (possible patterns E2 and E3) were not observed.

ST segment analysis

Calibrated tapes (Oxford Z.M-2) were replayed at 60 times normal speed under the visual control of the operator (Oxford PB 4). A reference point within the PQ segment and a point 80 ms after the J point within the ST segment were preselected by the operator at the beginning of the playback. The difference between the two points and the heart rate were averaged over periods of 9 s and simultaneously plotted on a strip chart recorder (Trend System, Reynolds Medical). ST segment elevations resulted in positive deflections, ST segment depressions in negative deflections of the ST trend. 1 cm of vertical deflection corresponded to 0.2 mV of deviation of the ST segment. A paper speed of 6 cm/h was selected for all trend recordings. Ventricular ectopic beats, detected by the Reynolds Pathfinder ECG Analyser, were excluded from ST segment analysis. During each episode with ST segment deviations ⩾ 0.1 mV electrocardiograms were printed out at a paper speed of 25 mm/s for 25 s. ST segment elevations and horizontal or downsloping ST segment depressions ⩾ 0.1 mV, persisting for at least 30 s, were regarded as ischemic episodes. These episodes were classified as follows (Figs. 1 and 2):
EO/DO = Abrupt (⩾ 0.1 mV/15 s) ST segment elevation (E)/depression (D)
E1/D1 = ST segment elevation/depression without significant heart rate increase (⩾ 15%) within 240 s before and 120 s after onset of ST deviation

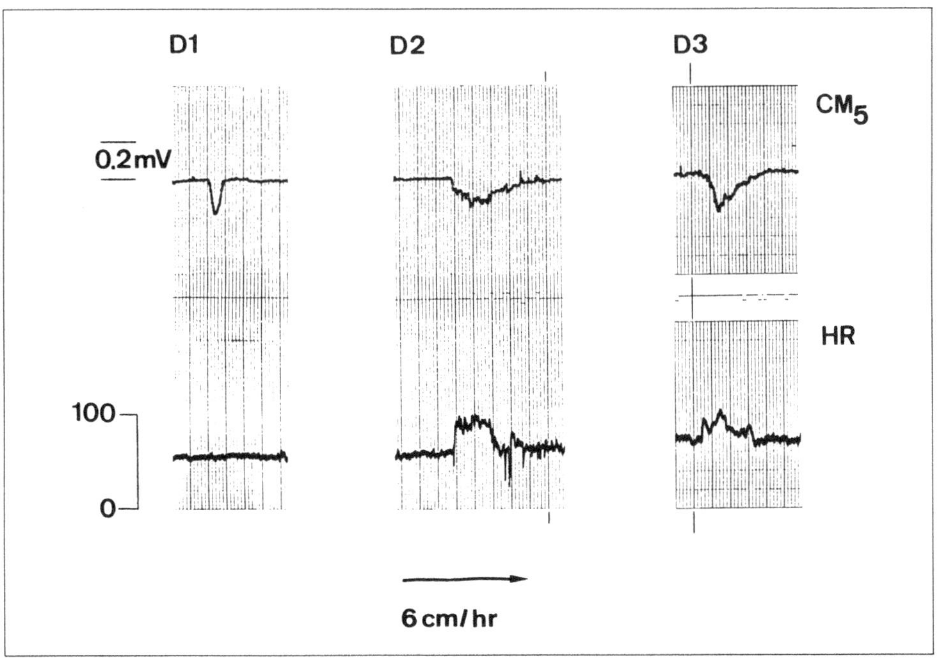

Fig. 2. Patterns of ST segment depression. D1 = ST segment depression without significant change of heart rate; D2 = ST segment depression with an increase in heart rate accompanying the onset of ST depression; D3 = ST segment depression with a rise in heart rate before the onset of ST depression.

E2/D2 = ST segment elevation/depression with significant heart rate increase parallel to ST deviation (within 30 s before to 120 s after onset of ST deviation)
E3/D3 = ST segment elevation/depression with significant heart rate increase before (30—240 s) ST deviation

Results

Ischemic episodes in patients with stable angina

Of the 20 patients with stable angina, 18 developed at least one episode with significant ST segment deviation. In nine patients only asymptomatic episodes were detected and in one patient only symptomatic episodes. Abrupt ST segment elevations (EO) due to postural changes were seen in five patients with stable angina. Such deviations occurred only at night and were always followed by corresponding abrupt deflections to baseline (Fig. 1). Episodic ST segment elevations (E1) were rare: in each of three patients, two such episodes were detected (Fig. 1). Patterns E2 and E3 did not occur.
Of the 122 episodes with horizontal or downsloping ST segment depressions, 99 (81.1%) remained asymptomatic. D2 episodes (heart rate increase parallel to ST depression) were the most common; there was no significant difference, however, in the relative frequency of the three different patterns of ST depression between symptomatic and asymptomatic ischemic episodes (Fig. 3).

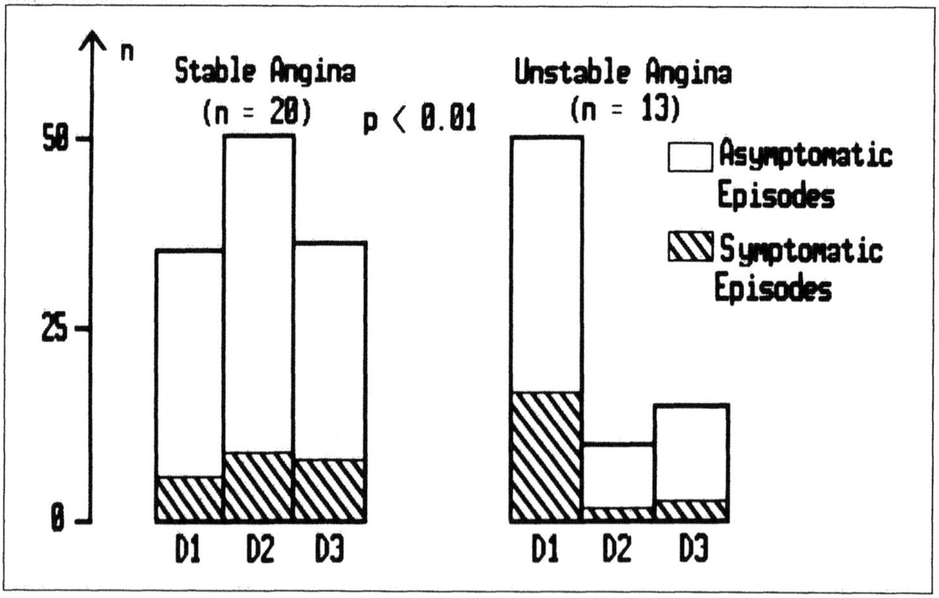

Fig. 3. Incidence of patterns D1, D2, and D3 in 20 patients with stable angina and in 13 patients with unstable angina. The incidence of the patterns did not differ significantly between symptomatic and asymptomatic ischemic episodes, but between patients with stable angina and patients with unstable angina ($p < 0.01$).

Ischemic episodes in patients with unstable angina

In four of the 13 patients with unstable angina, episodes with significant ST segment changes were not detectable. In another four patients, only asymptomatic episodes occurred. Abrupt ST segment elevations (EO) were found in one patient. As in stable angina, episodic ST segment elevations (E1) were very uncommon (one episode only), and patterns E2 and E3 did not occur. Again, the relative frequency of the three patterns of ST depression did not differ significantly between symptomatic and asymptomatic episodes (Fig. 3). The incidence of ST depressions without heart rate changes, however, was significantly higher in patients with unstable angina than in patients with stable angina (Fig. 3). Figure 4 shows a typical example of a patient with unstable angina, who developed ischemic episodes at low heart rates without significant heart rate changes before or during myocardial ischemia.

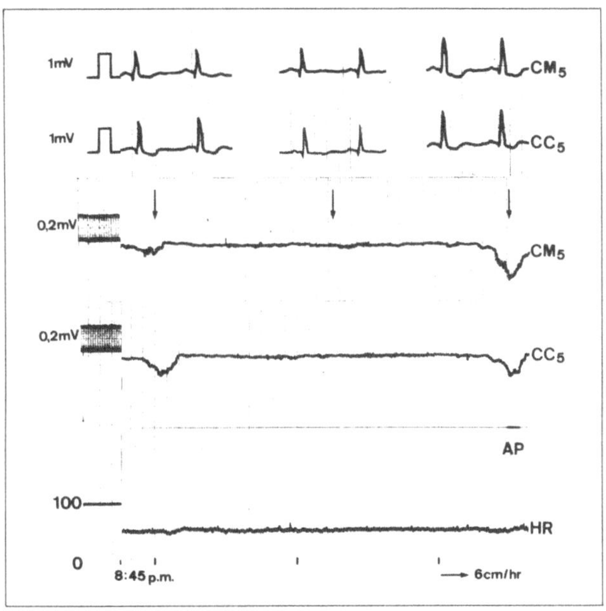

Fig. 4. Trend recordings of the heart rate and leads CM5 and CC5 in a 61-year-old man with 3-vessel coronary artery disease and unstable angina pectoris. At 9 p.m. an episode with descending ST segment depressions mainly in lead CC5 occurred without significant changes in heart rate (first arrow from the left). Similar to this asymptomatic episode a second episode of ST segment depression, without accompanying heart rate changes, was recorded 3 hours later (third arrow from the left). This episode was symptomatic, however. During the time interval between the two episodes the ST segment did not leave the isoelectric line (second arrow from the left).

Conclusions

1. Trend recordings of high temporal resolution offer the possibility of easy characterization of ischemic episodes with respect to accompanying heart rate changes.
2. Ischemic episodes without heart rate changes are more frequent in patients with unstable angina than in patients with stable angina. In this way the view is supported that, in contrast to stable angina, in unstable angina myocardial ischemia may be frequently induced by a spontaneous decrease in oxygen supply (5).

3. As in a previous Holter monitoring study by Quyyumi et al. (9) episodic ST segment elevations were very rare. By the high resolution trend recordings they could be easily differentiated from the more common posture-related ST elevations.
4. Symptomatic and asymptomatic ischemic episodes did not differ with regard to the relative frequency of the three ST segment depression/heart rate patterns. Thus, the extent and severity of ischemia (1, 2, 8), rather than the different pathophysiological mechanisms, seem to influence the occurrence of anginal pain.

References

1. Cecchi AC, Dovellini EV, Marchi F, Pucci P, Santoro GM, Fazzini PF (1983) Silent myocardial ischemia during ambulatory electrocardiographic monitoring in patients with effort angina. J Am Coll Cardiol 1: 934—939
2. Chierchia S, Lazzari M, Freedman SB, Brunelli C, Maseri A (1983) Impairment of myocardial perfusion and function during painless myocardial ischemia. J Am Coll Cardiol 1: 924—930
3. Cocco G, Braun S, Strozzi C, Leishman B, Chu D, Rochat N (1982) Asymptomatic myocardial ischemia in patients with stable and typical angina pectoris. Clin Cardiol 5: 403—408
4. Deanfield JE; Selwyn AP, Chierchia S, Maseri A, Riberio P, Krikler S, Morgan M (1983) Myocardial ischemia during daily life in patients with stable angina: its relation to symptoms and heart rate changes. Lancet 1: 753—758
5. Figueras J, Singh BN, Ganz W, Charuzi Y, Swan HJC (1979). Mechanism of rest and nocturnal angina: observations during continuous hemodynamic and electrocardiographic monitoring. Circulation 59: 955—968
6. Gallino A, Chierchia S, Smith G, Croom M, Morgan M, Marchesi C, Maseri A (1984) Computer System for analysis of ST segment changes on 24 hour Holter monitor tapes: Comparison with other available systems. J Am Coll Cardiol 4: 245—252
7. Hoberg E, Schwarz F (1985) Sensitivity of Holter monitoring for the detection of myocardial ischemia in one vessel disease. Circulation III-162 (abstr)
8. Hoberg E, Voggenreiter U, Schwarz F (1986) ST segment analysis of Holter monitoring: Evidence for more severe myocardial ischemia during symptomatic than during asymptomatic ischemic episodes. Circulation II-401 (abstr)
9. Quyyumi AA, Mockus L, Wright C, Fox KM (1985) Morphology of ambulatory ST segment changes in patients with varying severity of coronary artery disease. Br Heart J 53: 186—193
10. Schang SJ, Pepine CL (1977) Transient asymptomatic ST segment depression during daily activity. Am J Cardiol 39: 396—402
11. Stern S, Tzivoni D (1974) Early detection of silent ischemic heart disease by 24-hour electrocardiographic monitoring of active subjects. Br Heart J 36: 481—486

Author's address:
Dr. E. Hoberg
Medizinische Universitätsklinik III
Bergheimer Str. 58
6900 Heidelberg

Silent ischemia and coronary anatomy

P. Nikutta, D. Hausmann, W. G. Daniel, P. Wenzlaff, C.-A. Hartwig, P. R. Lichtlen

Department of Cardiology, Medical School of Hannover, West Germany

Introduction

During recent years, numerous studies have shown that in patients with coronary artery disease the majority of transient ischemic episodes, as documented by ambulatory electrocardiographic ST-segment monitoring, remain asymptomatic (2, 5, 7, 13, 14, 15). Thus, anginal pain alone has to be regarded as an insufficient parameter for assessing the incidence and duration of myocardial ischemia during daily life (4, 10, 14).
The characteristics of symptomatic and asymptomatic episodes of transient ST depression have been analyzed extensively (2, 5, 7, 14, 15); so far, however, only a few data are available correlating symptomatic and asymptomatic ischemic episodes with the extent and localization of coronary artery disease (9, 11).
Therefore, it was the purpose of the present study to analyze ST-segment changes during Holter monitoring in correlation with the underlying coronary anatomy.

Material and methods

Patients

The study included 101 patients, 84 males and 17 females, with a mean age of 54.7 $\pm$10.0 years (range: 32—74 years), who underwent coronary angiography for diagnostic reasons. All patients had a history of typical or atypical chest pain; 32 patients had suffered from one or more myocardial infarctions (anterior 19, inferior 10, lateral 5). Patients with manifest heart failure, previous coronary bypass surgery, atrioventricular or bundle branch block, atrial fibrillation or ventricular hypertrophy on the resting ECG, as well as patients with valvular heart disease, electrolyte disturbances and those under digitalis or β-blocker treatment were excluded. However, seventy patients treated with nitrates and Ca-antagonists were included; the therapeutic regimen remained unchanged during the complete study period.

Stress testing

Prior to coronary angiography, all patients underwent an exercise test (bicycle ergometry) with stepwise increase in work load up to a maximum, defined by heart rate, sex, age and body length (3). Stress tests were considered positive when ST-segment depression of $\geq$ 0.1 mV in at least two ECG leads was present.

Coronary angiography

All patients underwent diagnostic right and left heart catheterization including biplane left ventricular and selective coronary angiography using the Sones or Judkins technique. Right and left coronary arteries were visualized in multiple projections and stenoses $>$ 70% were considered as significant obstructions (visual estimation).
Minor coronary artery lesions (stenoses $<$ 30%) were found in 13 patients (12.9%). These patients served as a control group (minimal coronary artery disease; group I). In 88 patients (87.1%), significant stenoses in at least one major coronary branch were observed (advanced coronary artery disease; group II).

Holter monitoring

Ambulatory Holter recordings were registered for periods of 24 (61 patients), 48 (12 patients) or 72 consecutive hours (28 patients) using a direct recording system with two bipolar channels (recorder: Reynolds "tracker"; replay unit: "Pathfinder 3"). After preparation of the skin, two reference electrodes were attached to the upper and midright sternal border (at the level of the 2nd and 4th intercostal space). The exploring electrodes were positioned just below and slightly lateral to the apex. The position of the exploring electrodes was occasionally modified on the basis of exercise electrographic findings in order to register a lead optimal for ST-segment changes. Stability of the QRS-complex and ST-segment was verified in supine, left and right lateral and in upright body position. Patients with evidence of a marked postural vector shift were excluded from further analysis.
All patients filled in a detailed record of their daily activities and especially on the occurrence of anginal events. After each recording period, the patient was interviewed by the investigator.
The tapes were scanned visually at 60 times real speed for ST-segment changes occuring. On the screen of the replay unit, 128 s of the recording were displayed continuously. For quantitative measurements, all suspected ST-deviations were printed by a thermoprinter (paper speed of 25 mm/s). Horizontal or downsloping ST depression of $\geq$ 0.1 mV, 80 ms after the J-point, lasting for at least 1 min was considered as representing an ischemic event. For each episode, duration, maximal extent of ST depression and the maximal heart rate during or shortly before the ST depression were determined; heart rate was also measured at the onset of ST depression. Each episode was analyzed with regard to an increase in heart rate of $\geq$ 10 beats per min occurring within an interval from 3 min before onset until maximal ST depression. Symptomatic episodes were defined as significant ST depression accompanied by angina pectoris or its equivalents.

Results

Patients with minimal coronary artery disease (Group I)

Four (30.8%) of the 13 patients with minimal coronary artery disease developed episodes of transient ST depression during Holter monitoring. All of them were females with a positive exercise electrocardiogram. The remaining 9 patients without ST depression had negative exercise tests. Episodes of transient ST depression were significantly less frequent (7 episodes in 4 patients; 3 episodes associated with chest pain) in this group than in group II. In addition, the mean duration per episode (7.1 $\pm$ 4.9 min) and the mean duration of ST-segment depression per day (12.4 $\pm$ 15.4 min) were shorter than in group II ($p < 0.05$).

Patients with advanced coronary artery disease (Group II)

Coronary angiography

Of the 88 patients with stenoses > 70%, 39 (44.3%) had single vessel disease, 26 patients (29.5%) had double vessel disease and in 17 patients (19.3%) triple vessel disease was present. Six patients (6.8%) showed an isolated high-grade left main stem stenosis. From the 32 patients with prior myocardial infarction, 17 showed regional akinesia and 15 hypokinesia in the left ventricular angiogram.

ST-segment analysis

In the 88 patients with significant coronary lesions, Holter ECGs were recorded over a total period of 156 days. Sixty-four patients (72.7%) developed transient episodes of ST-depression $\geq$ 0.1 mV lasting for at least 1 min; a total number of 494 ischemic episodes was recorded with an average duration of 13.2 $\pm$ 14.4 min (range 1—90 min); 447 (90.5%) of these episodes were preceded by an increase in heart rate of at least 10 beats/min. No episodes of ST elevation were recorded. All 64 patients had positive exercise electrocardiograms; in the remaining 24 patients without episodes of ST depression on Holter monitoring, exercise tests were positive in 11 cases and negative in 13.
In the 64 patients with a positive stress test and episodes of ST depression during Holter monitoring, the maximal heart rate reached during the 24 hour recording period was significantly higher (125 $\pm$ 16 beats/min) than in the 11 patients with a positive stress test but without episodes of transient ST depression (112 $\pm$ 16 beats/min; $p < 0.05$).
The number of patients showing ischemic episodes on Holter monitoring was lowest in the group with single vessel disease (20 of 39 patients; 51.3%) and increased to 80.8% in double vessel disease (21 of 26 patients), whereas all patients with triple vessel disease (17 patients) and left main stem stenosis (6 patients) had episodes of transient ST depression (Table 1).

Table 1. Incidence of ischemic episodes documented by continuous ST-segment monitoring in patients with significant coronary artery disease (stenoses > 70%).

	1-vessel	2-vessel	3-vessel	LMCA
no. of pts	39	26	17	6
no. of pts without episodes of ST dep	19	5	0	0
no. of pts with episodes of ST dep	20 (51.3%)	21 (80.8%)	17 (100%)	6 (100%)
no. of recorded days in pts with episodes of ST dep	36	44	35	10
no. of pts with exclusively asymptomatic episodes	17 (85.0%)	11 (52.4%)	3 (17.6%)	1 (16.7%)
no. of pts with exclusively symptomatic episodes	0 (0%)	0 (0%)	1 (5.9%)	4 (66.7%)
total no. of episodes of ST dep	114	196	162	22
total no. of silent episodes of ST dep	104 (91.2%)	153 (78.1%)	119 (73.5%)	6 (27.3%)

1-, 2-, 3-vessel disease = single, double, triple vessel disease, respectively (stenoses > 70%); LMCA = isolated left main stem stenosis > 70%; pts = patients; ST dep = ST depression

Extent of coronary artery disease in patients with documented episodes of transient ST depression

The results of ST-segment analysis in the 64 patients with advanced coronary artery disease and transient ST depression on Holter monitoring are listed in Tables 1 and 2, with regard to single, double and triple vessel disease and left main stem stenosis.
The relative number of completely asymptomatic patients during the recording period declined as the number of diseased vessels increased (Fig. 1). Thus, less than 20% of the patients with episodes of ST depression and triple vessel disease or left main stem stenosis were completely asymptomatic during Holter monitoring; in contrast, more than 80% of the patients with single vessel disease had only asymptomatic episodes. On the other hand, none of the patients with single and double vessel disease had exclusively symptomatic episodes, whereas 4 of the 6 patients with left main stem stenosis had only symptomatic episodes. The percentage of silent episodes decreased with the number of vessels involved (Table 1).
Patients with double and triple vessel disease showed the highest incidence of ischemic episodes per day (Table 2). The lowest incidence was observed in left main stem stenosis, however, the majority of these episodes were symptomatic.
The mean duration of transient ST-segment depression per episode and per day was not significantly different in patients with single, double or triple vessel disease, but was significantly shorter in patients with left main stem stenosis (Table 2). Almost identical mean values in all four subgroups were found for the maximum ST depression, the heart rate at the onset of ST depression and the maximal heart rate during the episode.

Table 2. Incidence and morphology of ischemic episodes in patients with significant coronary artery disease (stenoses > 70%) and documented episodes of ST depression during ST-segment monitoring.

	1-vessel	2-vessel	3-vessel	LMCA
no. of pts with episodes of ST dep	20	21	17	6
no. of episodes of ST dep per day*	3.2±2.3	4.5±3.1	4.6±2.6	2.2±1.5
(range)	(1–9)	(1–13)	(1–11)	(1–5)
duration of ST dep per episode* (min)	13.5±13.9	14.1±14.5	13.1±15.1	8.5±4.5
(range)	(1–88)	(1–81)	(1–90)	(2–25)
total duration of ST dep per day* (min)	42.8±40.8	62.8±78.9	60.6±65.7	18.6±13.9
(range)	(2–136)	(3–241)	(2–328)	(3–39)
max. ST dep* (mV)	0.21±0.07	0.23±0.09	0.23±0.09	0.20±0.06
(range)	(0.1–0.42)	(0.1–0.49)	(0.1–0.46)	(0.1–0.25)
max HR* (1/min)	112±15	111±22	113±18	113±14
HR at the onset of ST dep* (1/min)	99±11	97±14	98±11	96±14

1-, 2-, 3-vessel disease = single, double, triple vessel disease, respectively (stenoses > 70%); LMCA = isolated left main stem stenosis > 70%; pts = patients; ST dep = depression; HR = heart rate; max. = maximal; * = mean value ± standard deviation

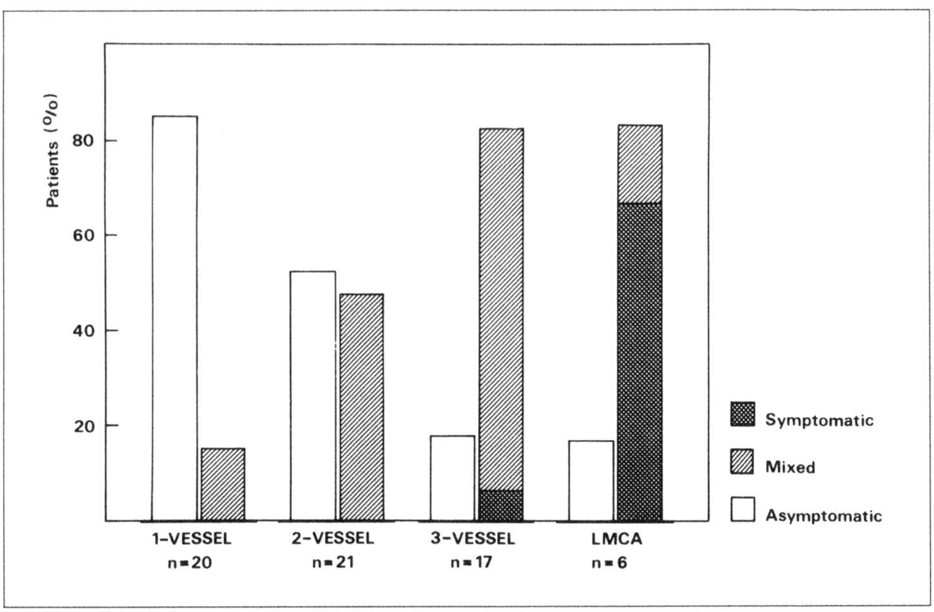

Fig. 1. Patients with exclusively asymptomatic, mixed (asymptomatic and symptomatic) or exclusively symptomatic episodes of ST depression during the recording period in single, double, triple vessel disease (1-, 2-, 3-vessel; stenoses > 70%) and isolated left main stem stenosis > 70% (LMCA).

Fig. 2. Total duration of transient ST depression per day in patients with single, double, triple vessel disease (1-, 2-, 3-vessel stenoses > 70%) and isolated left main stem stenosis > 70% (LMCA).

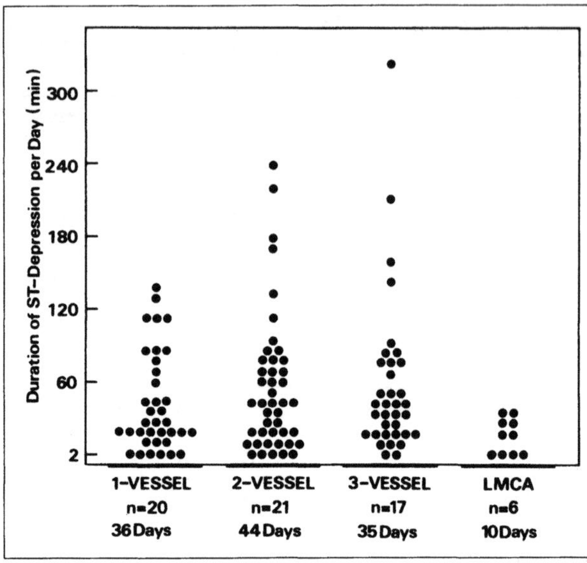

When comparing the distribution of values in patients with different extents of coronary atherosclerosis, considerable overlap was observed with regard to the duration of ST-segment depression per day (Fig. 2). Similar results were found for all parameters listed in Table 2. Furthermore, a combination of various parameters did not allow a clear differentiation between the subgroups.

Transient ST-segment depression in patients with single vessel disease

As indicated in Table 3, the number of patients with single vessel disease and documented ischemia on Holter monitoring was highest in patients with an isolated stenosis of the

Table 3. Incidence of ischemic episodes during continuous ST monitoring in patients with isolated LAD, CX and RCA stenoses > 70%.

	LAD	CX	RCA
no. of pts	23	8	8
no. of pts with episodes of ST dep	16 (69.7%)	2 (25%)	2 (25%)
no. of recorded days in pts with episodes of ST dep	24	6	6
total no. of episodes of ST dep	82	14	18
total no. of silent episodes of ST dep	74 (90.2%)	14 (100%)	16 (88.9%)
mean no. of episodes of ST dep per day*	3.4±2.7	2.3±0.6	3.0±1.2

LAD = left anterior descending artery; CX = circumflex coronary artery; RCA = right coronary artery; pts = patients; ST dep = ST depression; * = ± standard deviation left anterior descending coronary artery (LAD) (16 of 23 patients; 69.6%); only in 25% of the patients with a stenosis of the circumflex or right coronary artery transient ischemic episodes could be detected during the recording period. The episodes were predominantly silent regardless of the localization of the stenosis.

Importance of LAD involvement for the incidence of transient ST-segment depression in single and double vessel disease

Almost 70% of the patients with isolated high-grade LAD stenoses developed episodes of ST-segment depression during Holter monitoring. Of the 26 patients with double vessel disease the LAD was involved in 21 cases; in 18 of these patients (85.7%) ischemic episodes could be detected (Table 4). Altogether, LAD stenoses of > 70% were present in 34 of the 41 patients (82.9%) with single or double vessel disease and documented episodes of ST-segment depression during the recording period; in contrast, only 10 of the 24 coronary patients (41.7%) without ischemic episodes had a marked stenosis of the LAD ($p < 0.001$).

Table 4. LAD involvement and frequency of documented ischemic episodes during ST-segment monitoring in patients with single and double vessel disease.

ST depression		present	absent
no. of pts with LAD involvement	1-vessel	16	7
	2-vessel	18	3
	total*	34 (82.9)	10 (41.7%)
no. of pts without LAD involvement	1-vessel	4	12
	2-vessel	3	2
	total*	7 (17.1%)	14 (58.3%)
	total	41 (100%)	24 (100%)

1-, 2-vessel = single, double vessel disease, respectively (stenoses > 70%); LAD = left descending coronary artery; pts = patients. * = Chi square = 15.95; $p < 0.001$

Summary and Comments

1. ST depression provoked by stress tests or observed during Holter monitoring suggests ischemia without indicating its cause, which can be anatomical (high-grade fixed obstruction) or functional (increase of vasomotor tone) (12). However, in the presence of minimal coronary artery disease, ST depression is also occasionally documented (1, 6, 9, 11); 4 of our patients with positive exercise tests and documented episodes of transient ST depression during Holter ECG had only minimal stenoses of < 30%. Patients with ST-segment depression should undergo further evaluation by coronary angiography.
2. A comparison of the incidence and morphology of ischemic episodes in patients with single, double or triple vessel disease clearly shows that it is not possible to predict the extent of coronary atherosclerosis on the basis of Holter findings.

3. However, the percentage of patients with ischemic episodes during 24 h ST-segment recording increases with the number of severely diseased coronary arteries (11). This might be explained by an increased probability of detecting ST-segment depression by the Holter technique in patients with a larger amount of myocardium at risk of developing ischemia (as in patients with triple vessel disease).
4. Most episodes of ST depression remain silent in patients with single and multiple vessel disease. Patients with multiple vessel disease, however, have relatively more symptomatic episodes and less totally asymptomatic periods than patients with single vessel disease.
5. Patients with left main stem stenosis have a high incidence of symptomatic episodes of ST depression; the overall incidence of ischemic episodes, however, was relatively low in our corresponding subgroup of patients. This might be explained by the phenomenon that a low angina threshold usually reduces the amount and duration of physical activity (8).
6. The observation of a high incidence of ischemic episodes in patients with high-grade LAD stenoses might be partly due to a more sensitive recording over the anterior myocardium compared to the inferior wall. The large area of myocardium usually jeopardized by LAD stenoses might equally be contributing.

References

1. Armstrong WF, Jordan JW, Morris SN, McHenry PL (1982) Prevalence and magnitude of S-T segment and T wave abnormalities in normal men during continuous ambulatory electrocardiography. Am J Cardiol 49: 1638—1642
2. von Arnim T, Höfling B, Schreiber M (1985) Characteristics of episodes of ST elevation or ST depression during ambulatory monitoring in patients subsequently undergoing coronary angiography. Br Heart J 54: 484—488
3. Bühlmann A (1951) Oxymetrie, Arbeitsversuche und Bestimmung der Arbeitsfähigkeit. Schweiz Med Wschr 16: 374—376
4. Campbell S, Barry J, Rocco MB, Nabel EG, Mead-Walters K, Rebecca GS, Selwyn AP (1986) Features of the exercise test that reflect the activity of ischemic heart disease out of the hospital. Circulation 74: 72—80
5. Cecchi AC, Dovellini EV, Marchi F, Pucci P, Santoro GM, Fazzini PF (1983) Silent myocardial ischemia during ambulatory electrocardiographic monitoring in patients with effort angina. J Am Coll Cardiol 1: 934—939
6. Crawford MH, Mendoza CA, O'Rourke RA, White DH, Boucher CA, Gorwit J (1978) Limitations of continuous ambulatory electrocardiogram monitoring for detecting coronary artery disease. Ann Int Med 89: 1—5
7. Deanfield JE, Selwyn AP, Chierchia S, Maseri A, Ribeiro P, Krikler S (1983) Myocardial ischemia during daily life in patients with stable angina: its relation to symptoms and heart rate changes. Lancet II: 753—758
8. Hausmann D, Nikutta P, Hartwig C-A, Daniel WG, Lichtlen PR (1987) ST-Streckenanalyse im 24-Stunden Langzeit-EKG bei Patienten mit stabiler Angina pectoris und angiographisch nachgewiesener Koronarsklerose. Z Kardiol (in press)
9. Kunkes SH, Pichard AD, Smith Jr H, Gorlin R, Herman MV, Kupersmith J (1980) Silent ST segment deviations and extent of coronary artery disease. Am Heart J 100: 813—819

10. Quyyumi AA, Wright CM, Mockus LJ, Fox KM (1985) How important is a history of chest pain in determining the degree of ischemia in patients with angina pectoris? Br Heart J 54: 22—26
11. Quyyumi AA, Mockus L, Wright C, Fox KM (1985) Morphology of ambulatory ST segment changes in patients with varying severity of coronary artery disease: investigation of the frequency of nocturnal ischemia and coronary spasm. Br Heart J 53: 186—193
12. Rafflenbeul W, Lichtlen PR (1982) Zum Konzept der „dynamischen Koronarstenose". Z Kardiol 71: 439—444
13. Schang SJ, Pepine CJ (1977) Transient asymptomatic S-T segment depression during daily activity. Am J Cardiol 39: 396—402
14. Shea MJ, Deanfield JE, Wilson R, DeLandsheere C, Jones T, Selwyn AP (1985) Transient ischemia in angina pectoris: frequent silent events with everyday activities. Am J Cardiol 56: 34E—38E
15. Tzivoni D, Gavish A, Benhorin J, Keren A, Stern S (1986) Myocardial ischemia during daily activities and stress. Am J Cardiol 58: 47B-50B

Authors' address:
Dr. P. Nikutta
Department of Cardiology
Medical School of Hannover
Konstanty-Gutschow-Str. 8
3000 Hannover 61
West Germany

Dedicated ST-segment monitoring in the CCU after successful coronary angioplasty: incidence and prognosis of silent and symptomatic ischemia

M. W. Krucoff, J. E. Pope, R. K. Bottner, I. M. Adams,
G. S. Wagner, and K. M. Kent

Georgetown University Medical Center, Washington DC., Bowman Gray School of Medicine, Winston-Salem, NC., Duke University Hospital, Durham, NC.

Introduction

Following successful coronary angioplasty (PTCA) patients are usually taken to the Coronary Care Unit (CCU) for intensive monitoring, which, in most institutions, consists of arrhythmia monitoring and close clinical observation for angina. In patients with known coronary artery disease, however, transient ischemic episodes (TIE) may occur in the absence of arrhythmias or anginal symptoms (1—5, 11—13).
Successful PTCA disrupts intimal tissue, creating a potentially unstable state susceptible to spasm and thrombosis (14). In one study, electrocardiographically detectable silent and symptomatic TIE were associated with poorer prognosis amongs patients with unstable angina resistant to medical therapy (6). Since the incidence and significance of TIE immediately following successful PTCA has not previously been explored, we performed continuous ST-segment monitoring in our patients after PTCA.

Methods

Patients included in this study were consecutively undergoing elective coronary angioplasty. Exclusions included: total coronary occlusion; acute MI; bundle branch block or ventricular pacemaker. PTCA was performed in the standard manner for our institution, including antiplatelet therapy and either a calcium channel blocker or a beta blocker. Heparin was continued for 24 h in patients with severe intimal dissections. „Successful“ PTCA was defined as a $> 20\%$ reduction of the original stenosis to a residual stenosis of $< 50\%$ when averaged over two angiographic views.
All patients were monitored with a precalibrated 3-channel Holter monitor (Scole Engineering) for continuous recording during, and 18—24 h after, PTCA. This system has been previously validated for low frequency response and phase shift through the entire record/playback loop (8, 9) when paired with the Marquette 8000 Holter playback computer. This playback computer was then interfaced to a DEC PDP 11/34 mainframe for variable playback resolution from every 10 min to every 10 s of ST data. Bipolar lead

configurations addressed true anterior (V2), inferolateral (V5), and true inferior (AVF) bipolar vectors. Radiolucent electrodes (Quinton) were used to avoid interfering with fluoroscopy during PTCA.

During the latter part of this study, patients were additionally monitored with a portable programmable computer assisted real-time 12-lead electrocardiograph (Mortara EL-I). This device acquires and analyses standard 12-lead ECG in real time, comparing them to a previously acquired template ECG every 30 s. ECG's are stored digitally in the fashion standard to recently built ECG carts, and can be downloaded to floppy discs, then decompresed on a mainframe for more detailed analysis. Graphic representation of ST changes over time in all 12 leads may be visually inspected in multiple rotations (Fig. 1).

ST criteria for a TIE were taken as: ≥ 1.0 mm flat or downsloping ST depression lasting more than 60 s or ≥ 1.0 mm ST elevation lasting more than 60 s. TIE were taken as „new" when separated by more than 30 min between offset and subsequent onset. All patients were at full bedrest during the entire recording period.

The presence or absence of TIE's was correlated to the following clinical endpoints over the first 24 h: angina (defined as any symptoms leading to the urgent administration of an antianginal agent) and myocardial infarction (defined as elevation of CPK-MB isoenzymes).

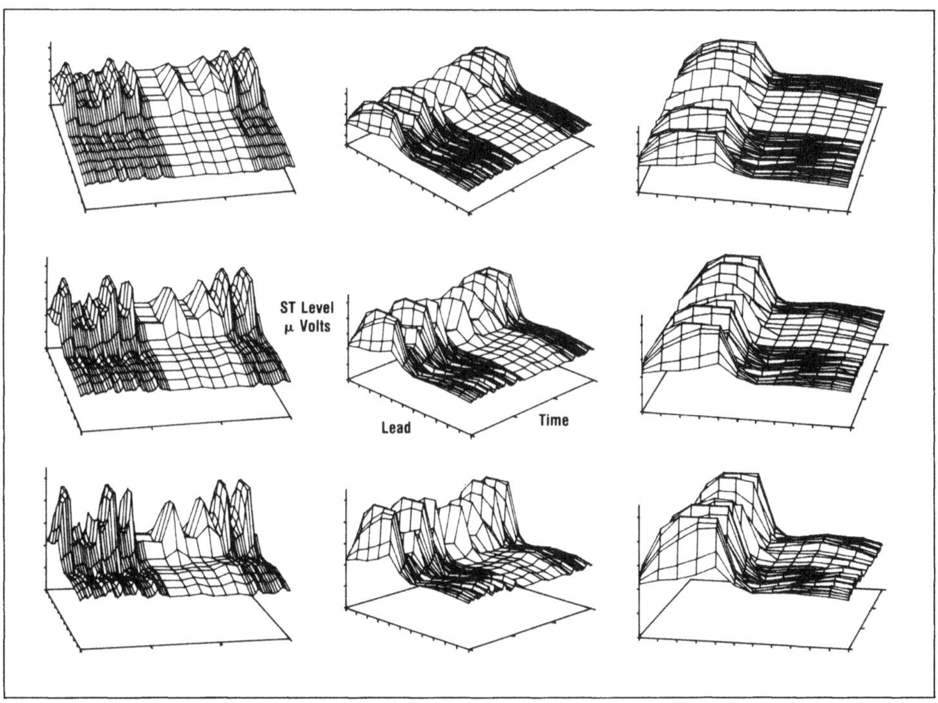

Fig. 1. Multiple rotations from one patient during PTCA of output from bedside monitor (Mortara EL-I) showing ST deviations in all 12 standard leads over time. As illustrated in center, y-axis shows ST level, x-axis shows 12 standard leads, and z-axis shows time (min). More detail on this patient in Fig. 2.

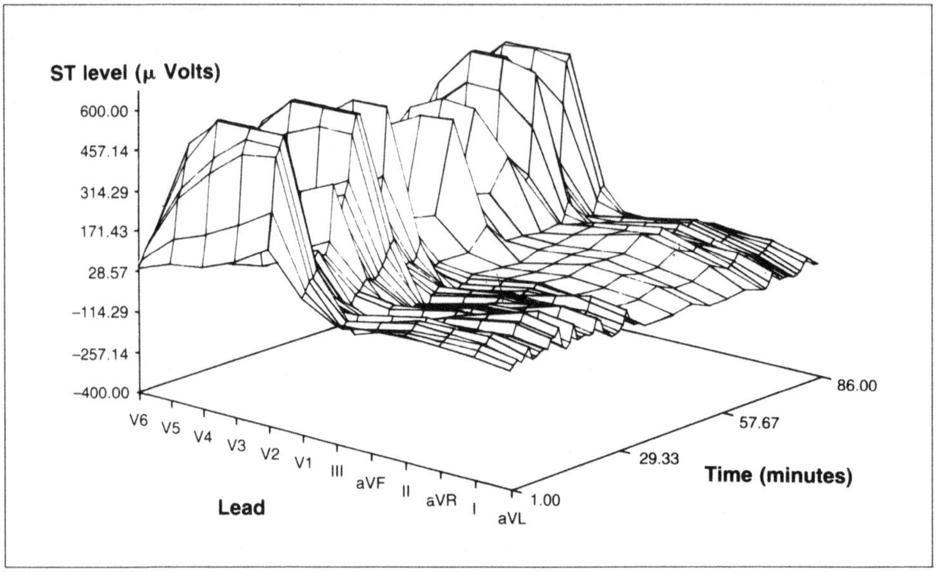

Fig. 2a

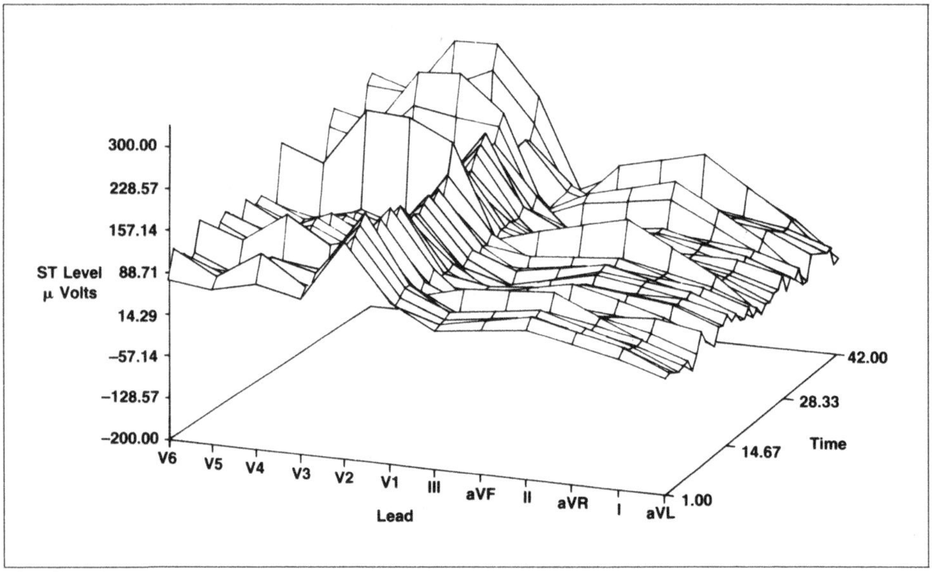

Fig. 2b

Fig. 2. (A) Detail of one rotation from patient shown in Fig. 1 during multiple transient LAD occlusions during angioplasty. ST elevation in anterior leads with reciprocal ST depression in inferior leads is highly reproducible over 7 dilatations. (B) Same patient during 3 episodes of angina preceded by ST elevation in CCU. Geographic distribution of injury current and reciprocal changes are almost identical to controlled occlusions in A, suggesting intermittent closure of the PTCA site.

Results

A total of 3940 h of continuous monitoring were completed in 200 patients after successful PTCA. Of these 200 patients, mean age was 54 years; 21 were females, 179 males; 78 had some angiographically visible collaterals prior to the procedure; 89 had some degree of intimal dissection with well preserved flow across the PTCA site. A mean of 2.2 sites were dilated per patient. Breakdown of sites dilated was: left anterior descending, 41%; right coronary artery, 34%; circumflex artery, 24%; bypass grafts (all), 1%.

Using our lead configurations, significant ischemia was detected during brief coronary occlusions during PTCA in 76% of patients. When patients with visible collaterals were excluded, 89% of patients had marked ST deviation during brief coronary occlusion. Of the patients with ST deviation, 94% had ST elevation. Geographic patterns of ST elevation and reciprocal depression across the leads monitored were quite reproducible over serial dilatations (Fig. 2A).

From our population, 22% of patients displayed a total of 173 TIE's lasting from 3—300 min per episode, with a range of 1—18 episodes per patient over a mean period of 19 h of continuous monitoring in the CCU after PTCA. There were no obvious angiographic predictors (especially the presence of a dissection) that correlated with either the occurrence of TIE's or other measured endpoints (angina, MI). Of the patients with TIE's, 20% had an MI, while there were no MI's amongst the patients with no ST changes ($p < 0.00001$).

Overall, 16% of patients were clinically treated for angina. Of these patients, 74% had electrocardiographically detectable ischemia at the time that they had angina. Of these 74%, 39% had associated MI. Of the remaining patients who were treated for symptoms in the absence of ST changes, none had associated MI ($p > 0.05$).

When the group of patients who had TIE's were examined alone, ST elevation had very different implications from ST depression. ST elevation was seen in 23% of patients with any ST deviation; in the remaining 67%, only ST depression was seen. Geographic location of ST elevation was almost identical to patterns seen in the catheterization laboratory during brief controlled coronary occlusion in 90% of episodes of late ST elevation (Fig. 2b). Geographic location of late episodes of ST depression was similar to changes seen with controlled coronary occlusions in only 29% of episodes ($p < 0.01$). Episodes of ST elevation were eventually accompanied by angina in 90% of cases, whereas only 41% of episodes of ST depression were accompanied by angina. CPK-MB isoenzymes were diagnostic of MI in 90% of patients with ST elevation and in 3% of patients with ST depression ($p < 0.01$).

Amongst patients with ST elevation, detectable ST changes preceded angina by a mean of 45 min (range 5—150 min). One additional patient had a classical inferior injury current, ultimately forming Q waves and with CPK-MB elevation, for 300 min in the complete absence of symptoms (Fig. 3).

Discussion

PTCA is assuming an ever growing role in the acute and elective management of coronary artery disease. The mechanism of successful PTCA includes traumatic disruption of the plaque and coronary endothelium, with subsequent intense platelet deposition (10, 14).

Thus, as with reperfusion therapy, this intracoronary therapy is mediated through the iatrogenic creation of a potentially unstable milieu.

While monitoring in most CCU's after successful PTCA consists of arrhythmia monitoring and attention to symptoms, TIE may not produce either (1-5, 11—13). While we have reported the impact of successful angioplasty on patients with silent ischemia or very mild symptoms (7) the frequency and significance of TIE in the CCU after successful PTCA have never been delineated. Where dedicated ST-segment monitoring was performed in patients with unstable angina, electrocardiographically detectable TIE's had a strong correlation with an adverse outcome (6).

Sixteen percent of our patients had symptoms that were treated as angina, while 22% had TIE's. In 74% of patients with angina, ST-segment abnormalities were detectable. Of patients with any TIE's, 48% had no angina during their CCU stay.

MI was documented in 4.5% of our patients. Using dedicated ST-segment monitoring, no patient had an MI in the absence of ST changes. One patient had an MI in the absence of angina, associated with marked ST-segment elevation (Fig. 3).

If only symptoms and arrhythmias had been monitored, 16% of our overall population would have caused alarm, 25% of whom had no accompanying ST changes and no complications. Thus, 4% of our entire patient population had worrying chest pain in the CCU with no ECG changes and no MI. Conversely, 11% of our whole patient population had ST changes in the complete absence of chest pain. Of this 11%, 10% had MI.

Most notable in patients with detectable ST changes in the CCU was the difference in clinical significance between TIE characterized by ST depression vs ST elevation. Observations in patients with known coronary disease and primary reduction in coronary flow have described a range of clinical manifestations within single patients, from focal transmural ischemia to diffuse subendocardial ischemia expressed variously as ST ele-

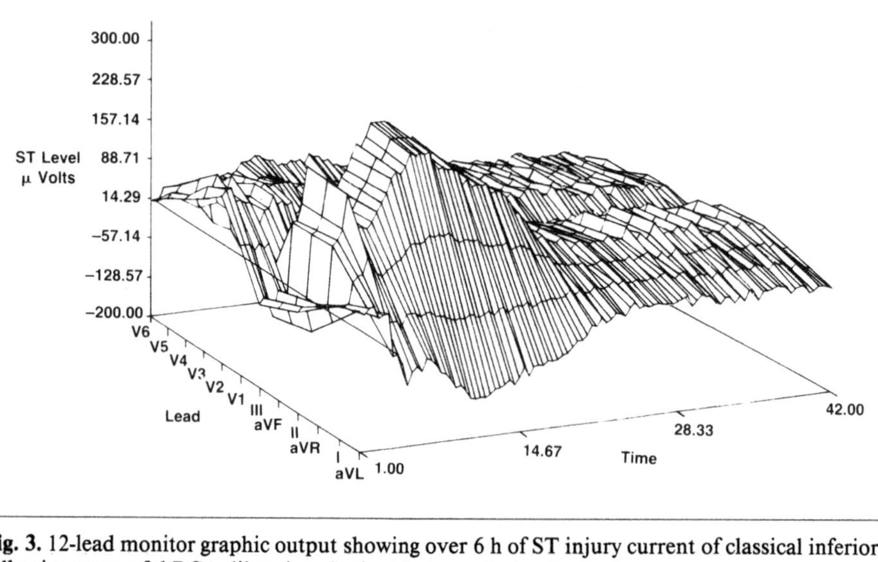

Fig. 3. 12-lead monitor graphic output showing over 6 h of ST injury current of classical inferior MI following successful RCA dilatation. Patient had no chest pain.

vation or ST depression, respectively (1, 3). In patients undergoing intracoronary thrombolysis, we found resolution of ST-segment elevation to be a sensitive and specific indicator of a change in coronary patency (8, 9). In our PTCA patients, patterns of injury current were first recorded in the controlled environment of brief coronary occlusion during PTCA, ie. with known coronary anatomy. ST elevation in this setting was seen in 94% of patients who had any significant ST deviation.

Of the patients with ST deviation in the CCU, 23% had ST elevation. Of the patients with ST elevation, 90% had ST elevation in lead locations essentially identical to their injury current during brief coronary occlusion at PTCA, strongly implying occlusion of the dilatation site during the CCU course. All patients with ST elevation in the CCU in a geographic pattern identical to their PTCA had MI. All of these patients also evolved angina, however, ST abnormalities preceded angina, often by more than 30 min and occasionally by hours.

While closure of a dilatation site from intimal dissection almost certainly requires mechanical revascularization to prevent or interrupt MI, platelet deposition may lead to either thrombus formation or coronary spasm through the release of mediators such as ADP and thromboxane. These latter events may have an early reversible phase that is more amenable to medical therapy. Real-time dedicated ST-segment monitoring appears to offer an "early warning" system for the detection of such events after PTCA. Insofar as angiographic predictors, arrhythmia detection, and attention to symptoms remain relatively insensitive and nonspecific. We have adopted real-time ST-segment monitoring as a standard of post-PTCA care. While the full impact of such monitoring on patient outcome awaits further study in a randomized trial, we feel that ST segment elevation in the CCU in the geographic distribution of injury current seen during PTCA brief occlusions merits aggressive therapy, medical and/or mechanical, for presumed closure of the dilatation site.

References

1. Biagini A, Mazzei MG, Carpeggiani C, Testa R, Antonelli R, Michelassi C, L'Abbate A, Maseri A (1982) Vasospastic ischemic mechanism of frequent asymptomatic transient ST-T changes during continuous electrocardiographic monitoring in selected unstable angina patients. Am Heart J 103: 13—19
2. Cecchi AC, Dovellini EV, Marchi F, Pucci P, Santoro G, Fazzini PF (1983) Silent myocardial ischemia during ambulatory electrocardiographic monitoring in patients with effort angina. J Am Coll Cardiol 1: 934—939
3. Chierchia S, Brunelli C, Simonetti I, Lazzari M, Maseri A (1980) Sequence of events in angina at rest: primary reduction in coronary flow. Circulation 61: 759—768
4. Chierchia S, Lazzari M, Freedman B, Brunelli C, Maseri A (1983) Impairment of myocardial perfusion and function during painless myocardial ischemia. J Am Coll Cardiol 1: 924—930
5. Cohn PF (1980) Silent myocardial ischemia in patients with a defective anginal warning system. Am J Cardiol 45: 697—702
6. Gottlieb SO, Weisfeldt ML, Ouyang P (1986) Silent ischemia as a marker for early unfavorable outcomes in patients with unstable angina. N Engl J Med 314: 1214—1219
7. Kent KM, Krucoff MW, Satler LF (1987) Angioplasty in asymptomatic and mildly symptomatic patients. Circulation (in press)
8. Krucoff MW, Green CE, Satler LF, Miller FC, Pallas RP, Kent KM, Del Negro AA, Pearle DL, Fletcher RD, Rackley CE (1986) Noninvasive detection of coronary artery patency using continuous T-segment monitoring. Am J Cardiol 57: 916—922

9. Krucoff MW, Satler LF, Green CE, Rackley CE, Kent KM (1987) ST segment changes during early myocardial infarction. In: Califf RM, Wagner GS (eds), Acute Coronary Care 1987, Martinus Nijhoff Publishing, Boston
10. Lam JYT, Chesebro JH, Steele PM, Dewanjee MK, Badimon L, Fuster V (1986) Deep arterial injury during experimental angioplasty: relation to a positive Indium-111-labelled platelet scintigram, quantitative platelet deposition and mural thrombosis. J Am Coll Cardiol 8:1380—1386
11. Selwyn A, Fox K, Eves M, Oakley D, Dargie H, Shillingford J (1978) Myocardial ischemia in patients with frequent angina pectoris. Br Med J 2: 1594—1595
12. Stern S, Tzivoni D (1973) Dynamic changes in the ST-T segment during sleep in ischemic heart disease. Am J Cardiol 32: 17—20
13. Stern S, Tzivoni D (1974) Early detection of silent ischemic heart disease by 24-hour electrocardiographic monitoring of active subjects. Br Heart J 36: 481—486
14. Waller BF, Gorfinkel J, Rogers FJ, Kent KM, Roberts WC (1984) Early and late morphologic changes in major epicardial coronary arteries after percutaneous transluminal coronary angioplasty. Am J Cardiol 53: 42C—47C

Authors' address:
M. W. Krucoff, M.D.
Georgetown University Hospital
Division of Cardiology
3800 Reservoir Road
Washington D.C. 20007
U.S.A.

Hemodynamics of painless ischemia

H. P. Krayenbühl, H. Hirzel, O. M. Hess, J. Schneider, M. Turina

Medical Policlinic, Division of Cardiology, Institute of Pathology and Clinic of Cardiovascular Surgery, University Hospital, Zürich, Switzerland

1. Introduction

It is well established that symptomatic ischemia is associated with abnormalities of systolic and diastolic left ventricular (LV) function (1, 2). The derangements of systolic function occur in the form of hypokinesia of the myocardial area supplied by the stenotic coronary artery. Diastolic abnormalities produced by ischemia encompass delayed and incomplete LV relaxation, as well as alterations of chamber stiffness associated with a massive increase in LV end-diastolic pressure.

In patients admitted to the coronary care unit because of angina at rest, Chierchia et al. (3) have monitored LV pressure and have found an increase of LV end-diastolic pressure and a reduction of peak positive and negative dP/dt not only during symptomatic but also during asymptomatic episodes of myocardial ischemia (Table 1). Impairment of LV function was significantly less during asymptomatic as compared to symptomatic ischemia. Iskandrian and Hakki (7) evaluated left ventricular ejection dynamics by radionuclide ventriculography at rest and during exercise, in patients with coronary artery disease who gave a history of angina pectoris. During exercise the patients who developed angina showed a decrease of LV ejection fraction whereas in those who exercised without pain ejection fraction increased. Workload, duration of exercise, frequency of multivessel

Table 1. Left ventricular function during episodes of symptomatic and asymptomatic ischemia (ST-T wave changes) in patients with unstable angina.

	Increase in LV filling pressure (mmHg)	Fall in peak pos dP/dt (mmHg/s)	Fall in peak neg dP/dt (mmHg/s)
Symptomatic episodes ($n = 46$)	+ 16.5	- 395	- 413
	*	*	*
Asymptomatic episodes ($n = 247$)	+ 5.9	- 252	- 259

* $p < 0.001$. Data taken from ref. (3).

Supported by a grant of the Swiss National Science Foundation disease, age, sex, frequency of diabetes and previous myocardial infarction did not differ between the two groups. In contrast, Cohn and coworkers (4) performed radionuclide ventriculography in truly asymptomatic patients with coronary artery disease who showed ST-segment depression at graded exercise test. For comparison, radionuclide angiography was also carried out in a group of symptomatic patients with coronary artery disease and ST-segment depression at stress testing. In both groups, global ejection fraction decreased by 6% during exercise (Table 2) and the percent of regions with normal ejection fraction at rest that demonstrated a decrease during exercise was identical. There were no intergroup differences as to age, sex, prevalence of multivessel disease and previous myocardial infarction. Hence, this study suggested that abnormalities in regional and global LV function are similar in patients with coronary artery disease with symptomatic and silent myocardial ischemia.

Table 2. Radionuclide angiographic ejection fraction (%) at rest and during exercise.

		Rest		Exercise
Group 1: ($n = 16$)	Asymptomatic patients; ST ↓ at graded exercise test	60	Δ–6%	54
Group 2: ($n = 24$)	Stable, chronic angina; ST ↓ at graded exercise test	53	Δ–6%	47

Note: No intergroup differences as to age, sex, previous MI, prevalence of multivessel disease. Data taken from ref. (4).

2. Exercise left ventricular cineangiography in matched patients with coronary artery disease with and without stress-induced angina

In order to have full insight into the hemodynamic alterations accompanying silent ischemia, we compared the LV cineangiograms obtained during dynamic exercise in 36 asymptomatic patients with proven coronary artery disease (10 without and 26 with previous infarction) with those of 36 carefully matched patients (10 without and 26 with previous infarction) whose exercise was limited by angina (6). The asymptomatic patients had had anginal episodes four to eight months prior to admission; at non-invasive bicycle ergometry they elicited however no pain. Matching was done with respect to age, number of vessels involved, extent of stenosis (Levine index), LV end-diastolic pressure at rest, ejection fraction and site of prior myocardial infarction. On admission, all medication was discontinued except for short-acting nitrates.

Comparisons between asymptomatic and symptomatic patients were made separately for the cohorts without and with prior infarction (Table 3). During the non-invasive upright bicycle stress test, the patients without angina exercised at a significantly higher workload than those in whom angina occurred. At bicycle exercise during catheterization the asymptomatic and the symptomatic patients within both cohorts exercised to the same workload, reached a similar rate-pressure product at the end of the stress test, showed a similar increase of LV end-diastolic pressure and similar changes of LV end-

Table 3. Exercise-induced hemodynamic changes in patients with proven coronary artery disease with and without previous myocardial infarction.

	Patients without MI		Patients with MI	
	Without AP	With AP	Without AP	With AP
n	10	10	26	26
Upright bicycle exercise (watts)	131	98*	129	97*
ST ↓ > 0.1 mV	3	6	12	13
Workload at cath (watts)	115	94	107	99
Ex HR × pressure (bpm · mmHg)	19'508	19'247	19'665	17'701
Ex LVEDP (mmHg)	36	29	32	36
EF rest → ex (%)	59 → 50	60 → 52	54 → 47	55 → 50
EDVI rest → ex (ml/m²)	100 → 116	100 → 103	121 → 130	111 → 125

Abbreviations: Ex = exercise during catheterization (cath); MI = myocardial infarction; AP = angina pectoris; HR = heart rate (beats per min = bpm); LVEDP = left ventricular end-diastolic pressure; EF = left ventricular biplane ejection fraction; EDVI = left ventricular end-diastolic volume index; ST = ST-segment depression at non-invasive upright bicycle stress testing; *n* = number of patients; * $p < 0.05$.
Data are taken from ref. (6).

diastolic volume (Table 3). In the cohort without previous infarction, LV ejection fraction decreased from 59% to 50% in the asymptomatic and from 60% to 52% in the symptomatic group. In the cohort with previous infarction, LV ejection fraction decreased from 54% to 47% and from 55% to 50%, respectively. Regional de novo hypokinesia appeared in all patients without prior infarction and in 25/26 asymptomatic and 22/26 symptomatic patients, respectively, of the two cohorts with prior infarction.

3. Myocardial structure of left ventricular segments with exercise-induced wall motion abnormalities

Although exercise-induced symptomatic as well as asymptomatic ischemic events appeared to be fully reversible based on the normalization of ST-segment depression and wall motion abnormalities upon termination of exercise, it is not clear, whether repeated bouts of ischemia will not eventually lead to an alteration of myocardial structure. Thus, intraoperative biopsies from the region of transiently ischemic myocardium and from the region supplied by nonstenosed coronary artery were taken in 17 patients with de novo exercise-induced wall motion abnormalities. Left ventricular ejection fraction at rest was normal in all patients although two had had a previous inferior infarction with small localized hypokinesia at rest. All 17 patients developed de novo wall motion abnormalities during bicycle exercise at catheterization; 12 patients had angina pectoris during the exercise-induced ischemia, whereas in 5 patients ischemia was silent. The morphometric analysis of the transmural biopsies was performed as described previously (5).

Table 4. The morphological data are given for the subendocardial mural third ("endocardium") and the subepicardial mural third ("epicardium").

Endo/epicardial morphological data	Endocardium		Epicardium	
	MFD (µ)	IF (%)	MFD (µ)	IF (%)
Normokinetic Region at Ex	28.1	18.2	27.0	16.2
		*		
Region with Ex-induced Hypokinesia	29.2	28.6	27.9	18.6
		** (28.6 vs 18.6)		

Abbreviations: Ex = dynamic exercise at catheterization; MFD = muscle fibre diameter ; IF = interstitial fibrosis; * $p < 0.05$; ** $p < 0.01$.

Table 4 presents the morphological findings for the inner mural third ("endocardium") and the outer mural third ("epicardium") of the normo- and the hypokinetic regions at bicycle LV cineangiography. At both regions, in the subendocardial as well as the subepicardial portion, there was cellular hypertrophy, the muscle fiber diameter (MFD) ranging between 27.0 and 29.2 µm (normal ≦ 20 µm). Interstitial fibrosis (IF) was markedly increased in the subendocardial region of the segments with exercise-induced hypokinesia, as compared to the subendocardial region of normokinetic segments, as well as to the subepicardial region of the segments with exercise-induced hypokinesia. It should be noted that even in the normokinetic segments interstitial fibrosis was increased (normal ≦ 5%) whereby this increase appeared commensurate with the degree of muscle hypertrophy.

4. Conclusions

From our cineangiographic investigations in symptomatic and asymptomatic patients with coronary artery disease during dynamic exercise, and from the morphometric assessment of intraoperative biopsies of wall regions with normo- and hypokinesia during exercise, it is concluded that:

1. Under similar physical stress conditions, comparable hemodynamic alterations indicative of ischemia are present in symptomatic and asymptomatic patients with coronary artery disease of similar severity
2. Angina pectoris cannot be considered a prerequisite for hemodynamically significant ischemia during exertion
3. Structural alterations with considerable interstitial fibrosis develop in the transiently ischemic myocardium with normal function at rest and hence anti-ischemic measures, i.e. revascularization or vigorous medical treatment, appear mandatory in patients with silent ischemia.

References

1. Carroll JD, Hess OM, Studer NP, Hirzel HO, Krayenbuehl HP (1983) Systolic function during exercise in patients with coronary artery disease. J Am Coll Cardiol 2: 206–216
2. Carroll JD, Hess OM, Hirzel HO, Krayenbuehl HP (1983) Exercise-induced ischemia: The influence of altered relaxation on early diastolic pressures. Circulation 67: 521–528
3. Chierchia S, Lazzari M, Freedman MB, Brunelli C, Maseri A (1983) Impairment of myocardial perfusion and function during painless myocardial ischemia. J Am Coll Cardiol 1: 924–930
4. Cohn PF, Brown EJ Jr, Wynne J, Holman BL, Atkins HL (1983) Global and regional left ventricular ejection fraction abnormalities during exercise in patients with silent myocardial ischemia. J Am Coll Cardiol 1: 931–933
5. Hess OM, Ritter M, Schneider J, Grimm J, Turina M, Krayenbuehl HP (1984) Diastolic stiffness and myocardial structure in aortic valve disease before and after valve replacement. Circulation 69: 855–865
6. Hirzel HO, Leutwyler R, Krayenbuehl HP (1985) Silent myocardial ischemia: Hemodynamic changes during dynamic exercise in patients with proven coronary artery disease despite absence of angina pectoris. J Am Coll Cardiol 6: 275–284
7. Iskandrian AS, Hakki A (1984) Left ventricular function in patients with coronary heart disease in the presence or absence of angina pectoris during exercise radionuclide ventriculography. Am J Cardiol 53: 1239–1243

Authors' address:
H. P. Krayenbühl, M.D.
Medical Policlinic
Division of Cardiology
University Hospital
CH-8091 Zürich

Discussion on Prevalence and Detection

Chairmen: P. R. Lichtlen and H. P. Krayenbühl

Droste started with the question of whether ST-segment depression, which can be observed on ambulatory ECG recordings sometimes for several hours, does actually represent ischemia. V. Arnim pointed out that in these instances it is especially important to scrutinize carefully the beginning and end of each episode of ST depression. Often, these very prolonged changes represent motion artifacts, which can be be identified by the sudden change in ECG configuration at the beginning or the end of such an "episode". On the other hand, it is certainly not impossible for ischemia to last for several hours.

Fox raised the question of what the changes are that should be the target for detection. Is it evidence for ischemia or is it detecting coronary artery disease, which would be different goals. Berman defined his testing as measurement of an imbalance between myocardial oxygen supply and oxygen demand. This could be achieved by monitoring lactate metabolism, with PET scanning or exercise thallium testing. Distante mentioned regional asynergy, detected by echocardiography, as an optimal definition of ischemia. He referred to the close relation between regional wall motion and blood flow, which would make transient asynergy a highly specific marker for transient ischemia. Fox and Resnekov, however, maintained that there must be other causes for regional asynergy apart from ischemia.

When asked on which sequence of tests he would base further diagnostic and therapeutic decisions, Berman pointed out that, especially in a population with a low prevalence of disease, e.g. 5%, even a test with 90% specificity would, with a positive result, be 20% true positive versus 80% false positive. Only with further testing could the post-test probability with a positive result be then brought to the 90% range, where, as Berman said, in his institution one would proceed to coronary angiography followed by interventional therapy. Krayenbühl added that among the tests performed to determine whether a patient has ischemia or not, he would also try antianginal treatment, which, if successful, would be further proof of ischemia. The value of thallium stress testing was questioned by Rutishauser and Lichtlen who pointed to the difficulties of defining ischemic regions, for instance in triple-vessel disease. In these cases under exercise conditions perfusion goes down uniformly in all regions without producing regional defects. As had been mentioned in earlier discussions, it was emphasized that conformation of silent ischemia in totally asymptomatic patients requires two independent objective markers of ischemia. Here Distante proposed echocardiography, because mechanical dysfunction is a good marker of ischemia and, in his hands, more sensitive than recording the ECG. Other participants mentioned the inherent problems of echocardiographic testing, precluding some patients and some regions of the heart from proper documentation.

The notion presented by Roskamm that in multi-vessel coronary disease the presence of angina is an effect of the size of the ischemic myocardium, was supported by Fassbender who mentioned a greater drop in ejection fraction in his group of patients in those with anginal symptoms.

While Berman reported that with his approach of sequential testing, a group of patients with a high prevalence of subsequent events can be defined, Lichtlen mentioned patients who can be stable for many years on drug treatment alone. Here would possibly lie the future application of Holter monitoring; that is, determining the activity of disease after the presence of disease has been defined by other methods. Holter monitoring in the current technological situation cannot be seen as a screening tool. Defining the level of disease activity by defining the amount of ischemia during daily life may have prognostic implications. As Krucoff pointed out for the Cass study and Rutishauser for the European Coronary Surgery study, a positive exercise test, demonstrating provocable ischemia, was a very strong marker of a subsequently bad prognosis.

Slight differences in experiences came out over the question of whether ischemia on Holter monitoring is as severe when it is silent as when it is symptomatic. Arnim would equate the two, as would Hausmann with respect to ST depression where, as Hoberg thinks, the amount of myocardium involved plays a decisive role. Distante found silent episodes less severe mechanically, in contrast to Krayenbühl, who found in matched patients, no differences in wall motion abnormalities for ischemia with and without pain. Accordingly, Berman also reported a large overlap between symptomatic and asymptomatic ischemia in exercise thallium testing.

Höfling and Krucoff discussed the ECG evidence of ischemia during PTCA. ST-segment elevation was seen as a clear sign of occlusion during PTCA as well as afterwards, during follow-up. The case of ST depression seems less clear; it may represent only subendocardial ischemia, as during exercise testing with a non-occluded artery, but may also represent reciprocal changes during severe transmural ischemia in the opposite left ventricular wall. Roskamm then asked, what the consequences would be of regular electrocardiographic monitoring during PTCA. Krucoff said he would normally extend his monitoring periods for around 20 h after PTCA. He would see a purpose for automated 12-lead ECG monitoring after PTCA, in providing the chance of early intervention in sudden occlusion of a coronary artery. ST-segment elevation in identical leads, which had been positive during PTCA, would prompt immediate review of such a patient in the catheterization laboratory.

The next point in the discussion was the presence of patchy fibrosis which Krayenbühl had demonstrated with biopsy studies. Droste asked how many of the 17 patients with biopsies were free from angina; there were five such patients. Tzivoni mentioned the study of Geft and Ganz on repeated coronary occlusions in dogs, which, in this experimental model, also led to patches of interstitial fibrosis. Lichtlen preferred to call these patches small focal infarcts, which, as Arnim pointed out, may be the result of distal embolization coming from an exulcerated plaque in a proximal coronary artery. For Krayenbühl, the development of fibrosis, which may not yet be harmful for contraction but may already be for diastolic function, would also be a clear indication for treatment in the patients with silent ischemia.

Against a trend towards treatment out of a feeling of necessity, Fox strongly proposed the initiation of a randomized study in patients with totally asymptomatic ischemia. Such a study should mainly address the question of whether treatment of silent ischemia — be it medically or by interventions — would improve the prognosis of the patient. As the number of such patients is not very high in most referral centers, this would have to be either a multi-center trial or a study in a large center where a large amount of screening is performed.

Medical and surgical therapy of patients with asymptomatic ischemia

K. Schnellbacher, C. Droste, and H. Roskamm

Rehabilitationszentrum für Herz- und Kreislaufkranke Bad Krozingen
(Medical Director: Prof. Dr. H. Roskamm)

Summary

Asymptomatic myocardial ischemia presents two different clinical pictures:

1. "Asymptomatic ischemia episodes": symptomatic patients with additional asymptomatic episodes in daily life.
2. "Asymptomatic ischemia patients": patients in whom ischemic episodes are always asymptomatic.

Study I, a randomized, double blind, placebo controlled study in 19 angina pectoris patients, demonstrates the efficacy of medical therapy (3×20 mg IS-5-MN or 3×60 mg diltiazem) on exercise induced ischemia (prolongation of exercise duration at onset of angina by 24% and 39%, respectively; at onset of ST-segment depression by 30% and 40% respectively) as well as on ischemic episodes during Holter monitoring (reduction of incidence and duration of ischemic episodes by 65% and 77%, respectively, on the first day of medication and 69% and 65%, respectively, on the seventh).

Study II shows the results of aortocoronary bypass surgery in 22 totally asymptomatic patients: a decrease of ST-segment depression from 0.31 mV preoperatively to 0.03 mV postoperatively; decrease of PCP at maximal exercise from 29 mm Hg preoperatively to 22 mm Hg postoperatively.

The studies demonstrate that in patients with asymptomatic myocardial ischemia, both medical therapy and surgical therapy are effective; special aspects regarding the indications for aortocoronary bypass surgery are discussed.

Introduction

Asymptomatic myocardial ischemia presents two different clinical pictures (2, 5, 7, 17, 18):

1. Many patients with symptomatic angina pectoris in the presence of exercise related objective signs of ischemia may also have additional asymptomatic episodes in their daily life: "asymptomatic ischemia episodes"
2. In some patients ischemic episodes are always asymptomatic not only in daily life, but also during exercise testing: "asymptomatic ischemia patients".

Study I describes the effects of medical therapy with two widely used antianginal drugs on asymptomatic ischemia episodes (20); Study II summarizes the effects of surgical therapy on asymptomatic ischemia patients (6).

Study I

After a placebo period of 3 days, 19 patients with exercise induced angina were randomized into two different treatment groups: one group received 3×20 mg IS-5-MN at 8 a.m., 2 p.m., and 8 p.m., the other group 3×60 mg diltiazem. This drug regimen was applied over 7 days.

Exercise tests were taken at the end of the placebo period, on the first day of treatment 2 h after the first medication, on the seventh day of treatment at 9 a.m., i.e. 13 h after the last medication, and once more 2 h after the first medication on the seventh day of treatment. Symptom-limited exercise tests were performed on the bicycle ergometer in the supine position. Starting with 25 W, the workload was increased by 25 W steps every 2 min. 24-hour Holter monitoring was performed on the third day of the placebo period, and on the first and seventh days of treatment. The ECG was recorded in leads CM_4 and CM_5 with a two-channel device of Diagnostic Medical Instruments (DMI), type Eclipse (0.05—100 Hz, amplitude modulation).

The parameters of pretest exercise testing, coronary angiographic findings, and hemodynamics at rest and during exercise were not significantly different for the two groups (20).

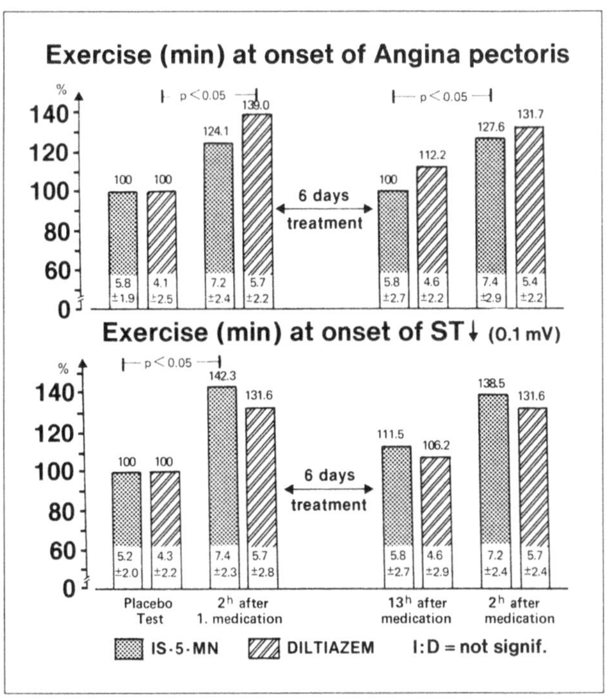

Fig. 1. Duration of exercise (min) at onset of angina pectoris and at onset of ST-segment depression (0.1 mV) under placebo (100%), and under acute and chronic drug regimen with 3 × 20 mg IS-5-MN and 3 × 60 mg diltiazem, respectively, at 8 a.m., 2 p.m., and 8 p.m.

Exercise testing

Duration of exercise at onset of angina in the first exercise test at the end of the placebo period was taken as 100%. This period was prolonged to 124% or 139% 2 h after the first medication of IS-5-MN or diltiazem, respectively. After 6 days of treatment and 13 h after the last medication, this effect was no longer present. Two hours after the following medication, however, the acute effects of either during were as impressive as after the first medication. There was a similar effect on exercise duration at the onset of ST-segment depression, and no differences between the drugs (Fig. 1).

Holter monitoring

At the end of the placebo period, a total of 26 ischemic episodes were registered during 24 h; 85% of these were asymptomatic. Taking these as 100%, the prevalence of ischemic episodes decreased to 34.6% and 30.7% on the first and seventh days of medication respectively (Fig. 2). Figure 3 depicts the prevalence of ischemic episodes during the

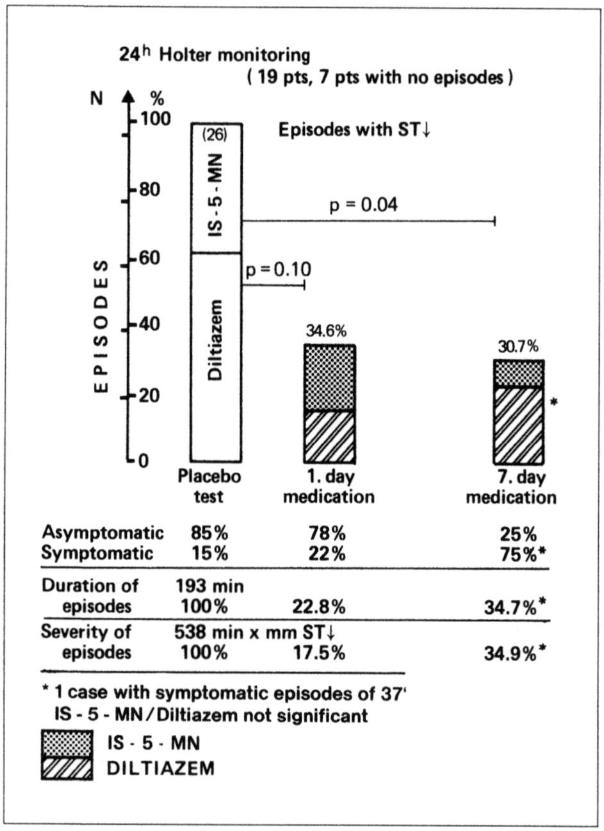

Fig. 2. Incidence, duration and severity of episodes with ischemic ST-segment depression during 24 h Holter monitoring (placebo, 1st and 7th days of medication).

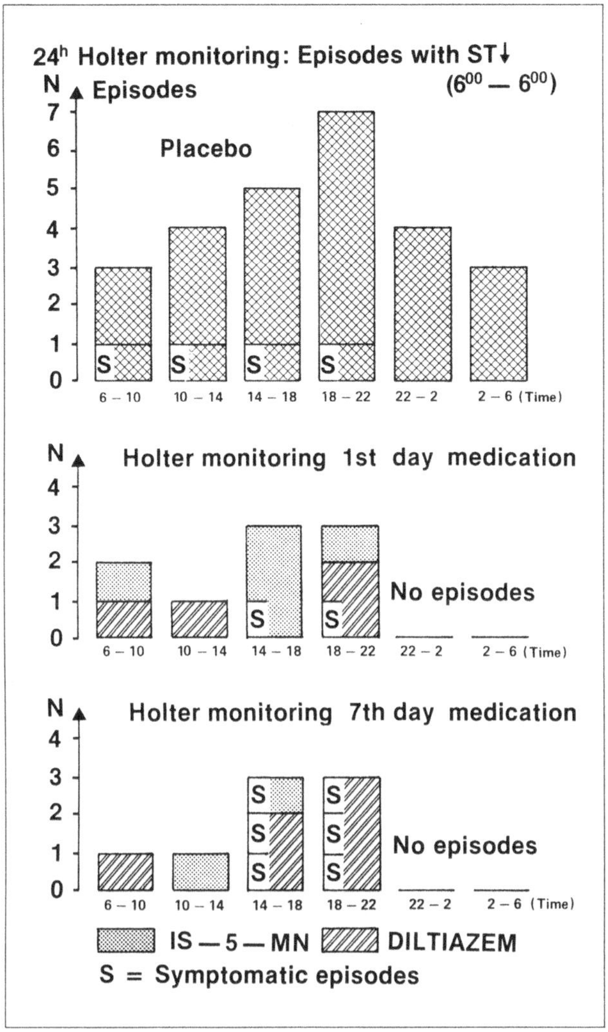

Fig. 3. Spontaneous ischemic episodes during 24 h Holter monitoring between 6 a.m. and 6 a.m. (placebo, 1st and 7th day of medication).

course of a day. After medication, nocturnal ischemic episodes (between 10 p.m. and 6 a.m.) vanished.

For this study we did not control the individual plasma levels of mononitrate; instead we performed computer simulation of the plasma concentrations after repeated application of our drug regimen (on the basis of data obtained in normals; Fig. 4). This stimulation shows a decrease of the IS-5-MN plasma concentration to approximately 100 ng/ml at the end of the 12 h night interval; for about 6 h, the concentration remained below 250 ng/ml. Apparently, under this drug regimen, the concentrations are low enough to avoid development of nitrate tolerance, but, on the other hand, these low concentrations are obviously sufficient for effective treatment of nocturnal ischemic episodes.

Fig. 4. Computer simulation reflecting the plasma concentrations of IS-5-MN after repeated application of 3 × 20 mg IS-5-MN daily at 8 a.m., 2 p.m., and 8 p.m.

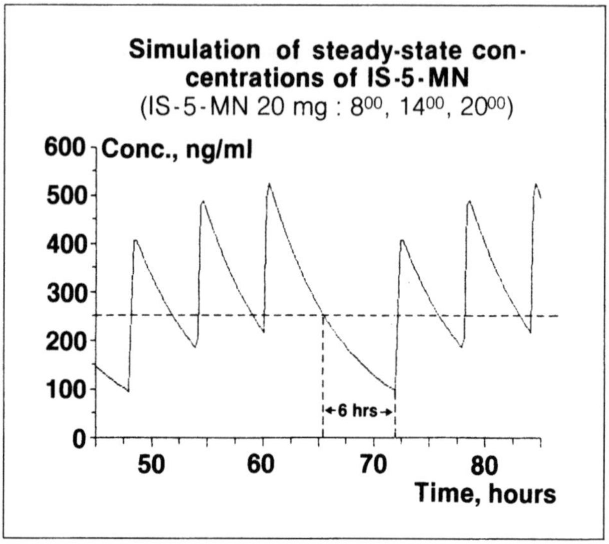

Study II

Twenty-two patients with completely asymptomatic ischemia underwent coronary bypass surgery. Their mean age was 49 years, mean exercise tolerance 76 ± 34 W, mean ST-segment depression 0.3 mV, and mean pulmonary capillary wedge pressure 29 ± 7 mm Hg; six patients had double vessel disease and sixteen had triple vessel disease; three patients had left main stem disease.

As expected, after bypass surgery, ST-segment depression was no longer present (mean 0.03 mV), the maximal pulmonary capillary wedge pressure decreased to 22 ± 9 mmHg; the maximal exercise tolerance increased to 113 ± 35 W (Fig. 5).

Discussion

The question whether asymptomatic ischemia should be treated generally or only in certain subgroups cannot be fully answered today. Prognostic studies on silent myocardial ischemia are currently in progress. It is widely indicated that recurrent myocardial ischemia is a prognostically negative factor, independent of the presence or absence of angina pectoris pain (1, 8, 10, 11, 13—16, 21). A patient's total ischemic burden, i.e. the sum of ischemic episodes with or without pain, is of prognostic relevance and should be the criterion for medical or surgical management of the individual patient (3).

Morphological studies show that intermittent periods of ischemia have a cumulative effect on subendocardial necroses (9, 19); this has currently also been shown for asymptomatic ischemic periods (12).

The studies mentioned above indicate that in asymptomatic patients with advanced disease, an active therapy should follow the same principles as in symptomatic patients.

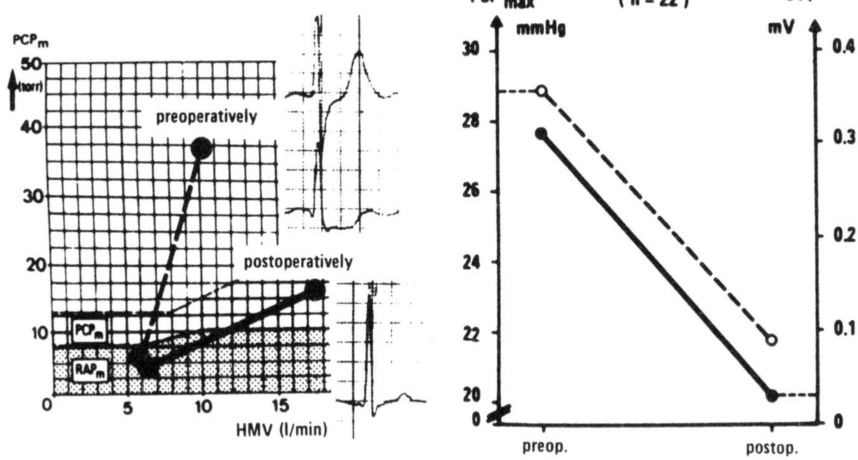

Fig. 5. Normalization of exercise-induced ST-segment depression and of pathologically increased pulmonary capillary wedge pressure after bypass surgery, in patients with asymptomatic myocardial ischemia (left: one patient with left main stem stenosis; right: 22 patients).

Our studies I and II demonstrate that medical, as well as surgical, therapy of these patients is effective. With respect to the indication of medical or surgical therapy, the following points should be particularly considered:

1. Severity of ischemia
2. Efficacy of medical therapy on exercise ECG and repeated Holter monitoring
3. Coronary morphology (left main stem disease, triple vessel disease)
4. Technical feasibility of bypass surgery
5. Additional factors such as age, secondary diseases etc.

Medical therapy

a) Asymptomatic ischemia episodes
Medical treatment should aim at the elimination of myocardial ischemia. Recently, the more or less favourables effects of the three antiischemic drugs (nitrates, betablockers, calcium channel blockers) have been widely discussed. We believe that most drug regimen that apply to patients with symptomatic ischemia are also effective in patients with asymptomatic ischemia. The possibilities of verifying drug efficacy by repeated monitoring of exercise ECG and ambulatory Holter-ECG, and eventually to titrate intensity of treatment, should be more widely used (17).
b) Asymptomatic ischemia patients
Totally asymptomatic patients with myocardial ischemia should be treated medically if asymptomatic ischemia has been proven (exclusion of false positive effects on exercise

ECG or Holter monitoring). In doubtful cases, ischemia should be stated by further investigations (nuclear medical methods, floating catheter, echocardiography).
Urgency and aggressiveness of therapy depend on the severity of ischemia and on the exercise level at which it can be provoked. A patient with ST-segment depression of 0.1 mV at 150 W will not need as intensive a therapy as a patient with ST-segment depression of 0.3 mV at 50 W.
If a totally asymptomatic patient has already suffered myocardial infarction, the decision to treat medically is much easier, because secondary prevention (betablockers, antiplatelets) is, in this case, indicated as much as in symptomatic patients.

Coronary angiography

The more pronounced the indicators of ischemia (ST-segment depression), and the lower the exercise level on which ischemia starts, the earlier the patient should undergo coronary angiography. This is especially valid if medical therapy is proven ineffective in eliminating silent ischemia.
If the coronary angiogram is positive (e.g. proximal LAD stenosis), and the presence of myocardial ischemia is obvious, despite the lack of symptoms, coronary angioplasty might be indicated or even necessary in these asymptomatic patients (see Rutishauser, this volume).

Surgical therapy

The indications for surgical therapy in asymptomatic patients are similar to those in symptomatic patients:
- significant left main stem stenosis (> 75%)
- Triple vessel disease, if ischemia has been proven (further investigation if doubtful)
- Ischemia on low or medium exercise levels
- Lacking effect of medical therapy (repeated test under medication)
- Coronary morphology suitable for surgical treatment.

References

1. Bruce RA, BeRousen Ta, Hossack KF (1980) Value of maximal exercise tests in risk assessement of primary coronary heart disease events in healthy men: five years' experience of the Seattle Heart Watch Study. Am J Cardiol 46: 371
2. Cohn PF (1986) (ed) Silent myocardial ischemia and infarction. Basic and clinical cardiology, Vol 5, Marcel Dekker, New York Basel
3. Cohn PF (1986) Total ischemic burden: experimental and clinical aspects of myocardial ischemia. Am J Med 81 (Suppl 4A): 1
4. Cohn PF, Harris P, Barry WH, Rosati RA, Rosenbaum P, Watrenaux C (1981) Prognostic importance of anginal symptoms in angiographically defined coronary artery disease. Am J Cardiol 47: 233
5. Deanfield JE, Shea MJ, Selwyn Ap (1985) Clinical evaluation of transient myocardial ischemia during daily life. Am J Med 79 (Suppl 3A): 18

6. Droste C, Roskamm H (1982) Normalisierung einer asymptomatischen Myokardischämie durch Revaskularisations-OP (Abstract). Z Kardiol 9: 632
7. Droste C (1984) Asymptomatische Myokardischämie, In: Roskamm H (Hrsg) Koronarerkrankungen, Handbuch der inneren Medizin Bd IX/3, Springer, Berlin Heidelberg New York, S. 613
8. Erikssen J, Thaulow E (1984) Follow-up of patients with asymptomatic myocardial ischemia. In: Rutishauser W, Roskamm H (eds) Silent Myocardial Ischemia, Springer, Berlin Heidelberg New York Tokyo, p 156
9. Geft IL, Fishbein MC, Ninomiyal K, et al (1982) Intermittent brief periods of ischemia have a cumulative effect and may cause myocardial necrosis. Circulation 66: 1150
10. Hickman JR Jr, Uhl GS, Cook RL, Engel PH, Hopkirk A (1980) A natural history study of asymptomatic coronary disease (abstract). Am J Cardiol 45: 422
11. Kent KM, Rosing DR, Ewels CJ, Kipson L, Bonow R, Epstein SE (1982) Prognosis of asymptomatic or mildly symptomatic patients with coronary artery disease. Am J Cardiol 49: 1823
12. Krayenbühl HP (1987) Hämodynamik bei stummer Ischämie. Vortrag beim 9. Österreichischen Kardiologentreffen, Bad Gastein 8—11 January 1987 (in press)
13. Langou RA, Huang EK, Kelley MJ, Cohen LS (1980) Predictive accuracy of coronary artery calcification and abnormal exercise test for coronary artery disease in asymptomatic men. Circulation 62: 1196
14. Lipid Research Clinics Coronary Primary Prevention Trial (1984) I. Reduction in incidence of coronary heart disease. JAMA 251: 351
15. Multiple Risk Factor Intervention Trial Research Group (1985) Exercise electrocardiogram and coronary heart disease mortality in the multiple risk factor intervention trial. Am J Cardiol 55: 16
16. Passamani E, Davis KB, Gillespie MJ, Killip T and the CASS Principal investigators and their associates (1985) Coronary artery surgery (CASS): a randomized trial of coronary artery bypass surgery. Survival of patients with a low ejection fraction. N Engl J Med 312: 1665
17. Pepine CJ (1986) (ed) Silent myocardial ischemia, in Cardiology Clinics, Vol. 4, No. 4, WB Saunders, Philadelphia
18. Rutishauser W, Roskamm H (1984) (eds) Silent myocardial ischemia. Springer, Berlin Heidelberg New York Tokyo
19. Schaper W (1987) Pathophysiologie der stummen Ischämie. Vortrag beim 9. Österreichischen Kardiologentreffen, Bad Gastein 8—11 January 1987 (in press)
20. Schnellbacher K, Samek L, Blaschke HJ, Roskamm H (1987) Efficacy of isosorbide-5-mononitrate and diltiazem in patients with myocardial ischemia. II International Symposium on Mononitrates, Berlin, 11—13 December 1986 (in press)
21. Theroux P, Waters DD, Halphen C, Debaisieux JC, Mizgala HF (1979) Prognostic value of exercise testing soon after myocardial infarction. N Engl J Med 301: 341

Authors' address:
Dr. K. Schnellbacher
Rehabilitationszentrum für
Herz- und Kreislaufkranke
Südring 15
7812 Bad Krozingen

Coronary angioplasty in silent myocardial ischemia

L. Finci, B. Meier, G. Steffenino, A. Righetti, J.-J. Bodenmann, W. Rutishauser

Cardiology Center, University Hospital, Geneva, Switzerland

Introduction

Silent myocardial ischemia is defined as the absence of anginal symptoms in patients with significant coronary disease with proved ischemic episodes (1). Two types of silent ischemia have been identified (2): a totally asymptomatic type, and a partially asymptomatic type with sometimes angina and sometimes painless episodes of myocardial ischemia. Based on data from angiography and necropsy, the prevalence in middle aged males is about 2—4% for the totally asymptomatic, and 20—30% for the partially asymptomatic type (3). Patients without anginal pain but with angina equivalents, such as an abnormal exertional dyspnea, arrhythmia and fatigue may be classified separately.
Percutaneous transluminal coronary angioplasty has been accepted as a therapeutic method in selected patients with symptomatic coronary artery disease. Present indications, however, do not consider patients with silent myocardial ischemia. The patients discussed in this report were accepted for coronary angioplasty, because of silent myocardial ischemia documented by the combination of electrocardiographic stress testing and/or scintigraphic data, and corroborated angiographically by the presence of a severe stenosis of the coronary artery of the respective myocardial area.

Patients and methods

Patients

Between August 1983 and October 1985, 426 patients were accepted for coronary angioplasty at our institution, and a one year follow-up was solicited in all. Of these, 35 had silent ischemia according to the following criteria: (1) absence of chest pain (2) objective evidence of myocardial ischemia and (3) angiographically significant coronary lesion(s). There were 31 males and 4 females. Their mean age was 54 ± 11 years (range 24 to 66 years). The patients were divided into three main groups (Table 1). Group I (n = 5): patients with significant coronary lesion(s) but no angina, myocardial infarction, arrhythmia, or congestive heart failure on admission, and no anginal symptoms during a stress test. Group II (n = 11): patients who were asymptomatic following a myocardial infarction and still showed ischemia. Group III (n = 19): patients with significant coronary lesion(s), no history of myocardial infarction, but angina equivalents such as abnormal

Table 1. Patient characteristics.

Group	I (n = 5)	II (n = 11)	III (n = 19)
Age (years)	52±15	56±8	53±9
Males	4 (80%)	11 (100%)	16 (84%)
Prior myocardial infarction (months)	–	1.5±1.0	–
Total coronary occlusion	–	5 (45%)	–

Groups of patients: I = totally asymptomatic, II = asymptomatic after myocardial infarction, III = with angina equivalents.

exertional dyspnea, arrhythmia, or fatigue induced by ischemia. We excluded all patients that were asymptomatic after myocardial infarction and had no signs of ischemia according to the tests mentioned below.

Exercise testing

Exercise tests were carried out according to a bicycle exercise protocol, using a Marquette Electronics Inc. computer-assisted system in all cases. All tests were started at a workload of 25 watts with increments of 25 watts every 3 min up to the maximal calculated target heart rate or workload, unless significant ST-segment depression (> 0.1 mV), or an angina equivalent appeared. The 12 standard electrocardiographic leads or at least leads V1, V5, and aVF in patients with radionuclide tests were recorded before, during, and after exercise. The time from the start of exercise until > 0.1 mV horizontalor descending ST-segment depression (0.08 s from the J point) was recorded.

Radionuclide testing

Exercise Thallium-201 or Technetium-99m scintigraphy was performed in 10 and 4 patients, respectively. Sequential imaging for Thallium-201 was performed according to a standard protocol (4) immediately after a heart rate limited exercise test, and again 4 hours later. During exercise, electrocardiogram was monitored and analyzed. The scintigraphic images were processed on a DEC gamma-11 system. Basically, circumferential profiles were computed in three projections (anterior, 45 degree and 90 degree left anterior oblique) within the automatically detected contour of the left ventricle after background subtraction. The circumferential profiles, the processed images, and the analog Polaroid images were interpreted by two observers unaware of angiographic data. Ischemia was considered to be present if both observers found a redistribution score higher than the early postexercise score. The Technetium-99 scintigraphy was performed using the same exercise protocol; the resting and exercise left ventricular ejection fractions were calculated. If no increment of > 5% in exercise ejection fraction was noted, ischemia was considered to be present. The following signs of ischemia were documented in the three groups: symptoms (angina equivalents) in 0, 0, and 8 (42%) patients, ST-segment depression in 2 (40%), 8 (73%), and 6 (32%) patients, and positive radionuclide testing in 3 (60%), 3 (27%) and 5 (26%) patients respectively.

Coronary angioplasty

The coronary angioplasty procedure was considered successful if the angiographic aspect of the stenosis was improved (residual stenosis < 50%), the transstenotic gradient was reduced (< 30 mm Hg), and no electrocardiographic or enzymatic evidence of myocardial infarction or need for bypass surgery occurred. The transstenotic pressure gradient was defined as the difference between the mean pressures at the tip of the guiding catheter in the coronary ostium and at the tip of the balloon catheter distal to the stenosis. Pressure gradients were not available in 9 patients. Restenosis was defined as a loss of 50% or more of the gain in luminal diameter achieved at angioplasty. Stenoses were estimated and averaged independently by two experienced angiographers in at least two projections. Coronary wedge pressure was defined as the pressure measured distal to the stenotic site during balloon inflation at 2 bar for at least 15 s. Recruitable collaterals were demonstrated by opacification of the vessel distal to the stenosis during injection of contrast in the contralateral or ipsilateral coronary artery while the balloon was inflated, or assumed in the presence of a coronary wedge pressure ≥ 30 mm Hg (8). Angioplasty was performed with balloon inflation pressures up to 12 bar and maximal time of 90 s. During balloon inflation, patients were questioned about symptoms. Three to four standard electrocardiographic leads were monitored during angioplasty in all cases, and the intracoronary electrocardiogram (9) in most of them.

Statistics

The results were expressed as mean values ± 1 standard deviation. Students t-test for paired data was used to evaluate statistical significance.

Results

Group I

Coronary angioplasty was successful in all 5 patients. The mean diameter stenosis was reduced from 77 ± 13% to 25 ± 15% and the mean transstenotic pressure gradient from 55 ± 8 mm Hg to 13 ± 5 mm Hg. Three patients had had previous successful angioplasty at the same site; one had double vessel angioplasty during the same procedure. All patients showed significant ST-segment changes within the first 20 s of balloon inflation (Table 2) (Fig. 7).

Exercise stress tests (Table 3) showed no significant functional improvement after angioplasty, since the predicted workload values had already been reached before angioplasty. Clinical follow-up (mean 6 months, range 3—12 months) was satisfactory in all 5 patients.

Table 2. Data during coronary angioplasty.

Group	I (n = 5)	II (n = 11)	III (n = 19)
Symptoms*	0	1 (9%)	7 (37%)
ST-segment elevation	5 (100%)	4 (36%)	16 (84%)
Coronary wedge pressure (mm Hg)	27±16	31±13	28±8
Collaterals	1 (20%)	6 (54%)	2 (11%)

* angina equivalents
Groups of patients: I = totally asymptomatic, II = asymptomatic after myocardial infarction, III = with angina equivalents.

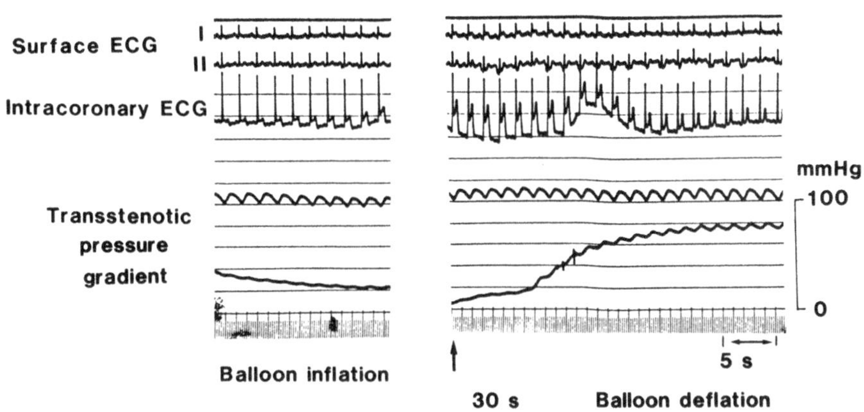

Fig. 1. Early ischemic response in a 58-year-old male patient who underwent coronary angioplasty of the proximal left anterior descending artery. Standard leads, I, II, and intracoronary electrocardiogram with aortic and coronary pressure recordings. There is ST-segment elevation within 10 s of balloon inflation with prompt return to baseline after deflation.

Group II

Coronary angioplasty was successful in 9 of 11 patients, with a mean reduction of the stenosis from 90 ± 10% to 21 ± 14%, and of the transstenotic pressure gradient from 58 ± 12 mm Hg to 19 ± 11 mm Hg. In 5 patients the involved artery had previously been totally occluded. Collaterals were present in 6 patients. During angioplasty ST-segment elevation occurred in 4 patients (36%) (Table 2).
The exercise test before angioplasty (Table 3) was positive in 8 patients (73%), and ischemia was documented on myocardial scintigraphy in 3 patients (27%). The workload, the exercise time, and the double product improved significantly after successful angioplasty. Clinical follow-up (mean 8 months, range 1—12 months), available in 8 of 11 patients was satisfactory in 7 patients; one patient underwent elective coronary artery bypass surgery for progression of coronary artery disease.

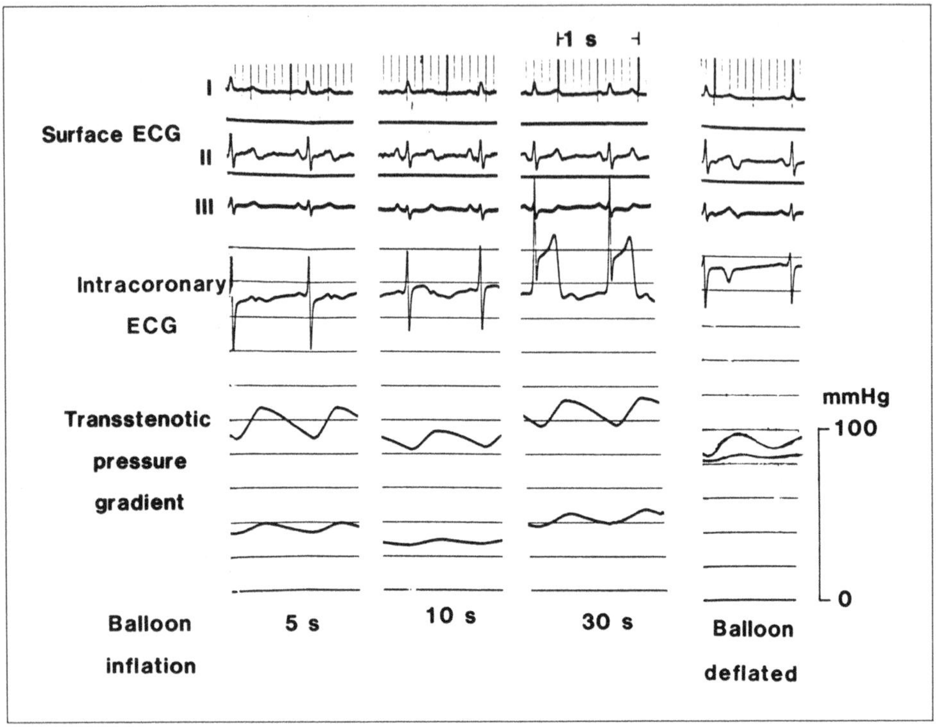

Fig. 2. Late ischemic response in a 65-year-old male patient who underwent double lesion coronary angioplasty of the left anterior descending artery. Standard leads I, II and III, and intracoronary electrocardiogram with aortic and coronary pressure recordings. Functional collaterals were demonstrated by both previous contrast injection and a coronary wedge pressure of 40 mm Hg. ST-segment elevation only at 30 s of balloon inflation.

Group III

Coronary angioplasty was successful in 17 of 19 patients. The mean diameter stenosis was reduced from 77 ± 10% to 25 ±13% and the transstenotic pressure gradient from 55 ± 17 mm Hg to 13 ± 7 mm Hg. Sixteen patients (84%) had significant ST-segment changes during angioplasty which were accompanied by angina equivalents in 7 patients. Two out of 17 patients had collaterals (Table 2). These patients showed only late (> 25 s) signs of ischemic during balloon inflation (Fig. 2).

Before angioplasty, 6 patients (32%) had electrocardiographic signs of ischemia during exercise test, and 5 patients (26%) in radionuclide tests. These signs were still present in the 2 patients with unsuccessful angioplasty. At the exercise test after successful angioplasty (Table 3), the workload, the exercise time, and the double product were significantly improved in all patients with successful angioplasty.

Clinical follow-up (mean 6 months, range 4 to 12 months) available in 7 of 17 patients with primary success was satisfactory in 5 patients. None of them had electrocardiographic or clinical evidence of a myocardial infarction, and repeat stress tests were un-

Table 3. Data of exercise tests before and after angioplasty.

Group	I (n = 5)		II (n = 11)	III (n = 19)
Symptoms				
before	0		0	8 (42%)
after	0		0	1 (5%)
ST-segment depression				
before	2 (40%)		8 (73%)	6 (32%)
after	0		0	2 (11%)
Radionuclide testing ischemia				
before	3 (60%)		3 (27%)	5 (26%)
after	0		1 (9%)	1 (5%)
Workload (watts)				
before	138±93		103±36	82±36
after	156±87	N.S.	142±30**	112±38**
Exercise time (min)				
before	17±7		12±4	10±4
after	17±9	N.S.	17±4**	13±5**
Double product (beats/min × mm Hg/100)				
before	229±74		230±56	265±75
after	234±43	N.S.	270±36**	292±60*

* $p < 0.05$, ** $p < 0.01$, N.S. = not significant.

Double product = heart rate × blood pressure in beats/min × mm Hg/100. Groups of patients: I = totally asymptomatic, II = after myocardial infarction, III = with angina equivalents.

changed from immediately after angioplasty. Two patients underwent elective coronary artery bypass surgery for recurrence.

Discussion

Myocardial ischemia is usually equated with angina pectoris, but angina is merely one of the subjective manifestations of ischemia. Typical chest pain, or any other recognised anginal equivalents need not occur during ischemic episodes. Electrocardiographic abnormalities, Thallium-201 myocardial perfusion defects, unimproved radionuclide left ventricular ejection fraction or absent rise of blood pressure with exercise (1—6) may be signs of myocardial ischemia.

Coronary angioplasty is a treatment primarily used to alleviate angina, which is obviously absent in silent ischemia. Most of our patients had unequivocal ST-segment changes during balloon inflation, representing transient myocardial ischemia. There were, however, certain differences between the groups. Totally asymptomatic patients with no previous myocardial infarction (group I) responded promptly to balloon occlusion, within 20 s by significant ST-segment changes. Patients with angina equivalents (group III) responded to balloon occlusion with electrocardiographic changes as well, while most patients with previous myocardial infarction (group II) did not. In group II therefore, collateral blood flow was sufficient to prevent significant ischemia, as indicated by the coronary wedge pressure. In one patient, no ischemia could be induced, even when balloon inflation was prolonged to 90 s. Nevertheless, the patient improved his exercise performance after successful coronary angioplasty proving that the dilated artery still served viable myocardium. The role of collaterals is crucial to the understanding of ischemic changes during coronary angioplasty. Coronary blood flow supplied by collaterals is usually adequate at rest, but inadequate during exercise. As the balloon was inflated only during the resting state, patients with good collaterals, either functional or recruitable, showed no signs of ischemia.

The issue is unsettled as to whether patients with single-vessel disease and silent myocardial ischemia should be treated with an invasive procedure, such as coronary angioplasty. There is growing evidence that patients who repeatedly have silent ischemia, may be at increased risk for serious cardiac events (10). This concern is based on the large number of patients with coronary artery disease whose first clinical manifestation is sudden death or myocardial infarction (11).

Droste and Roskamm (12) have suggested that these individuals display true albeit unexplained alterations in pain threshold and tolerance. This conclusion was based on various tests comparing pain threshold and tolerance in patients with and without silent myocardial ischemia. In each type of test, the group with silent ischemia showed a significantly different response from symptomatic patients. If some patients have alterations in pain threshold and tolerance, on eventual defect in their anginal warning system mightrepresent an added risk for myocardial infarction or sudden death, especially during exertion (1, 13). In the study of Sharma (14), many patients surviving out-of-hospital ventricular fibrillation had no anginal history and no symptoms during subsequent tests provoking ischemia.

The identification of these individuals remains an important problem. In patients with coronary risk factors, a stress test is a convenient and reasonable first procedure. Positive responders should also have a radionuclide exercise test to corroborate the result. The combination of a positive exercise electrocardiogram and an abnormal radionuclide test in the absence of symptoms markedly increases the probability of identifying asymptomatic coronary disease (15). Any combination of ST-segment depression greater than 1 mm, hypotension during the test, Thallium defects, or decrease in exercise radionuclide ejection fraction strongly suggests significant coronary artery disease. These patients should undergo coronary arteriography, and in selected patients coronary angioplasty or coronary bypass surgery should be considered. Patients with infarctions should have low level exercise tests done before discharge (16). An adverse one year prognosis in patients with abnormal responses to low-level exercise has been shown (17), and coronary arteriography and an optimal therapeutic approach was advocated (18), whether or not angina accompanies the ST-segment depression.

In conclusion, patients with silent myocardial ischemia do not differ from others with classical angina in terms of ischemic responses to angioplasty. The degree and onset of ischemia is related to the presence of collaterals. We believe that coronary angioplasty should be performed if a significant coronary artery lesion is accompanied by objective evidence of myocardial ischemia, since functional improvement could be demonstrated in most of the successful cases.

References

1. Roskamm H (1984) Closing Remarks. In: Rutishauser W, Roskamm H (eds) Silent myocardial ischemia. Springer-Verlag, Berlin, Heidelberg, New York, Tokyo, p 201

2. Cohn PF (1985) Silent myocardial ischemia: classification, prevalence, and prognosis. Am J Med 79 (suppl 3A): 2—9
3. Cohn PF (1980) Silent myocardial ischemia in patients with a defective anginal warning system. Am J Cardiol 45: 697—702
4. Righetti A, Ratib O, El-Harake B, Rutishauser W (1984) Thallium-201 myocardial scintigraphy and electrocardiographic findings in asymptomatic coronary patients during exercise. In: Rutishauser W, Roskamm H (eds) Silent myocardial ischemia. Springer-Verlag Berlin, Heidelberg, New York, Tokyo, pp 77—83
5. Pepine CJ (1986) Clinical aspects of silent myocardial ischemia in patients with angina and other forms of coronary heart disease. Am J Med 80 (suppl 5C): 25—34
6. Deanfield JE, Shea M, Ribiero P, De Landsheere CM, Wilson RA, Horlock P, Selwyn AP (1984) Transient ST-segment depression as a marker of myocardial ischemia during daily life. Am J Cardiol 54: 1195—1200
7. Cohn PF (1984) Time for new approach to management of patients with both symptomatic and asymptomatic episodes of myocardial ischemia. Am J Cardiol 54: 1358—1359
8. Meier B, Luethy P (1984) Coronary wedge pressure as predictor of recruitable collateral arteries. Circulation Suppl II 70: 1062 (Abstr)
9. Meier B, Killisch JP, Adatte JJ, Casalini P, Rutishauser W (1985) Intrakoronares Elektrokardiogramm während transluminaler Koronarangioplastie. Schweiz med Wschr 115: 1590—1593
10. Cohn PF (1984) When is concern about silent myocardial ischemia justified? Ann Intern Med 100: 597—599
11. Kannel WB, Abbott RD (1984) Incidence and prognosis of unrecognized myocardial infarction. An update on the Framingham Study. N Engl J Med 311: 1144—1147
12. Droste C, Roskamm H (1983) Experimental pain measurement in patients with asymptomatic myocardial ischemia. J Am Coll Cardiol 1: 940—945
13. Uhl GS, Froelicher V (1983) Screening for asymptomatic coronary artery disease. J Am Coll Cardiol 1: 946—955
14. Sharma B, Francis G, Hodges M, Asinger R (1981) Demonstration of exercise-induced ischemia without angina in patients who recover from out-of-hospital ventricular fibrillation. Am J Cardiol 47: 445 (Abstr)
15. Cohn PF (1984) Silent myocardial ischemia: concern is justified for the patients with known coronary artery disease. Ann Intern Med 100: 599—601
16. Cohn PF (1983) The role of noninvasive cardiac testing after an uncomplicated myocardial infarction. N Engl J Med 309: 90—93
17. Fioretti P, Brower RW, Simoons ML, Bos RJ, Baardman T, Beelen A, Hugenholtz G (1985) Prediction of mortality during the first year after acute myocardial infarction from clinical variables and stress test at hospital discharge. Am J Cardiol 55: 1313—1318
18. FitzGibbon GM, Keon WJ, Burton JR (1984) Aorto-coronary bypass in patients with coronary artery disease who do not have angina. J Thorac Cardiovasc Surg 87: 717—724

Authors' address:
Prof. Dr. W. Rutishauser
Cardiology Center
University Hospital
1211 Geneva 4
Switzerland

Alleviation of silent ischemia by PTCA

B. Höfling, A. Stäblein, Th. v. Arnim

Medizinische Klinik I der Universität München, Klinikum Großhadern

Introduction

Generally, PTCA is indicated in patients with symptomatic angina, refractory to medical therapy, if the underlying stenosis is suitable for balloon dilatation (4, 7, 8). Following the guidelines of the Council on Scientific Affairs "relatively asymptomatic patients with strong objective evidence of myocardial ischemia . . . may also be considered for PTCA" (3). In these cases „silent ischemia" represents a substantial factor for the indication of PTCA.

In this paper we investigate whether PTCA can alleviate signs of silent ischemia in the above mentioned category of patients. The phenomenon of silent ischemia can also be seen during PTCA, i.e. signs of severe ischemia appear in ECG without anginal symptoms (1). We tested whether these signs of ischemia can be alleviated by intracoronary applied drugs, such as Nifedipine i.c.

Methods

We report on the phenomenon of "silent ischemia" related to

- PTCA indication (positive stress test and T1 201-SPECT in relatively asymptomatic patients),
- PTCA monitoring (balloon inflation induced ischemic changes (in 12-lead ECG appearing prior to angina).

Thallium-201 SPECT

T1-SPECT according to the following protocol (2) was performed in 17 asymptomatic patients:

- Bicycle exercise up to ST depression ($\geq$ 0.2 mV) or age-standardized maximum workload.
- Injection of 2 mCi T1-Chloride i.v. during the last minute of exercise.
- The measurements were performed immediately after stress-test and 3 h later.
- For data acquisition, the patient was lying on a couch with the heads of the gamma camera rotating around the chest.
- After data acquisition (22 min) the transverse slices were reconstructed using filtered backprojection, followed by the calculation of the sagittal, frontal and oblique-frontal planes.

The same procedure was repeated after PTCA and the results were compared.

12-lead ECG monitoring

During routine PTCA we continuously recorded a complete ECG with 12 chest and limb leads using X-ray transparent electrodes and wires, which we designed in our laboratory. We registered the appearance-time of significant ST-T-changes after balloon inflation, the number of involved chest leads, the duration of the ischemic changes and the interval between balloon deflation and recovery of ECG. The appearance times of ECG and anginal pain were compared.
We then studied the effect of 0.2 mg Nifedipine intracoronary (Adalat intrakoronar®) on the described ECG parameters. These investigations were started after previous repetitive balloon dilatations, when the appearance time of ECG changes proved to be constant.

Results and Discussion

PTCA-induced changes of T1-SPECT in asymptomatic patients

Seventeen patients with high-grade stenoses in major vessels and presumably a high amount of myocardium at risk, who were in clinical class I or II (CHC) and showed no chest pain during stress test were analyzed. According to the images in T1-SPECT stress test, we always subdivide our patients into five groups:

Group 1. No Thallium defect (by definition "silent ischemia" none of the described patients fell into this group).

Group 2. Minor* T1-defects immediately after stress with total redistribution after 3 h at rest. None of our patients with silent ischemia fell into this category.

Group 3. Major* T1-defects immediately after stress, with total redistribution after 3 h rest ($n = 4$). All these patients had an infarction prior to PTCA.

Group 4. Major* T1-defects immediately after stress, with partial redistribution after 3 h at rest ($n = 2$). Both patients had a history of myocardial infarction.

Group 5. T1-defects after stress test, persisting over 3 h at rest ($n = 11$). Ten of these patients had had a previous myocardial infarction.

After PTCA the distribution of the patients was as follows:

Group 1. $n = 8$ with 8 cases of infarction prior to PTCA.
Group 2. $n = 1$ with myocardial infarction prior to PTCA.
Group 3. $n = 2$ one of them had an infarction pre-PTCA.
Group 4. $n = 2$ with 2 cases of infarction prior to PTCA.
Group 5. $n = 4$ with 4 cases of infarction prior to PTCA.

The course of the individual patients can be seen in Fig. 1. Of 17 patients, 12 had an improved T1-score after PTCA, four remained unchanged and one deteriorated according to the T1-scan. This latter patient had a temporary occlusion during PTCA (10 min) and could be recanalized. There was no residual stenosis in the final result and no clinical event between PTCA and post-PTCA T1-scan.

---

* The terms "minor" and "major" defects correspond to a non-quantitative visual evaluation of TI-images. This classification proved to correlate roughly with sophisticated quantitative coefficients (5, 6).

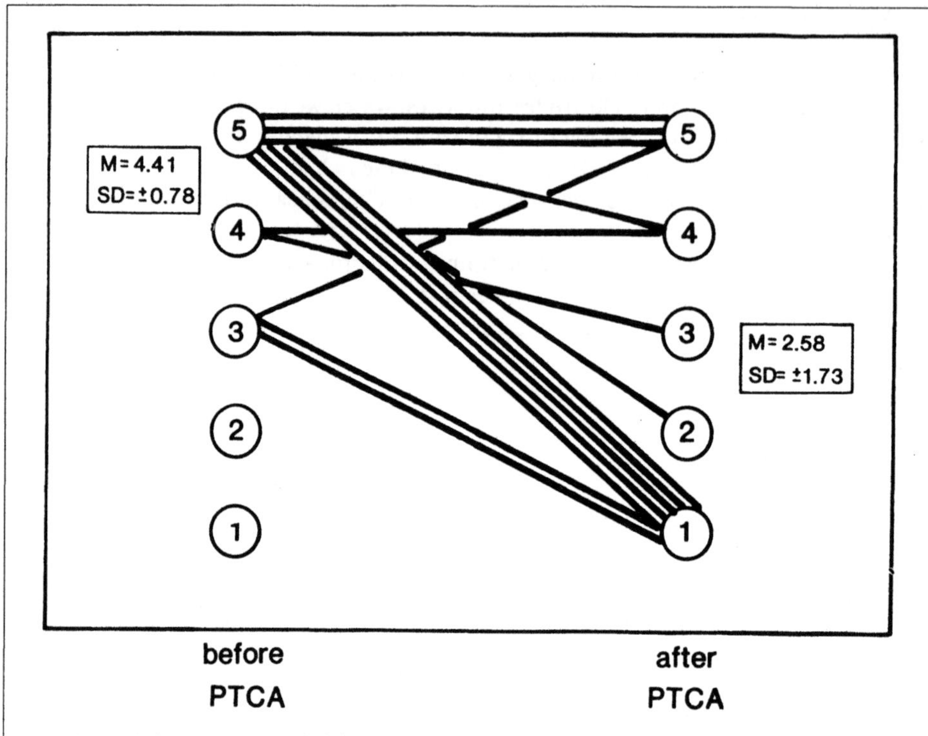

Fig. 1. Graduation of ischemia as detected by T1-201-SPECT in 17 asymptomatic patients and the fluctuation towards lower scores after PTCA. ① = no Thallium defect after exercise ② = minor-, ③ = major T1-defect after stress with redistribution after 3 h ④ = with partial-, ⑤ = without redistribution. M = mean score of the 17 patients before and after balloon dilatation.

It is noteworthy that 16/17 patients had a previous myocardial infarction which could be related to the stenosis in 15/16 cases. Nevertheless, asymptomatic objective signs of severe ischemia in the infarcted areas were documented pre-PTCA and improved by the intervention in the majority of cases. This analysis teaches us that infarcted areas may be composed of scarred tissue as well as of considerable amounts of vital, but jeopardized myocardium, which can be salvaged by an intervention. Furthermore a persisting T1-defect does not necessarily represent scar tissue, it can well signal most severe ischemia, reversible by PTCA.

PTCA-induced ECG changes and their alleviation by intracoronary Nifedipine

Continuous 12-lead ECG-registration during each single balloon-inflation in 104 patients showed the following results (see Fig. 2).
Eight patients had neither ECG changes, nor anginal pain during balloon inflation (duration 45 ± 23 s). Of these patients 7 (88%) had a myocardial infarction prior to PTCA, which could be related to the approached stenosis. ST-T-changes with an onset of

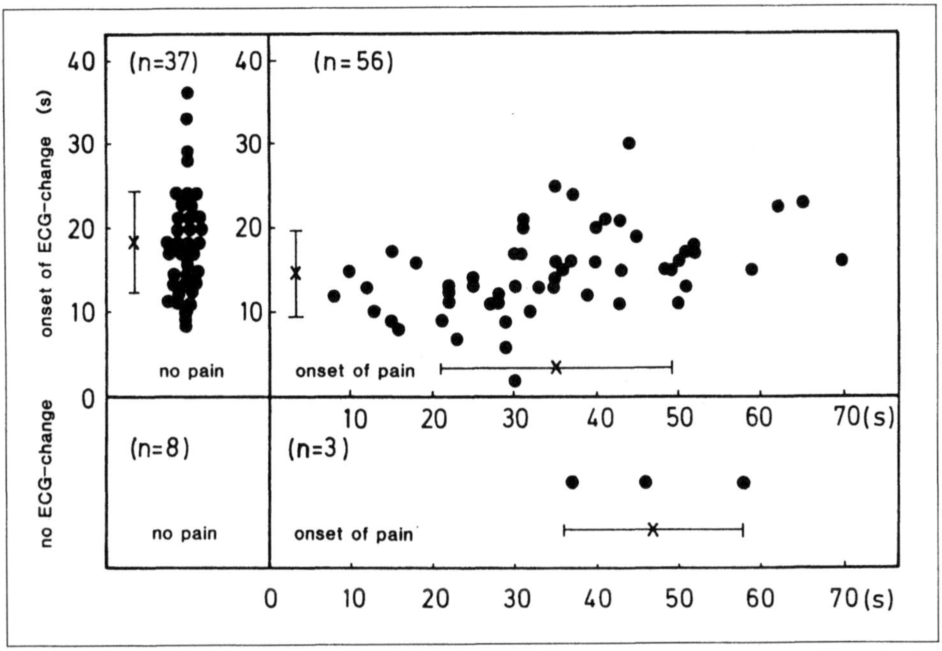

Fig. 2. Analysis of ECG changes and pain in 104 patients undergoing routine PTCA. Differentiation into four groups:

1. no pain, no ECG changes ($n = 8$)
2. no pain, but ischemic ECG changes ($n = 37$) (silent ischemia)
3. ECG changes and pain ($n = 56$) (interval of silent ischemia = 20 s)
4. subjective pain without ECG changes ($n = 3$)

18.5 ± 6.2 s after balloon inflation were seen in 37 patients, but no pain during dilatation over a period of 44 ± 17 s. The duration of the ST-T-changes was 49.8 ± 18.1 s. Of 37 patients, 20 (54%) showed a myocardial infarction prior to PTCA.

ST-T-changes with an onset of 14.7 ± 5.0 s after balloon inflation and anginal pain beginning 35 ± 14 s after dilatation were seen in 56 patients. The duration of balloon insufflation was 44 ± 12 s, while the duration of ECG changes was 50.2 ± 15.1 s. Of the 56 patients, 32 (57%) had a myocardial infarction before PTCA. Three patients had anginal pain, but no ischemic ECG changes during balloon inflation. The onset of pain was 47 ± 11 s, while the mean duration of the balloon insufflations was 54 ± 12 s. Two of these patients showed an infarction prior to PTCA.

In all four groups the balloon inflation time did not differ significantly. If no pain and no ECG changes occurred, the percentage of pre-PTCA infarctions was higher, compared to the groups where ECG changes, pain, or both could be seen.

Interestingly, if pain occurred, the onset of ECG changes was significantly earlier ($p < 0.005$) than in those cases where no pain was reported by the patient.

The second group (37/104) showed the phenomenon of silent ischemia and the third group (56/104) showed a period of transient silent ischemia (between 14.7 ± 5.0 and 35 ± 14 s).

In 16 patients, we tested whether 0.2 mg Nifedipine intracoronary can alleviate silent (ECG) and apparent (angina) signs of balloon-induced ischemia. Steady state was achieved by previous repetitive balloon inflations. The appearance time of ECG changes following balloon inflation was 17.1 ± 8.4 s without intracoronary pretreatment, and 20.5 ± 10.9 s after intracoronary application of 0.2 mg Nifedipine ($p > 0.1$) (see Fig. 3). The ischemic ECG changes due to balloon-induced vessel occlusion could be prevented by intracoronary injection of 0.2 mg Nifedipine in 5/16 patients; one patient had ECG changes only after Nifedipine intracoronary.

Fig. 3. Appearance time (s) of ECG changes (●) due to balloon-induced vessel occlusion before and after intracoronary Nifedipine. Note: 5 patients (○) who had ECG-changes before Nifedipin intracoronary did not show such ischemic signs after Nifedipine. One patient with no ECG-changes during dilatation before Nifedipine i.c. had ischemic ECG alterations after intracoronary injection of Nifedipine.

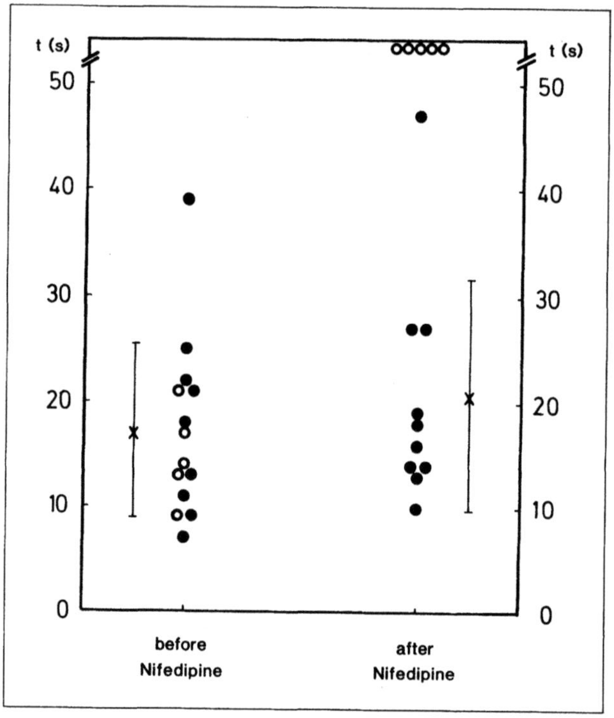

Furthermore we graduated the ST-segment changes (Fig. 4) and saw a shift towards lower grades after Nifedipine intracoronary. The appearance time of anginal pain was not influenced by intracoronary Nifedipine (40 ± 19 s vs 40 ± 16 s). The frequency of anginal pain induced by balloon inflation also was not influenced by intracoronary Nifedipine (pain in 49% of the inflations without Nifedipine vs 53% after Nifedipine i.c.), however anginal pain was less severe after Nifedipine, a repetitive statement of patients that cannot be objectively quantified.

Thus our results demonstrate that Nifedipine intracoronary barely affects the appearance time, if ECG changes are present; however, it clearly reduces the severity of ischemic signs.

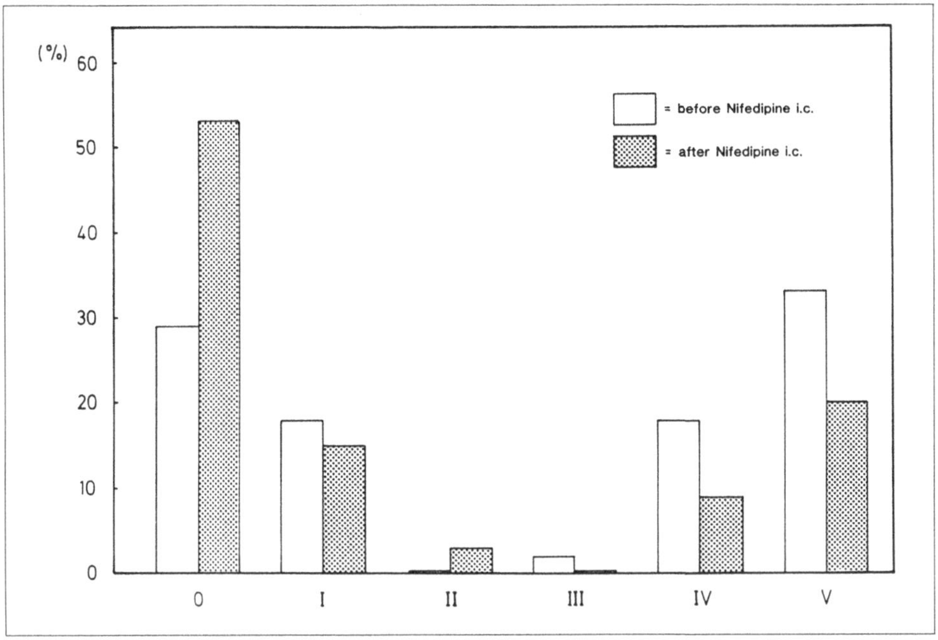

Fig. 4. ECG changes after balloon-induced vessel occlusion in 104 patients before (□) and after (□) Nifedipine intracoronary. Ordinate: Percentage of patients. Abscissa: 0 = no ECG-changes; I = T-changes (Amplitude changes $\geq$ 0.1 mV); II = ST depression $\leq$ 0.2 mV; III = ST depression $>$ 0.2 mV; IV = ST elevation $\leq$ 0.1 mV; V = ST elevation $>$ 0.1 mV.

Conclusions

We demonstrated that PTCA is able to decrease signs of silent ischemia. This finding supports the indication for PTCA as proposed by the Council on Scientific Affairs (3); however, it does not prove that PTCA is able to prolong life in asymptomatic patients. Intracoronary Nifedipine is able to alleviate signs of silent ischemia during PTCA. This result is significant for prolonging balloon inflation time and management of complications.

References

1. von Arnim T, Stäblein A, Höfling B (1986) Detection of Ischemia during PTCA with Extended Electrocardiographic Monitoring. In: Höfling B (ed) Current problems in PTCA. Steinkopff-Verlag Darmstadt, Springer Verlag New York
2. Büll U, Kirsch CM, Höfling B, Roedler HD (1986) Ergebnisse der 201-Thallium SPECT des Myokards zur Erfassung der Koronaren Herzkrankheit und zur Verlaufskontrolle bei PTCA. Nuklearmedizin 25: 71—77
3. Council on Scientific Affairs (1984) Percutaneous transluminal angioplasty. JAMA 251: 764
4. Höfling B, von Arnim T, Stäblein A, Kreuzer E, Kemkes B (1986) Current indications for PTCA. In: Höfling B (ed) Current problems in PTCA. Steinkopff-Verlag Darmstadt, Springer Verlag New York

5. Höfling B, Stäblein A, von Arnim Th, Werdan K, Graeven C, Kirsch CM, Moser E, Büll U (1987) Stellenwert der Thallium-201-SPECT bei Indikationsstellung und Erfolgskontrolle der Ballondilatation. In: Felix, Wolf, Zeitler (eds) Neues im Kontrastbild (in press)
6. Kanemoto N, Hör G (1985) Improvement of Regional Myocardial Perfusion Following Percutaneous Transluminal Coronary Angioplasty in Patients with Coronary Artery Disease. Jpn Heart J 26: 495–508
7. Kent KM (1985) Indications for Transluminal Coronary Angioplasty. Circulation 72 (suppl V): V166–V168
8. Meier B, Grüntzig A (1984) Indikationen der transluminalen Koronardilatation. Dtsch med Wschr 109: 673–675

Authors' address:
PD Dr. B. Höfling
Medizinische Kinik I
Klinikum Großhadern der
Universität München
Marchioninistraße 15
8000 München 70

Guiding anti-ischemic therapy by Holter monitoring

D. Tzivoni, A. Keren, A. Gavish, J. Benhorin, and S. Stern

Heiden Department of Cardiology, Bikur Cholim Hospital and the Hebrew University Hadassah Medical School, Jerusalem, Israel

The dynamic nature of ischemic changes during daily activities

Ischemic changes frequently occur in patients with coronary artery disease (CAD) during heavy or light exercise, mental stress, at rest or even during sleep (1—5). Most of the ischemic episodes, occur without any significant increase in heart rate or blood pressure, indicating that the main mechanism for these ischemic episodes is not an increase in MVO_2 but rather a decrease in coronary perfusion, or a combination of both. Continuous recording of the ECG of patients with CAD, at home, at work and under various conditions, provided important information on the characteristics of the ischemic changes. In our recent study (3) of 210 patients who had Holter monitoring for 24 hours, ischemic changes were detected in 97. These ischemic changes were much more frequent during the waking hours, and developed at a relatively low heart rate (94/min). These patients also had a treadmill stress test, during which the threshold of ischemia, (heart rate at which 1 mm of ST depression developed) was significantly higher (109/min) than during daily activities. The ischemic episodes lasted from 2 to 240 minutes, and the number of episodes also varied markedly from patient to patient. While some patients had only one episode per day, others had up to 15 per day, and the duration of ischemia varied accordingly from 2 minutes to 240 minutes per day. Thus, it seems that the activity of CAD varies markedly from patient to patient, and the true incidence and duration of ischemia during everyday life can be established only by Holter monitoring.

As early as 1974, we described ST depressions during daily activities in CAD patients which were not associated with any symptomatology (6—8) and attributed them to myocardial ischemia. These findings were confirmed in 1976 by Allen et al. (9) and by Schang et al. (10) in 1977. In our recent study (3), 97 patients had 351 ischemic episodes, of which 241 were silent and 110 were symptomatic. In 46 of the 97 patients all ischemic episodes were silent, in 15 all episodes were symptomatic, and in 36 both symptomatic and asymptomatic episodes were recorded. Thus, in only 15 of the 97 patients could the activity of the disease be correctly assessed by the symptoms, while in the others, chest pain was either not present at all, or was present in only part of the episodes. Some of our symptomatic patients with angina pectoris, who had several monitoring periods, were completely asymptomatic on other monitoring days. Holter monitoring revealed that they had the same number of ischemic episodes during the symptomatic and the asymptomatic days, indicating that symptoms are poor indicators of the activity of the ischemic process.

Von Arnim and coworkers (4) performed Holter monitoring during daily activity in 296 CAD patients. Seventy of these patients had 221 episodes of ST depression or elevation. Only 34% of these episodes were symptomatic. The duration of the episode, the heart rate at the beginning of the episode, or the extent of ST deviation were not related to the occurrence of pain.

The characteristics of silent and symptomatic ischemic episodes were studied by Stern et al. (11) who found that these episodes were identical with regard to their duration, degree of ST depression and the heart rate of appearance of ST depression. Patients with silent ischemic episodes were found to have a similar degree of coronary pathology. Deanfield and coworkers (5), using Rubidium 82 tomography, confirmed that silent ischemic episodes are similar to symptomatic ones, and that they are also similar to those induced by exercise with regard to location and extent of myocardial perfusion defects.

Today, anti-anginal therapy is guided mainly by the patient's symptoms. Patients with more severe and frequent symptoms receive more intensive anti-anginal therapy, while patients with rare symptoms usually receive only minimal therapy. Deterioration of anginal symptoms is usually regarded as an indication to increase anti-anginal therapy. This traditional concept, that one can judge the activity of the coronary disease by the patient's symptoms, has been challenged by the above reports and by many others. As a consequence of this new approach, in recent years many studies have utilized changes in frequency and duration of ischemic episodes during daily activities for evaluating the efficacy of anti-ischemic (not anti-anginal) drugs.

Nitrates and myocardial ischemia

Various forms of nitrates are used by most patients suffering from angina pectoris. It is the experience of every clinician that they are effective in reducing the frequency of anginal episodes. The question is, can they also reduce the frequency of silent ischemia? Schang and Pepine (10) found that hourly administration of sublingual nitroglycerin prevented or markedly reduced the frequency of silent and symptomatic ischemic episodes. Distante et al. (12) found that in patients with unstable angina and frequent silent ischemic episodes, continuous infusion of isosorbide dinitrate, eliminated all silent episodes of ST depression, and markedly reduced the frequency of ST elevation.

Shell (13) used Holter monitoring to study the effect of transdermal nitroglycerin on the number, duration and magnitude of ischemic events in 8 patients with chronic stable angina. They increased the dosage of the transdermal nitroglycerin in each patient until the disappearance of anginal symptoms. Thereafter, the 24-hour Holter monitoring was repeated. The number of symptomatic events decreased in all the 8 patients. The total number of events was reduced from 5.8 to 0.9/24 h. The duration of the ischemic episodes decreased from 110 to 21 minutes/24 h, and the magnitude of ischemia, as estimated by the ischemia-magnitude integral, was also significantly decreased.

Levin and coworkers (14), used programmable real time Holter monitoring for evaluating the effect of transdermal nitroglycerin in 26 patients. During 10 days on placebo, these patients had 69 ischemic episodes, while during 10 days on nitroglycerin they had only 33 ischemic episodes. The duration of ischemic was also reduced from 102 minutes to 46 minutes.

Beta blockers and myocardial ischemia

Glazier and coworkers (15) studied the efficacy of atenolol in 10 patients with angina pectoris. During a placebo period they had 264 ischemic episodes, 80% of which were silent. During atenolol therapy, there was a 63% suppression in the number of episodes. Atenolol was more effective in preventing ischemic episodes that were preceded by an increase in heart rate (72% suppression) than those that were not (49% suppression). Quyyumi et al. (16) compared the effects of two beta blockers on spontaneous ischemic episodes. They found that atenolol, a selective beta blocker, reduced the frequency of ischemic episodes from 8.0/24 h to 3.7/24 h, and their duration from 228 minutes /24 h to 66 minutes/24 h and also the magnitude of ischemic episodes; while pindolol, a non-selective beta blocker with intrinsic sympathomimetic activity, had only a minimal effect. Atenolol reduced the frequency of both symptomatic and silent episodes.

Rod et al. (17) evaluated the effect of acebutalol in 23 patients with coronary disease by treadmill stress testing and ambulatory ECG monitoring. The number of spontaneous episodes was significantly decreased, especially in patients who were beta blocked (had a significant reduction in heart rate). These patients also had a significant improvement in their exercise ST depression response. Holter monitoring had an advantage over treadmill testing only in patients who, because of weakness, were unable to complete the treadmill exercise.

Quyyumi and coworkers (18) in another study of 10 patients with coronary disease, evaluated the effects of labetalol, an alpha-beta blocking agent, on ischemic episodes. Labetalol reduced the frequency of ischemic episodes by 56% and their duration by 73%. This drug was effective in reducing both symptomatic and silent ischemic episodes.

Since some authors have cast doubts on the effectiveness of beta blocking agents in patients unstable angina, Gottlieb et al. (19) performed Holter monitoring in 81 such patients. Thirty-nine were assigned to placebo and 42 to propanolol therapy (at least 160 mg/day). All patients were also treated with vasodilators, nifedipine and long acting nitrates. The incidence of cardiac death, myocardial infarction, and the requirement for coronary bypass surgery or coronary angioplasty, did not differ between the two groups. However, during propanolol therapy the mean number of ischemic episodes per 48 hours of monitoring was 2.0, and during placebo 3.8 ($p = 0.03$). The mean duration of ischemic episodes was also lower in the propanolol group (43 min) than in the placebo group (104 min, $p = 0.039$). It seems therefore, that in patients with unstable angina, the addition of propanolol to nitrates and nifedipine has beneficial and not detrimental effects.

Calcium antagonists and myocardial ischemia

Calcium antagonists are expected to be efficacious especially in patients with spontaneous ischemic episodes. Since documentation of such episodes are best achieved by Holter monitoring, it is not surprising that many recent studies have evaluated the efficacy of calcium antagonists in different ischemic syndromes by this method. Cocco and coworkers (20) studied 12 patients with stable angina pectoris. During the monitoring day, in 6 of the 7 patients who had silent ischemic episodes, these episodes were reduced or eliminated by nifedipine, while only 1 out of 5 showed improvement with pindolol.

Fazzini et al. (21), studied the effect of diltiazem on spontaneous angina in a double-blind cross-over study of 20 patients. During treatment with diltiazem, the number of ischemic episodes was reduced from 357 to 100 ($p < 0.001$). Diltiazem was more effective in the morning hours than in the evening, and was also more effective in preventing ST elevation than ST depression.

The effect of verapamil and nifedipine was studied by Piccolo and coworkers (22) in 15 patients who were admitted to the coronary care unit for spontaneous angina. During the placebo period, 243 ischemic episodes were recorded. The number of ischemic episodes decreased to 129 during verapamil treatment (60 mg/day) ($p < 0.05$), and to 57 during nifedipine treatment (480 mg/day) ($p < 0.01$). Both drugs were especially effective in patients with the variant form of angina. The effect of verapamil was compared by Parodi and coworkers (23) to that of propanolol in patients with spontaneous angina. The mean number of ischemic episodes, as recorded by Holter monitoring, was 25/48 h. The frequency of ischemic episodes was not significantly reduced during two propranolol treatment periods (23 episodes 48 h), but was reduced significantly by treatment with verapamil (5 events; $p < 0.01$).

Oakley et al. (24) assessed the effects of propanolol, nifedipine and the combination of these drugs in 6 patients with angina pectoris. Each drug reduced the number of both symptomatic and asymptomatic ischemic episodes. However, the combination of the two drugs was significantly more effective than was each one alone. During the control period, the number of ischemic episodes was 47/day; during propanolol (480 mg/day), 20/day; during nifedipine (60 mg/day), 23/day; while during a combination of nifedipine and propranolol, only 10 episodes were observed per day.

Gelman and coworkers (25) studied the effects of nicardipine, a new calcium antagonist, on angina at rest. Among the 17 patients studied, 11 had previously unsatisfactory results with long acting nitrates or other calcium channel blockers. During nicardipine therapy, the frequency of angina decreased compared to placebo (0.47 vs 2.11 attacks/day; $p < 0.05$). There was a similar decrease in nitroglycerin requirements. Nicardipine was effective and safe in preventing both symptomatic and silent ischemic episodes.

Advantages of Holter monitoring in assessing anti-ischemic therapy

Exercise testing is the most widely-used method for evaluating efficacy of antianginal drugs. However, since many of the ischemic episodes occur during everyday life, without the provocation of a heavy physical stress, it seems logical to record the ECG under similar conditions and to evaluate the frequency, duration and severity of the ischemic episodes with and without therapy. Exercise testing is probably a faster and simpler method to assess drug efficacy in patients with effort induced ischemia only. These patients have heart rate-dependent ischemia, and therefore they will enjoy betablockers with or without additional medications. On the other hand, patients in whom ischemic changes are not induced by effort, Holter monitoring seems to be a logical method to assess therapy, especially if vasodilators are employed. Two patients may have the same response to a stress test, yet one may have 1—2 ischemic episodes per day, while the other may have very frequent episodes. We believe that patients with frequent and prolonged episodes required a more aggressive approach.

Day-to-day variability of myocardial ischemia

When trying to assess the efficacy of an anti-ischemic drug by Holter monitoring, one should take into consideration the marked day-to-day variability of myocardial ischemia. Recently we performed 72 hours of Holter monitoring in 18 patients with coronary heart disease and ischemic episodes during daily activity (26). We found marked variability between different patients in the frequency and duration of ischemic changes. This marked variability can be attributed to the differences in activity and severity of the coronary disease in different patients. Surprisingly, we also found, marked variability in individual patients on different days (Fig. 1). The day-to-day variability was 36% in the number of ischemic episodes and 51% in their duration. Slightly less variability was observed in the maximal degree of ST depression (31%) and only minimal variation was found in the heart rate at the beginning of ST depression (9%). We also evaluated the additional information of each of the 3 monitoring days for assessing the severity of ischemic changes. We came to the conclusion that during two monitoring days, 80—90% of the maximal severity of ischemic changes had already been detected, thus the third day added very little information. The number of ischemic episodes per 24 hours varied from 2 to 15 (mean = 6.5). The duration of ischemic episodes per 24 hours varied from 6 to 419 minutes (mean = 76 minutes). The maximal ST depression varied from 1 to 6 mm (mean = 3.4 mm).

Because of the marked variability of ischemic episodes, both between patients and in individual patients on different days, in order to prove the efficacy of an anti-ischemic drug by Holter monitoring, the reduction in the number of ischemic episodes and in their duration should exceed the day-to-day variation. We calculated that for a significant suppression ($p < 0.05$) in the number of ischemic episodes in a study group of 20 patients, with a mean number of ischemic episodes per day of 6.5, the number of ischemic episodes per day should be reduced by the anti-ischemic drug by an average of 2.3. If the total duration of ischemia per day is used, a significant anti-ischemic effect ($p < 0.05$) is achieved if the mean duration of ischemia is reduced by 68.5 minutes.

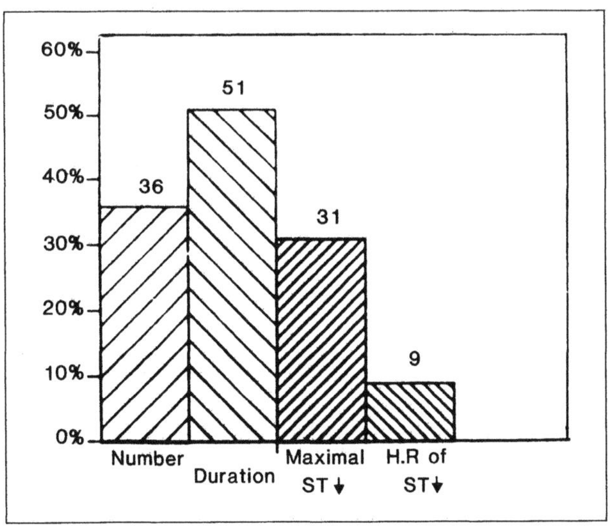

Fig. 1. The day-to-day variability (in percent) in individual patients in the number of ischemic changes, their duration, the maximal degree of ST depression and the heart rate at the beginning of ST depression.

For an individual patient, it is almost impossible to prove the anti-ischemic effect of a drug as the required reduction in the number of ischemic episodes is 7/day. Since most patients have less than 7 episodes per day, drug efficacy cannot be established in them. One can slightly reduce this figure by adding a second monitoring day. Thus for assessing efficacy of an anti-ischemic drug by Holter monitoring, a group study is required. The size of this group and the duration of monitoring will depend on the frequency and duration of ischemic episodes in the study group.

References

1. Stern S, Tzivoni D (1976) The dynamic nature of the ST-T segment in ischemic heart disease. Am Heart J 91: 820—822
2. Stern S, Tzivoni D (1973) Dynamic changes in the ST-T segment during sleep in ischemic heart disease. Am J Cardiol 32: 17—21
3. Tzivoni D, Gavish A, Benhorin J, Keren A, Stern S (1986) Myocardial ischemia during daily activities and stress. Am J Cardiol 58: 47B—50B
4. von Arnim T, Hofling B, Schreiber M (1985) Characteristics of episodes of ST elevation or ST depression during ambulatory monitoring in patients subsequently undergoing coronary angiography. Brit Heart J 43: 484—488
5. Deanfield JE, Shea M, Ribiero P, de Landsheere CM, Wilson RA, Horlock P, Selwyn AP (1984) Transient ST-segment depression as a maker of myocardial ischemia during daily life. Am J Cardiol 54: 1195—1200
6. Stern S, Tzivoni D (1974) Early detection of silent ischemic heart disease by 24 hour ECG monitoring of active subjects. Br Heart J 36: 481—486
7. Wolf E, Tzivoni D, Stern S (1974) Comparison of exercise test and 24-hour-ambulatory electrocardiographic monitoring in detection of ST-T changes. Br Heart J 36: 90—95
8. Stern S, Tzivoni D, Stern Z (1975) Diagnostic accuracy of ambulatory ECG monitoring in ischemic heart disease. Circulation 52: 1045—1049
9. Allen RD, Gettes LS, Phalan C, Avington MD (1976) Painless ST-segment depression in patients with angina pectoris. Chest 69: 467—473
10. Schang SJ, Pepine CJ (1977) Transient asymptomatic ST-segment depressing during daily activity. Am J Cardiol 39: 396—402
11. Stern S, Gavish A, Weisz G, Benhorin J, Tzivoni D (1986) Characteristics of silent and symptomatic myocardial ischemia during everyday activity (Abstr) Circulation 74(II): 57
12. Distante A, Maseri A, Severi S (1979) Management of vasopastic angina at rest with continuous infusion of isosorbide dinitrate: a double-crossover study in a coronary care unit. Am J Cardiol 44: 533—539
13. Shell WE (1985) Mechanisms and therapy of silent myocardial ischemia and the effect of transdermal nitroglycerin. Am J Cardiol 56: 231—271
14. Levin RI, Keller B, Campbell DQ (1986) Long-term ambulatory ECG monitoring for optimizing anti-ischemic therapy. (Abstr) Circulation 74(II): 190
15. Glazier JJ, Chierchia S, Gerosa S, Crean PA, Berkenboom G, Maseri A (1986) Atenolol prevents silent and painful ischemia in patients with mixed angina. Circulation (Abstr) 74(II): 45
16. Quyyumi AA, Wright C, Mockus L et al (1984) Effect of partial agonist activity in beta-blockers in severe angina pectoris. Br Med J 289: 951—953
17. Rod JL, Admon D, Kimchi A, Gotsman MS, Lewis BS (1979) Evaluation of the beta-blocking drug acebutol in angina pectoris. Am Heart J 98: 604—612
18. Quyyumi AA, Wright C, Mockus L et al (1985) Effects of combined alpha and beta-adrenoceptor blockade in patients with angina pectoris: a double-blind study comparing labetalol with placebo. Br Heart J 53: 47—52
19. Gottlieb SO, Weisfeld ML, Ouyang P, Achuff SC, Baughman KL, Traill TA, Brinker JA, Shapiro EP, Chandra NC, Mellits ED, et al (1986) Effect of the addition of propanolol to therapy with nifedipine for unstable angina pectoris: a randomized, double-blind, placebo — controlled trial. Circulation 73: 331—337

20. Cocco G, Strozzi C, Chu D et al (1979) Therapeutic effects of pindolol and nifedipine in patients with stable angina pectoris and asymptomatic resting ischemia. Eur J Cardiol 10: 59—69
21. Fazzini PF, Multino D, Zambaldi G (1985) Diltiazem in spontaneous angina: double blind cross over study with Holter monitoring. G Ital Cardiol 15: 1085—1089
22. Piccolo E, Cazzin R, Sartori F, Artusi L, Pascotto P (1982) Effects of oral calcium-antagonists in spontaneous angina. Verapamil and nifedipine in a double-blind cross-over trial. G Ital Cardiol 12: 359—364
23. Parodi O, Simonetti I, L'Abbate A, Maseri (1982) Verapamil versus propranolol for angina at rest. Am J Cardiol 50: 923—928
24. Oakley GDG, Fox KM, Dargie HJ, et al (1979) Objective assessment of treatment in severe angina. Br Med J 1: 1540
25. Gelman JS, Feldman RL, Scott E, Pepine CJ (1985) Nicardipine for angina pectoris at rest and coronary arterial spasm. Am J Cardiol 56: 232—236
26. Tzivoni D, Gavish A, Keren A, Stern S (1986) Day-to-Day variations of ischemic changes on Holter monitoring. (Abstr) Circulation 74(II): 507

Authors' address:
Dan Tzivoni, MD
Department of Cardiology
Bikur Cholim Hospital
P.O.B. 492
Jerusalem, Israel

Silent myocardial ischemia: Current concepts and management

L. Resnekov*

Department of Medicine, Section of Cardiology, University of Chicago, Chicago, Illinois

Introduction

Even when severe, myocardial ischemia may occur and symptoms be absent (1). In the same individual and at differing times, myocardial ischemia may occur with symptoms and at other times with apparently equivalent degrees of ischemia, symptoms are absent (2).

To unify these facts, it is important to recognize that although arterioslcerosis is an important cause of narrowings of the epicardial coronary artery, it is by no means the only mechanism by which ischemia can occur. Coronary artery spasm may also bring about a sudden reduction in blood supply to regions of the myocardium. It can affect both epicardial and intramyocardial arteries; the degree of ischemia associated can be profound and the duration variable (3—5). In addition, the role of platelets as they aggregate at the site of endocardial atherosclerotic plaques is yet another factor. Vaso-active chemical substances, such as thromboxane A2, are released and in atherosclerotic coronary arterial walls the effect of the dilating prostacyclin may be blunted. Other vaso-active chemical agents that are part of the arachadonic acid cycle and which may also help precipitate ischemia are the leukotrienes and breakdown products of a eicosatetraenoic acid. Also, mental stress may precipitate myocardial ischemia; long postulated, but only recently convincingly demonstrated (6).

Clinical presentation of myocardial ischemia

Myocardial ischemia occurs not only with angina pectoris as its major symptom but fatigue and breathlessness, particularly when paroxysmal, are equally important as symptoms. Their occurrence suggests associated left ventricular dysfunction, a result of the sudden precipitation of myocardial ischemia. On the other hand, ischemia may be silent (without there being any symptoms precipitated) and silent and symptomatic ischemia may vary. Contrary to classical teaching, there is, in fact, little relationship between the severity of ischemia and the degree or duration of symptoms. Furthermore, during an episode of otherwise asymptomatic myocardial ischemia, dangerous ventricular rhythm disturbances may be precipitated and sudden death can occur (1).

---

* Dr. Resnekov is the Rawson Professor of Medicine (Cardiology)

Diagnosis of silent myocardial ischemia

The following investigations may document that silent myocardial ischemia is occurring:

1. Long-term ECG Monitoring

As documented by Holter (7) ambulatory ECG monitoring can demonstrate ST-segment shift, suggesting ischemia both during episodes that are symptomatic and those that are silent. Subsequently, other investigators have confirmed these original observations (6, 8, 9). It must be recognized, however, that only meticulous attention to detail ensures the absence of false positives, since the ST-segment recording requires a capability of low-frequency capacity to about 0.6 hz at a time constant of 1.6 seconds and with appropriate phase shift (10). The use of liquid electrodes for skin contact, meticulous attention to detail of lead positioning, avoidance of undue movement of the connections to the recorder, integrity of the tape drive system and ensuring an absence of play-back artifact should provide reliable recordings. There is little evidence that FM recording systems provide more reliable recordings than AM. In addition, both disease states and physiological conditions, as well as medications, can all simulate ST-segment shift - a result of myocardial ischemia. Finally, there may well be a relationship between the voltage of R waves and subsequent ST-segment shift (11). The R wave amplitude may vary throughout the 24-hours with little relationship to ischemia. The use of Holter monitoring techniques in the diagnosis of myocardial ischemia has recently been reviewed by Feldman & Resnekov (12). No doubt in the future systems will be available for digital recording of the ECG signal with subsequent analog play-back as needed. Such electronically advanced systems should obviate many of the current technical problems.

2. Exercise testing

Myocardial ischemia may be demonstrated during standard exercise testings either at low or high levels and during both, typical ST-segment deviations may be recorded. At times, silent ischemia can be shown to occur soon after the onset of exercise with the angiographically proven precipitation of coronary artery spasm, usually at the site of an atherosclerotic plaque of an epicardial coronary artery branch and probably precipitated by the sudden adrenergic drive precipitated by effort (13). Hyperventilation with the start of exercise may also be a factor (14).

3. Isotopic evidence of myocardial hypoperfusion

During ST-segment depression, as recorded on the electrocardiogram, injecting isotopes to determine the state of myocardial perfusion may help in the diagnosis of silent ischemia. Thallium-201 has a half-life of 72 hours and is less than an ideal isotope for investigations of this sort. On the other hand, the generator-produced positron emitting rubidium-82 with a half-life of 75 seconds permits perfusion myocardial scintigrams to be obtained during a control state, an event and once the effects of the event are over.

Using this isotope, myocardial scintigrams have confirmed that the ST-segment shift of the electrocardiogram results from myocardial ischemia (9).

4. Demonstration of left ventricular dysfunction

Segmental left ventricular dysfunction precipitated by myocardial ischemia can be demonstrated by: a) radionuclide angiographic techniques or b) high quality 2-dimensional echocardiographic imaging. Both investigations aim to demonstrate an abnormality of ventricular function, usually segmental, that may affect total ventricular function as well during the occurrence of temporary myocardial ischemia.

5. Other provocative tests to precipitate myocardial ischemia

There appears to be an important relationship between mental stress and the precipitation of myocardial ischemia, symptomatic or silent. Its use as a cause of silent ischemia has been documented by Deanfield and his colleagues (6) who confirmed by rubidium-82 scintigrams that the associated ST-segment shift precipitated by mental stress was associated with myocardial ischemia.
The cold pressor test has also been used to bring about myocardial ischemia. Originally introduced into medical practice as a diagnostic test of abnormal vascular reactivity of hypertensive subjects (15), it precipitates vaso-constriction that affects the vascular system widely, including the coronary circulation. The ECG may record typical changes suggesting ischemia during the vaso-constrictor phase that can be confirmed as resulting from an inadequate blood supply to the myocardium, by rubidium-82 or thallium-201 scintigraphy.

Management of silent ischemia

Treatment may be required under the following circumstances (1):
1. The individual who has episodes of silent ischemia varying with symptomatic
2. Totally silent myocardial ischemia
3. Silent myocardial ischemia in the early months following acute myocardial infarction.

1. Silent myocardial ischemia varying with symptomatic

In this group decisions about management are less complex. Ischemia is always undesirable and patients may need protection against it whether it is silent or symptomatic. The physician should determine the degree of ischemia by the investigations listed above and, if severe, confirm the degree of atherosclerosis of the coronary arteries by selective coronary arteriography and its effects on ventricular function by left ventriculography. With this information to hand, a decision can then be taken about the need for aorto-coronary bypass graft surgery, percutaneous transluminal coronary angioplasty or medical management.

It should be recognized that in those in whom ischemia varies, being silent at times and at other times symptomatic, the episodes of silent ischemia are far more frequent than symptomatic, on average about four times (9).

2. Totally asymptomatic myocardial ischemia

The diagnosis here is usually fortuitous, possibly a result of an exercise test as part of fitness assessment. Alternatively, a long-term ECG ambulatory monitor may have recorded episodes of ST-segment shift suggestive of ischemia.

It is known that silent ischemia is more frequent in members of families in whom there is a history of premature and more severe coronary atherosclerosis. In addition, the presence of coronary risk factors, particularly in such family members, increases the likelihood that silent ischemia in association with atherosclerotic lesions of the coronary arteries may be found.

Part of the investigation leading to management in those with total silent ischemia therefore includes a careful history of family members. Coronary risk factors in the individual under consideration should be determined. Cigarette smoking, hyperlipidemia, hypertension and diabetes mellitus all significantly worsen the prognosis of all forms of myocardial ischemia, including silent ischemia and increase the likelihood of silent ischemia being manifest.

In this totally silent group a multiple stage exercise treadmill test should be undertaken and if positive, repeated with myocardial perfusion scintigraphy not only to document that the ST-segment depression precipitated by exercise is a result of myocardial ischemia, but also as a guide to its severity. In addition, an inability to achieve a predicted heart rate for age on exercise may have serious prognostic significance (16).

3. Silent ischemia following myocardial infarction

Following myocardial infarction the prognosis depends on the extent of myocardial damage and its effect on ventricular function as well as the degree of coronary artery atherosclerosis and the collateral circulation. A multiple stage exercise test should be done during the early recovery phase to document whether symptomatic or asymptomatic ST-segment shift occurs as a result of ischemia being precipitated (17). In those in whom ischemia is demonstrated in this way, the nature and extent of coronary artery lesions and their associated precipitation of left ventricular dysfunction should be determined.

It has been shown that in patients recovering from acute myocardial infarction, episodes of silent myocardial ischemia may occur in about 20% (1). During such episodes there may be dangerous ventricular rhythm disturbances precipitated that could lead to sudden death (1).

Medical management of silent ischemia

Decisions about treatment remain difficult and controversial. Myocardial ischemia has complex causes, there being an intimate inter-relationship between atherosclerosis, coronary artery spams, platelet aggregation, formation of thrombus, and the effects of the prostaglandin system on the coronary artery endothelium. In addition other vaso-constrictor substances may cause sudden coronary artery spasm to occur, as may mental stress.

Wherever possible and necessary coronary risk factors should be modified. There is an urgent need to stop the smoking; any hypertension should be treated, diabetes mellitus, when present, should be controlled and hyperlipidemias managed according to the abnormal lipid profile present.

Proposed drug therapy has included nitrates, beta-adrenergic blocking drugs, calcium blocking drugs, aspirin.

Nitrates

Although introduced into medicine more than 100 years ago, nitrates produce complex effects by mechanisms still not fully understood (18). Their dominant effect, however, is venodilation and in consequence the end-diastolic volume and pressure of the ventricle are reduced. These in turn reduce myocardial oxygen requirements. Unfortunately, nitrate therapy is associated with considerable tachyphylaxis and when used chronically, the effect achieved is less than when administering nitrates intermittently as with sublingual nitroglyerine. Even when skin patches of nitroglycerine are used, there is now evidence that it may be necessary to apply two or even three such patches every 24 hours to achieve a therapeutic blood nitrate level, even apart from the problem of tachyphylaxis (19). An addedifficulty regarding the use of chronic nitrate therapy is cross-tolerance that blunts the effects of sublingual nitroglyerine when used intermittently in patients on chronic nitrate therapy (20).

Beta-adrenergic blocking drugs

All beta-adrenergic blocking drugs, despite their individual properties (21) relieve myocardial ischemia by reducing the work of the heart. Heart rate and contractility are lessened, conduction across the AV node is slowed and blood pressure reduced. In consequence, myocardial oxygen requirements are less; myocardial ischemia is relieved.

Calcium channel blocking drugs

The three oral agents now available in the United States, namely nifedipine, verapamil and diltiazem are all powerful dilators of smooth muscle (22). Peripheral vaso-dilation follows their use, coronary flow is increased directly, myocardial collateral flow is enhanced and diastolic ventricular compliance improved. The three calcium blocking drugs are, however, very dissimilar chemical substances and the mechanism by which their effects are produced varies considerable, as do the side-effects that may be precipitated. It is likely that nifedipine is the most potent vasodilator of the three. Verapamil and diltiazem both have important electrophysiological effects that may cause sinus bradycardia and conduction disturbances, particularly at the AV nodal level. Verapamil is the most negatively inotropic of the three calcium blocking drugs, followed by diltiazem. Since there is usually an associated mild tachycardia because of peripheral vasodilation when nifedipine is given, it is less negatively inotropic than the other calcium blocking drugs.

Aspirin

Aspirin may help reduce abnormal platelet aggregation, lessening the risk of thrombus formation. An appropriate dose in an adult is 325 mg every 24 hours. Whether similar therapeutic effects can be achieved with reduced dosages is uncertain but under investigation at present.

The medical management of silent ischemia, as outlined above, therefore envisages patients being maintained on a combination of a calcium blocking drug that will reduce the precipitation of coronary spasm and help increase myocardial perfusion and a beta-adrenergic blocking drug to protect against inappropriate increases of heart rate on exercise in individuals who might have significant coronary atherosclerosis. Beta-adrenergic blocking drugs may also prevent ventricular premature beats or tachycardia from emerging, particularly on effort. Aspirin is used to help reduce abnormal platelet aggregation.

The choice of the individual drugs is determined by the individual requirements of the patient and the absence of bradycardia, conduction disturbances or incipient left heart failure that might be a contra-indication to using verapamil or diltiazem. With regard to the beta-adrenergic blocking drugs, once a day therapy is recommended since this will improve patient compliance. Once on a medical regimen, the Holter monitor or exercise test should be repeated to document that episodes of ischemia are being lessened.

Discussion

The need for protecting the patient against intermittent myocardial ischemia, even when asymptomatic, has been demonstrated by retrospective studies of follow-up in those in whom silent or near silent myocardial ichemic episodes were documented. Of 147 individuals followed-up, there was an incidence of 30.5% of an acute cardiac event occurring within 3 to 8.5 years follow-up after the original diagnosis (23—25). The acute cardiac events noted were precipitation of myocardial infarction, sudden death or a dangerous rhythm disturbance.

The beneficial effects of both beta-adrenergic blocking and calcium blocking drugs in patients with silent myocardial ischemia have been documented. Propranolol, atenolol and lobitalol have all been tried in association with nifedipine, verapamil or diltiazem (26—28). Randomized studies have been undertaken and have demonstrated that calcium blocking drugs as compared with placebo, successfully reduced episodes of silent myocardial ischemia (29).

Over a short period of follow-up, nitrate therapy reduces the frequency of silent ischemia (30) and similarly, infusions of isosorbide dinitrate may also be of short-term benefit (31).

It is very likely that the combination of calcium blocking and beta-adrenergic blocking drugs is very effective and that adding to the regimen isosorbide dinitrate does not increase benefit (32). In addition nifedipine may help preserve and improve ventricular performance at rest and during exercise when added to maximal beta-adrenergic blocking and nitrate therapy. It does not precipitate electrophysiological change and the emergence of acute left ventricular dysfunction is fortunately rare (33, 34).

Chierchia and colleagues (35) investigated the effects of aspirin administered intravenously, but no prevention of attacks of silent myocardial ischemia occurred. When nitrates and calcium blockers were added, a significant eduction in the episodes of silent ischemia followed.

It is apparent therefore that silent myocardial ischemia is a major diagnostic and therapeutic problem. It occurs more frequently than does symptomatic myocardial ischemia and in certain individuals its prognosis can be serious. Ischemia is always undesirable and potentially dangerous. Its severity should be determined and decisions about management as outlined in this article taken since it is the ischemia that may kill the patient; no patient dies because of symptoms. The absence of symptoms, on the other hand does not necessarily confer an absence of cardiac risk.

Medical management is aimed at reducing the episodes of ischemia by directing therapy against the pathophysiological mechanisms thought to be occurring. Although difficult, the diagnosis can be established and patients be managed successfully even when ischemia occurs without symptoms.

References

1. Resnekov L (1985) Silent myocardial ischemia: Therapeutic implications. Am J Med 79 Suppl 3A: 30—34
2. Stern S, Tzivoni D (1973) Dynamic changes in the ST segment during sleep in ischemic heart disease. Am J Cardiol 32: 17-20
3. Yasue H, Touyama M, Kato H (1976) Prinzmetal's variant form of angina as a manifestation of alpha-adrenergic receptormediated coronary artery spasm: Documentation by coronary arteriography. Am Heart J 91: 148—155
4. Maseri A, Severi S, Denes M (1978) "Variant" angina: One aspect of a continuous spectrum of vasospastic myocardial ichemia: Pathogenetic mechanisms, estimated incidence and clinical coronary arteriographic findings in 138 patients. Am J Cardiol 42: 1019—1035
5. Hillis LD; Braunwald E (1978) Coronary artery spasm. N Engl J Med 299: 695—702
6. Deanfield JE, Kensett M, Wilson RA (1984) Silent myocardial ischemia due to mental stress. Lancet ii: 1011—1015

7. Holter NJ (1961) New method for heart studies. Continuous electrocardiography of active subjects over long periods is now practical. Science 134: 1214—1220
8. Stern S, Tzivoni D (1974) Early detection of silent ischemic heart disease by 24-hour electrocardiographic monitoring of active subjects. Brit Heart J 36: 481—486
9. Deanfield JE, Selwyn AP, Chierchia S (1983) Myocardial ischemia during daily life in patients with stable angina: Its relation to symptoms and heart rate changes. Lancet ii: 753—758
10. Lambert CR, Imperi GA, Pepine CJ (1986) Low-frequency requirements for recording ischemia ST-segment abnormalities in coronary artery disease. Am J Cardiol 58: 225—229
11. Hollenberg M, Go M, Jr, Massie BM, Wisneski JA, Gertz EW (1985) Influence of R-wave amplitude on exercise-induced ST depression: Need for a "gain factor" correction when interpreting stress electrocardiograms. Am J Cardiol 56: 13—17
12. Feldman T, Resnekov L Ambulatory ECG monitoring in the diagnosis of myocardial ischemia. Cardiovasc Clin (in press)
13. Oliva PB, Pitts DE, Pluss RG (1973) Coronary arterial spasm in Prinzmetal angina: Documentation by coronary arteriography. N Engl J Med 288: 745—751
14. Donald DE, Shepherd JT (1978) Reflexes from the heart and lungs: Physiological curiosities or important regulatory mechanisms? Cardiovasc Res 12: 449—469
15. Hines EA Jr, Brown GE (1936) The cold pressor test for measuring the reactibility of the blood pressure: Data concerning 571 normal and hypertensive subjects. Am Heart J 11: 1—9
16. Reisman S, Ladenheim M, Staniloff HM, Rozanski A, Berman DS (1985) Asymptomatic patients with exercise T-201 hypoperfusion: Identification of a high-risk subset. Ciculation 72, Suppl 111: 111—445
17. Fioretti P, Brower RW, Simoons ML, Das SK, Bos RJ, Wijns W, Reiber JH, Lubsen J, Hugenholtz PG (1984) Prediction of mortality in hospital survivors of myocardial infarction. Comparison of predischarge exercise testing and radionuclide ventriculography at rest. Br Heart J 52: 292—298
18. Brunton TL (1857) Use of nitrite of amyl angina pectoris. Lancet ii: 97
19. Thompson RH (1983) The clinical use of transdermal delivery devices with nitroglycerin. Angiology 34: 23—31
20. Manyari DE, Smith ER, Spragg J (1985) Isosorbide dinitrate and glyceryl trinitrate: Demonstration of cross tolerance in the capacitance vessels. Am J Cardiol 55: 927—931
21. Thadani U, Davidson C, Singleton W, Taylor SH (1979) Comparison of drugs with different ancillary properties in angina pectoris. N Engl J Med 300: 750—755
22. Haeusler G (1972) Differential effect of verapamil on excitation — contraction coupling in smooth muscle and on excitation-secretion coupling in adrenergic nerve terminals. J Pharmacol Exp Ther 180: 672—682
23. Erikssen J, Thaulow E (1984) Follow-up of patients with asymptomatic myocardial ischemia. In: Rutishauser W, Roskamm H (eds) Silent myocardial ischemia: Springer-Verlag, 156—164
24. Hickman JR Jr, Uhl GS, Cook RL, Engel PJ, Hopkirk A (1980) A natural history study of asymptomatic coronary disease. Am J Cardiol 45: 422 (abstr)
25. Sharma B, Francis G, Hodges M, Asinger R (1981) Demonstration of exercise-induced ischemia without angina in patients who recover from out-of-hospital ventricular fibrillation. Am J Cardiol 47: 445 (abstr)
26. Oakley GDG, Fox KM, Dargie HJ (1979) Objective assessment of treatment in severe angina. Br Med J i: 1540
27. Quyyumi AA, Wright C, Mockus L (1984) Effect of partial agonist activity in β-blockers in severe angina pectoris. Br Med J ii: 951—953
28. Cocco G, Strozzi C, Chu D: Therapeutic effects of pindolol and nifedipine in patients with stable angina pectris and asymptomatic resting ischemia. Eur J Cardiol 1979, 10: 59—69.
29. Winniford MD, Johnson SM, Mauritson DR (1982) Verapamil therapy for Prinzmetal's variant angina: Comparison with placebo and nifedipine. Am J Cardiol 50: 913—918
30. Schang SJ Jr, Pepine CH (1977) Transient asymptomatic ST-segment depression during daily activity. Am J Cardiol 39: 396—402
31. Distante A, Maseri A, Severi S (1979) Management of vasospastic angina at rest with continuous infusion of isosorbide dinitrate a double-crossover-study in a coronary care unit. Am J Cardiol 44: 533—539

32. Morse JR, Nesto RW (1985) Double-blind cross-over comparison of the antianginal effects of nifedipine and isosorbide dinitrate in patients with exertional angina receiving propranolol. J Am Coll Cardiol 6: 1395—1401
33. Nesto RW, White HD; Ganz P, Koslowski J, Wynne J, Holman L, Antman E (1985) Addition of nifedipine to maximal beta-blocker-nitrate therapy: Effect on exercise and global left ventricular performance at rest and during exercise. Am J Cardiol 55: 3E-8E
34. Vetrovec GW, Parker VE (1985) Acute electrophysiologic, hemodynamic and left ventricular effects of nifedipine and beta-blocker interactions. Am J Cardio 55: 21E—30E
35. Chierchia S, DeCaterina R, Crea F (1982) Failure of thromboxane A_2 blockade to prevent attacks of vasospastic angina. Circulation 66: 702—705

Author's address:
Leon Resnekov, M.D., F.R.C.P.
Hospital Box 423
University of Chicago Medical Center
5841 South Maryland Avenue
Chicago, Illinois 60637

Importance of silent myocardial ischemia in therapy for unstable angina pectoris

W. Rafflenbeul, D. Hausmann

Division of Cardiology, Hannover Medical School, F.R.G

In the spectrum of acute ischemic syndromes, unstable angina pectoris is characterized by specific features in the patients history, including recent occurrence of angina at rest, or brought on by minimal exertion, as well as the deterioration of a chronic stable angina into more severe, prolonged or more frequent anginal attacks (crescendo angina). Typical electrocardiographic criteria include reversible ST-segment deviations and/or variable T-wave inversions. Cardiac enzymes are usually not elevated.

Of patients with unstable angina pectoris, 10%—12% develop myocardial infarction or die suddenly within 12 weeks of onset (42). Adverse outcome might be found in as many as 30% of patients (3, 18).

Coronary morphology

Patients afflicted with unstable angina have in general shown a similar pattern of coronary vessel involvement to that found in patients with chronic exertional angina, in terms of the number of diseases vessels and the degree of obstruction (33, 35). However, more detailed analysis of the lesion morphology has revealed distinctive differences in patients

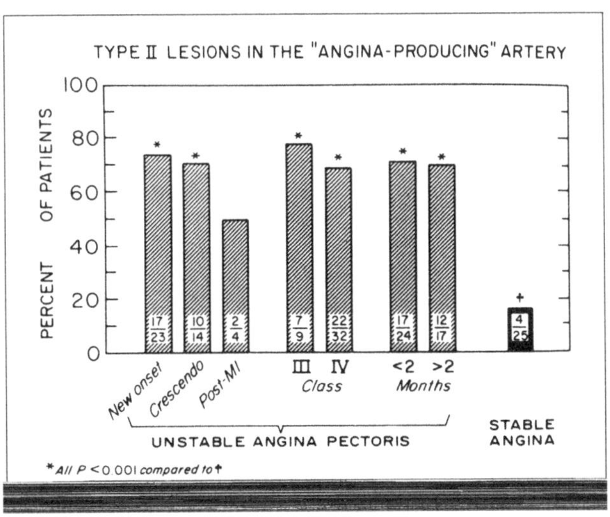

Fig. 1. Distribution of type II eccentric coronary lesions (asymmetric, convex intraluminal encroachment with narrow base, due to overhanging edges that are very irregular or scalloped) in different subgroups of patients with unstable angina. Numbers within the bars represent the number of type II lesions and the number of patients in each subgroup. MI = myocardial infarction (reproduced from [1] with permission).

catheterized *during* the phase of unstable angina (1). The majority of lesions (71%) are eccentrically located with irregular borders and overhanging edges, suggesting intraluminal thrombi (15). Postmortem analysis has confirmed that such eccentric lesions identified at angiography are frequently manifest as ruptured atherosclerotic plaques with thrombi attached (13, 20). This is in accordance with a recent study which presented evidence that the rate of progression of coronary artery disease is accelerated in unstable angina (27).

Pathophysiology

Since many patients with unstable angina have advanced obstructive coronary artery disease, sudden myocardial ischemia may be precipitated either by a relatively small rise

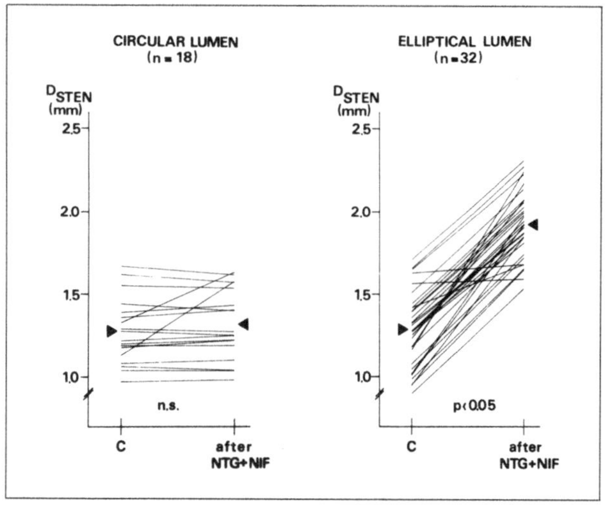

Fig. 2. Effect of 0.8 mg nitroglycerin (NTG) plus 20 mg nifedipine (NIF) sublingually on coronary stenoses diameter after separation according to angiographic morphology. A stenosis with the smallest diameter (D_{sten}) which measured less than 25% difference in multiple angiographic projection was called *circular;* with more than 25%, *elliptical* (reproduced from [39]).

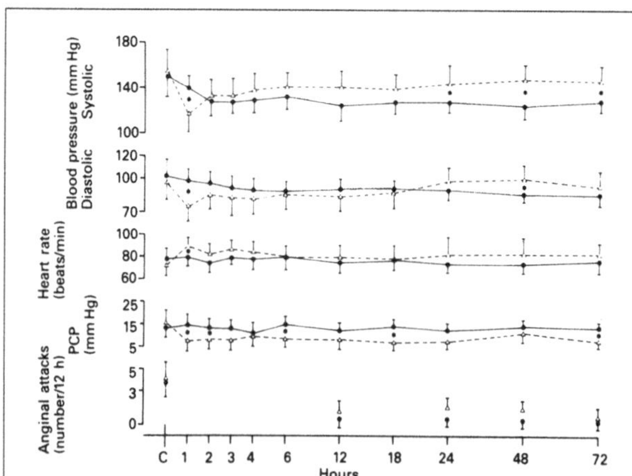

Fig. 3. Effects of intravenous nifedipine (15–30 mg/24 h) (●—●) vs intravenous nitroglycerin (30–60 mg/24 h) (Δ---Δ) in 20 patients with unstable angina. Results are mean values ± SD. C = control state before onset of infusion; PCP = pulmonary capillary pressure. Number of anginal attacks are indicated for the total interval, i.e. 1–12, 12–24, 24–48 and 48–72 h. * = significant differences ($p < 0.05$) between nifedipine and nitroglycerin values (reproduced from [40]).

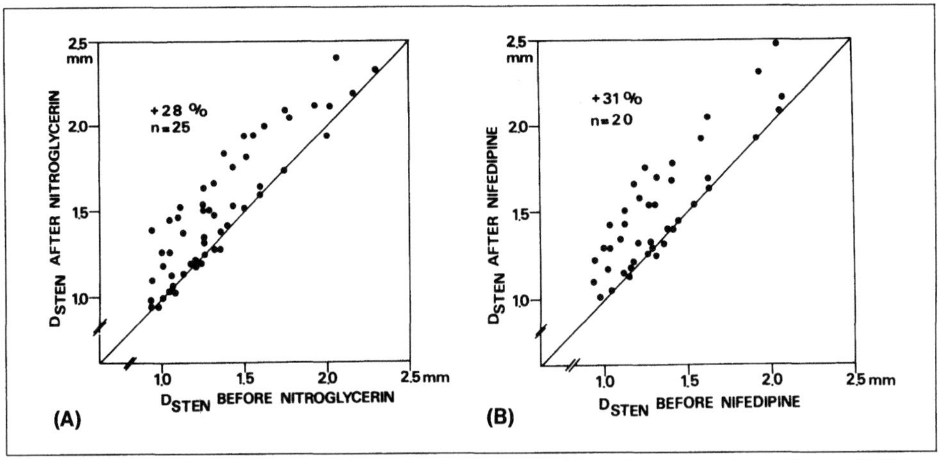

Fig. 4A and B. Dilatory effect of either 0.8 mg nitroglycerin sublingually (A) or 20 mg nifedipine sublingually (B) on the smallest diameter (D_{sten}) of $n = 42$ coronary artery stenoses. The mean increase of D_{sten} was + 28% and + 31% respectively (reproduced from [39]).

in oxygen demand surpassing severely restricted oxygen delivery, or by a sudden reduction in myocardial oxygen supply. A small increase of blood pressure and/or heart rate may already increase myocardial oxygen consumption, depleting the limited coronary reserve.

In recent years, however, numerous studies (2, 4, 5, 6, 7, 10, 11, 24, 26, 32, 44) have suggested that the primary mechanism of angina at rest in many patients is a reduction of oxygen supply in the presence of constant oxygen requirements. In addition, it has been established that ST-segment changes during such episodes reflect myocardial ischemia, as evidenced by myocardial perfusion deficits (12, 25, 31), an increase in left

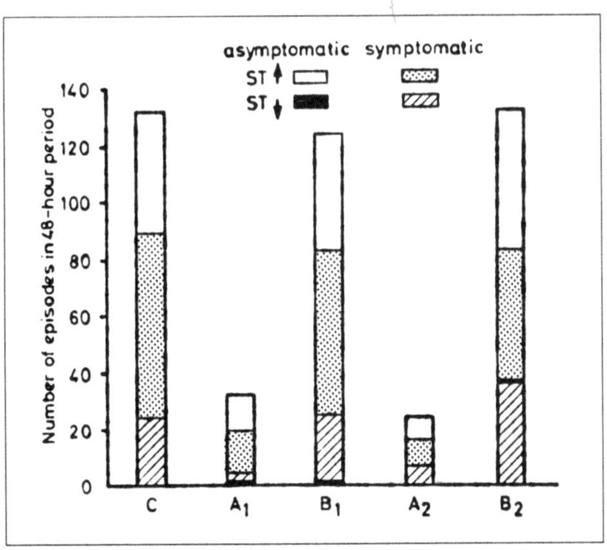

Fig. 5. Total number of ischemic episodes in 12 patients with angina at rest. C = run-in period; A_1, A_2 = verapamil periods; B_1, B_2 = placebo periods. Verapamil reduced the frequency of all types of episodes (reproduced from [30] with permission).

ventricular filling pressures (5), transient ventricular dysfunction (8) or a decrease in oxygen saturation of the coronary sinus blood (6). These types of ischemic events are triggered by an abrupt increase of coronary stenosis severity, due to enhanced vasomotor tone (24), platelet aggregation (13) and thrombus formation ("complicated atherosclerotic plaque") or a combination of both (15).
Such "secondary" phenomena, during the course of coronary artery disease, decrease coronary blood flow abruptly with subsequent myocardial ischemia. The increased vasoreactivity occurs predominantly in the area of an eccentric coronary lesion in the epicardial conductive vessels (37, 39).

Management

Patients with unstable angina pectoris should be referred to a coronary care unit where medical treatment should be initated immediately. Above all a vigorous antianginal therapy is mandatory in order to disrupt anginal symptoms as soon as possible and prevent the progress into myocardial infarction.
Symptomatic relief is accomplished in the majority of patients with intravenous infusion of powerful vasodilatory drugs, like nitroglycerin or calcium-antagonists. Both drugs lower myocardial oxygen requirements by different mechanisms (40) and at the same time improve oxygen supply, due to their vasodilatory potency in coronary artery stenoses (34, 39). The release of vasoconstrictor tone may attenuate stenosis severity, particularly with vasospasm superimposed on high-grade coronary obstructions.
A combination regimen has shown to be more efficacious in patients with refractory episodes of rest angina. In addition, drugs which inhibit further platelet aggregation should be administered (21). Following stabilization, coronary anatomy should be delineated and left ventricular function assessed.

Silent ischemia in unstable angina

Recent analyses of continuous electrocardiographic recordings in patients with unstable angina have revealed that the vast majority of transient ischemic episodes are painless. Biagini et al. (2) registered anginal symptoms in only 12% of ischemic attacks recorded in a coronary care unit. In 41 patients with unstable angina, only 20% of 781 ischemic events were accompanied by chest pain (29). Furthermore, in patients with rest angina due to coronary artery spasm only 7% of ischemic episodes recorded with Holter monitoring were associated with pain (9).
These data indicate that in unstable angina the largest number of episodes of transient myocardial ischemia are silent and are not initiated by increases in the major determinants of myocardial oxygen consumption.
It should be emphasized, however, that the extent and persistence of silent myocardial ischemia during a phase of unstable angina is of major prognostic relevance.
Kunkes et al. (19) reported that the severity of silent myocardial ischemia shows a close correlation with the severity of the underlying coronary artery disease. In patients with unstable angina that is obviously controlled with medical therapy, the persistence of silent ischemic attacks identified with Holter monitoring was associated with frequent

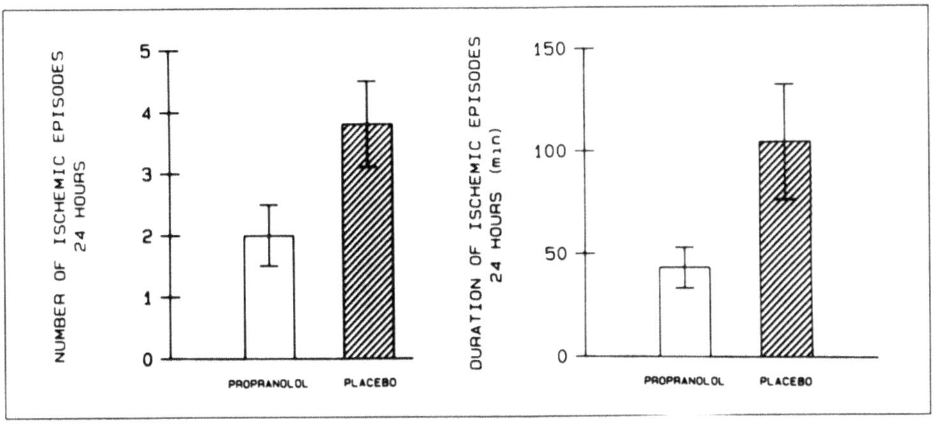

Fig. 6. Total number (left panel) and duration (right panel) of ischemic episodes per 24 h during the first 2 days in patients treated with additional propranolol vs patients on control treatment with nifedipine plus long-acting nitrates ("placebo") (reproduced from [17] with permission).

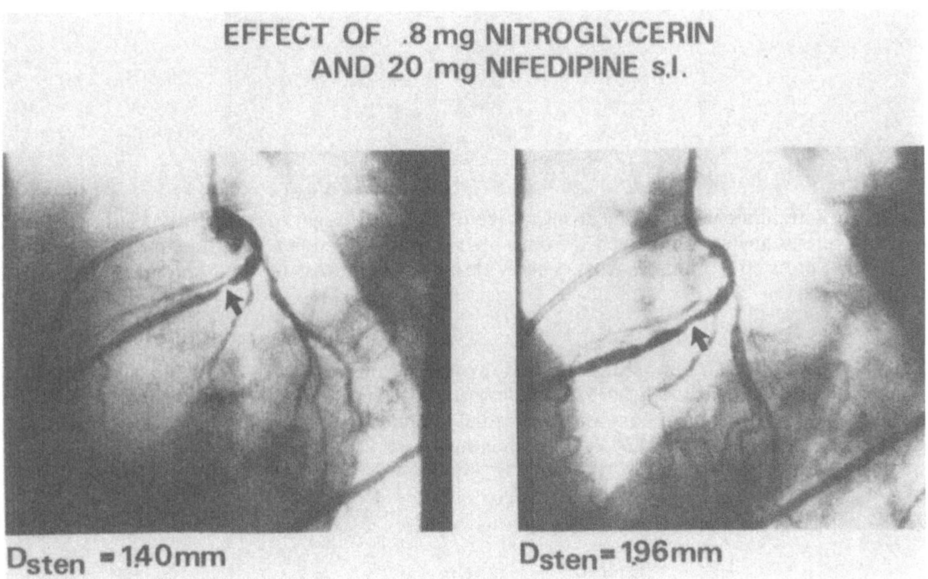

Fig. 7. Effect of combined sublingual application of 0.8 mg nitroglycerin and 20 mg nifedipine on a high-grade obstruction of the left anterior descending coronary artery. The smallest diameter (D_{sten}) dilated from 1.40 mm to 1.96 mm (~ 40%) (reproduced from [36]).

complications (28) or a higher incidence of myocardial infarction or early revascularization (16).

Unfortunately, the same antiischemic vasodilator drugs that proved sufficient to eliminate symptomatic ischemic attacks, are less effective in controlling asymptomatic ischemic episodes in unstable angina, as demonstrated by various study protocols:

In 12 patients with frequent daily attacks of angina at rest Verapamil (480 mg/day) only attenuated asymptomatic episodes of ST-segment changes (30). Furthermore, the addition of isosorbide dinitrate (300 mg/day) to Verapamil (240—400 mg/day) abolished all symptomatic attacks but asymptomatic transient ECG changes disappeared in only six out of ten patients with unstable angina monitored in a coronary care unit (2).
In nine patients with Prinzmetal's angina (multiple episodes of angina at rest), in whom coronary vasoconstriction is the most likely cause of ischemia, the combination of calcium-antagonists (either Verapamil or Nifedipine) and isosorbide dinitrate therapy was effective in reducing both symptomatic attacks and silent ST-segment deviations during Holter monitoring only to about 10% of control level (43).
In 81 patients with unstable angina pectoris treated with Nifedipine (80 mg/day) and topical nitrates, additional Propranolol (minimum 160 mg/day) further reduced the num-

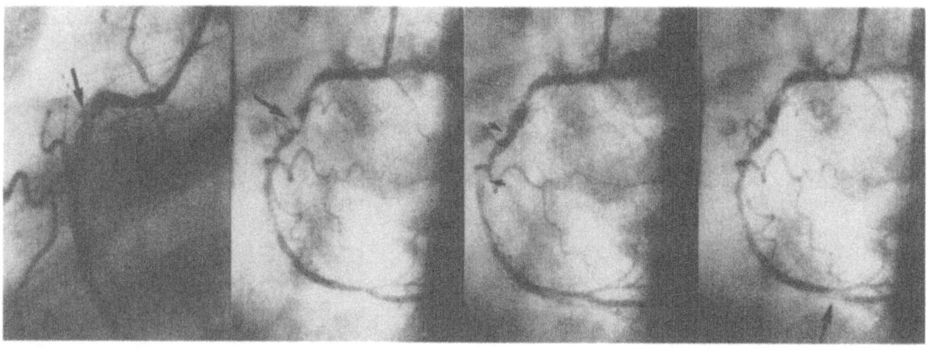

Fig. 8. An intraluminal filling defect suggestive of an intracoronary thrombus (far left panel) in a patient with rest angina, was detached from a high-grade obstruction after intracoronary application of 250 000 units streptokinase. Arrows show thrombus fragments on their way to the peripheral coronary artery.

Table 1. Frequency distribution of death and myocardial infarction in 1266 patients with unstable angina treated either with aspirin (324 mg/day) or with placebo over a 12-week study period. The reduction in death (—51%) or non-fatal myocardial infarction (—51%) in the aspirin group was highly significant (reproduced from [22] J with permission).

Event	No. of Patients*		Reduction in Aspirin Group	P Value Unadjusted	P Value Adjusted †
	Placebo (N = 641)	Aspirin (N = 625)	%		
Death or acute myocadial infarction	65 (10.1)	31 (5.0)	51	0.0005	0.0002
Fatal or nonfatal acute myocardial infarction	50 (7.8)	22 (3.5)	55	0.001	0.0003
Nonfatal acute myocardial infarction	44 (6.9)	21 (3.4)	51	0.005	0.002
Death	21 (3.3)	10 (1.6)	51	0.054	0.059

* Figures in parentheses represent percentage of group.

† Adjusted for base-line characteristics, using logistic regression model.

ber of ischemic events detected by continuous electrocardiographic monitoring from mean 3.8 to 2.0 and the duration from mean 104 to 43 min (17).
Vasoconstriction or enhanced vasomotor tone — particularly in high-grade artery stenoses — is regarded as a major pathophysiological mechanism triggering the onset of rest angina. With potent vasodilator drugs like nitroglycerin and/or Ca-antagonists vascular smooth muscle tone can be substantially diminished as demonstrated in Fig. 7. Therefore, it is most unlikely that recurrent coronary vasoconstriction superimposed on high-grade coronary artery stenoses is responsible for persistent silent ischemic attacks.
Recent angiographic (1) and angioscopic (41) studies demonstrated a high percentage of intracoronary thrombi in patients hospitalized with unstable angina. Fig. 8 shows an example of such an intracoronary thrombus in a patient with unstable angina successfully dissolved with intracoronary streptokinase. Consequently, persistence of silent ischemic attacks despite vigorous vasodilator therapy might be indicative of recurrent thrombus formation. Specific platelet aggregation inhibitors like ticlopidine have shown to be particularly successful in reducing the number of episodes of ST-segment depression occuring without an increase in heart rate and during the night (14). This is in accordance with the significant reduction of myocardial infarction and death in patients with unstable angina treated with aspirin (22, Table 1).
The prognostic importance and therapeutic consequences of persistent silent ischemia in patients with unstable angina are demonstrated on Fig. 9 to Fig. 11. In a 54-year-old

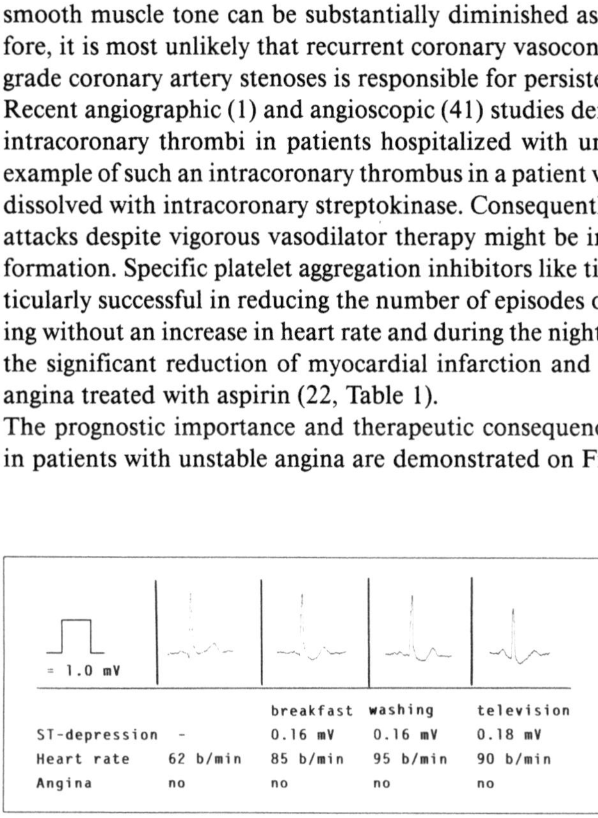

Fig. 9. Silent ischemic episodes detected by continuous electrocardiographic monitoring in a patient hospitalized with unstable angina. These recordings were obtained after complete cessation of anginal symptoms with vigorous medical treatment.

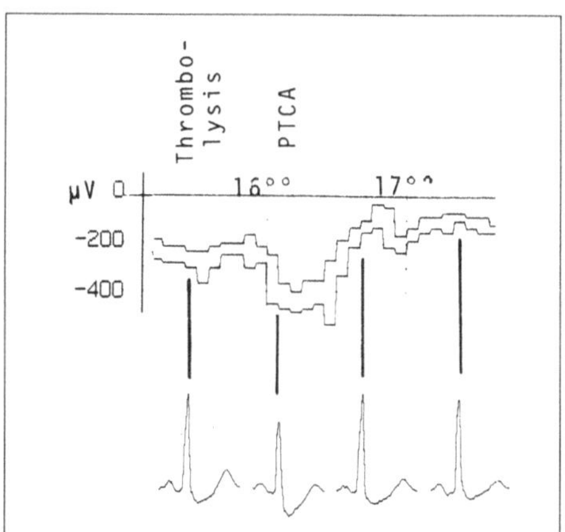

Fig. 10. Continuous printout of ST-segment depression (µV) during acute symptomatic myocardial infarction, immediate thrombolysis with 1.5 million units streptokinase and subsequent balloon dilatation (PTCA) in the same patient as Fig. 9.

Fig. 11. Repeated Holter-monitoring in the same patient as Fig. 9 after 3 days of recovery. No ST-depression could be detected at comparable heart rates; the patient was asymptomatic.

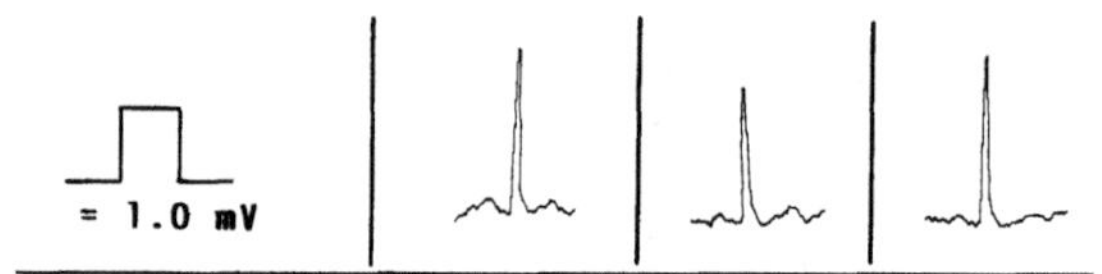

	walking	television	walking
ST-depression	-	-	-
Heart rate	100 b/min	85 b/min	90 b/min
Angina	no	no	no

patient hospitalized with angina at rest of recent onset, repeated ambulatory Holter recordings revealed recurrent silent ischemic attacks despite complete disappearance of anginal symptoms with vigorous combined application of nitroglycerin and Ca-antagonists. Silent ischemic attacks persisted concomitant with moderate increases of heart rate. The patient went into acute myocardial infarction within 24 h. Immediate intracoronary thrombolysis with streptokinase and balloon dilatation of a high-grade residual stenosis subsequently abolished ischemic events.

Therefore, taking into account the prognostic importance of persistent silent myocardial ischemia, symptomatic relief of ischemia in patients with unstable angina may not be an adequate therapy and our primary interest should be focussed on abolition of silent ischemic episodes as a more significant endpoint of therapy in unstable angina.

References

1. Ambrose JA, Winters SL, Stern A, Eng A, Teichholz LE, Corlin R, Fuster V (1985) Angiographic morphology and the pathogenesis of unstable angina pectoris. J Am Coll Cardiol 5: 609—616
2. Biagini A, Mazzei MG, Carpeggiani C, Testa R, Antonelli R, Michelassi C, L'Abbate A, Maseri A (1982) Vasospastic ischemic mechanism of frequent asymptomatic transient ST-T changes during continuous electrocardiographic monitoring in selected unstable angina patients. Am Heart J 103: 13—19
3. Bykerk VP, Haq A, Adelman AG (1985) Changing pattern of unstable angina, a review of 90 cases. Circulation 72 (Suppl III): III—113
4. Cannom DS, Harrison DC, Schroeder JS (1974) Hemodynamic observations in patients with unstable angina pectoris. Am J Cardiol 33: 173—178
5. Chierchia S, Lazzari M, Maseri A (1981) Hemodynamic monitoring in painless myocardial ischemia (abstr). Am J Cardiol 47: 446
6. Chierchia S, Sazzari M, Freedman B, Bruneli C, Maseri A (1983) Impairment of myocardial perfusion during painless myocardial ischemia. J Am Coll Cardiol 1: 924—930
7. Coccol G, Braun G, Strozzi C, Leishman B, Chu B, Rochat N (1982) Asymptomatic myocardial ischemia in patients with stable and typical angina pectoris. Clin Cardiol 5: 403—408
8. Cohn PF, Brown EJ, Wynne J, Holman BL, Atkins HL (1983) Global and regional left ventricular ejection fraction abnormalities during exercise in patients with silent myocardial ischemia. J Am Coll Cardiol 1: 931—933
9. Curry RC, Pepine CJ, Conti CR (1979) Ambulatory monitoring to evaluate therapy results in variant angina patients. Circulation 59/60 (Suppl II): II—190
10. Davies AB, Bala Subramanian V, Cashman PMM, Raftery EB (1983) Simultaneous recording of continuous arterial pressure heart rate, and ST segment in ambulant patients with stable angina pectoris. Br Heart J 50: 85—91

11. Deanfield JKE, Maseri A, Selwyn AP, Ribesito P, Chierchia S, Krikler S (1983) Myocardial ischemia during daily life in patients with stable angina: its relation of symptoms and heart rate changes. Lancet 2: 753—758
12. Deanfield J, Shea M, Wilson R, et al (1983) ST-segment change as a marker of ischemia in stable angina: a patient study using positron tomography (abstr) Circulation 68: suppl III: 22
13. Falk E (1985) Unstable angina with fatal outcome: Dynamic coronary thrombosis leading to infarction and/or sudden death. Autopsy evidence of recurrent mural thrombosis with peripheral embolization culminating in total vascular occlusion. Circulation 71: 699—708
14. Fox KM, Jonathan A, Selwyn AP (1982) Effects of platelet inhibition on myocardial ischemia Lancet 2: 727—730
15. Fuster V, Steele PM, Chesebro JH (1985) Role of platelets and thrombosis in coronary atherosclerotic disease and sudden death. J Am Coll Cardiol 5: 175B—184B
16. Gottlieb SO, Weisfeldt ML, Onyang P, Mellits ED, Gersenblith G (1986) Silent ischemia as a marker for early unfavorable outcomes in patients with unstable angina. Eng J Med 314: 1214—1219
17. Gottlieb SO, Weisfeldt ML, Onyang PJ, Aschuff SC, Baughman KL, Traill TA, Brinker JA, Shapiro EP, Chandra NC, Mellits ED, Townsend SN, Gerstenblith G (1986) Effects of the addition of propranolol to therapy with nifedipine for unstable angina pectoris; a randomized, double-blind, placebo-controlled trial. Circulation 73: 331—337
18. Julian DG (1985) The natural history of unstable angina. In: Hugenholtz PG, Goldman BS (eds) Unstable Angina. Schattauer, Stuttgart, pp 65—70
19. Kunkes SH, Pichard AD, Smith H, Gorlin R, Herman MV (1980) Silent ST-segment deviation and extent of coronary artery disease. Am Heart J 100: 813—816
20. Levin DC, Fallon JT (1982) Significance of the angiographic morphology of localized coronary stenoses. Histopathologic correlations. Circulation 66: 316—320
21. Lewin HD, Davies JW, Archibald DG, Steinke WE, Smitherman TC, Doherty JE, Schnaper HW, LeWinter MM, Linares E, Pouger JM, Sabbarwal SC, Chester E, DeMots H (1983) Protective effects of aspirin against acute myocardial infarction and death in men with unstable angina: results of a Veterans Administration Cooperative Study. N Eng J Med 309: 396—403
22. Lewis HD, Davis JKW, Archibald DG et al. (1983) Protective effects of aspirin against acute myocardial infarction and death in men with unstable angina. N Engl J Med 309: 396—403
23. MacAlpin KN, Kattus AA, Alvaro AB (1973) Angina pectoris at rest with preservation of exercise capacity. Circulation 47: 946—953
24. Maseri A, Mimmo R, Chierchia S, Marchkesi C, Pesola A, L'Abbate A (1975) Coronary spasm as a cause of acute myocardial ischemia in man. Chest 68: 625—633
25. Maseri A, Parodi O, Severi S, Pesola A (1976) Transient transmural reduction of myocardial blood flow, demonstrated by thallium-201 scintigraphy, a cause of variant angina. Circulation 54: 280—288
26. Maseri A, Severi S, De Nes M, L'Abbate A, Chierchia S, Marzili M, Ballestra AM, Parodi O, Biagini A, Distante A (1978) "Variant angina": one aspect of a continuous spectrum of vasospastic myocardial ischemia. Am J Cardiol 42: 1019—1025
27. Moise A, Theroux P, Taeymans Y, Descoings B, Lesperance J, Waters DD, Peletier GB, Bourassa MG (1983) Unstable angina and progression of coronary atherosclerosis. N Engl J Med 309: 685—689
28. Nademanee K, Intarachot V, Piontek M, Gaghaiwalla Mody F, Rieder D, Josephson MA, Singh BN (1984) Silent myocardial ischemia on Holter: has it clinical significance? (abstr) Circulation 70: suppl II: 451
29. Nademanee K, Intarachot V, Singh PN, Josephson MA, Singh BN (1986) Characteristics and clinical significance of silent myocardial ischemia in unstable angina. Am J Cardiol 58, 26B—33B
30. Parodi O, Maseri A, Simonetti I (1979) Management of unstable angina at rest by verapamil. A double-blind cross-over study in coronary care unit. Br Heart J 41, 167—174
31. Parodi O, Uthurralt N, Severi S, Bencivelli W, Michelasi C, L'Abbate A, Maseri A (1981) Transient reduction of regional myocardial perfusion during angina at rest with ST-segment depression or normalization of negative T-waves. Circulation 63: 1238—1247
32. Quyyumi AA, Mockus I, Wright C, Fox KM (1985) Morphology of ambulatory ST segment changes in patients with varying severity of coronary artery disease. Investigations of the frequency of nocturnal ischemia and coronary spasm. Br Heart J 50: 186—193

33. Rafflenbeul W, Smith LR, Rogers WJ, Mantle JA, Rackley CE, Russell RO (1979) Quantitative coronary arteriography. Coronary anatomy of patients with unstable angina pectoris reexamined 1 year after optimal medical therapy. Am J Cardiol 43: 699—707
34. Rafflenbeul W, Urthaler F, Russell RO, Lichtlen P, James TN (1980) Dilatation of coronary artery stenoses after isosorbide dinitrate in man. Br Heart J 43, 546—549
35. Rafflenbeul W, Russell RO, Lichtlen PR (1981) Angiographic anatomy of coronary arteries in unstable angina pectoris. In: Rafflenbeul W, Lichtlen P, Balcon R (eds) Unstable Angina pectoris. Stuttgart, Thieme, pp 51—57
36. Rafflenbeul W, Lichtlen PR (1982) Zum Konzept der dynamischen Koronarstenose. Z Kardiol 71: 439—444
37. Rafflenbeul W, Lichtlen PR (1983) Release of residual vascular tone in coronary artery stenoses with Nifedipine and nitroglycerin. In: Kaltenbach M, Neufeld HN (eds). V Adalat Symposium, Excerpta Medica, Amsterdam, pp 300—308
38. Rafflenbeul W (1983) Dilation of coronary artery stenoses with diltiazem i.v. In: Fleckenstein H, Hashimoto K, Herrmann M, Schwarz H, Seipel L (eds) New Calcium Antagonists, Stuttgart, Gustav Fischer, pp 181—182
39. Rafflenbeul W, Lichtlen PR (1983) Quantitative coronary angiography: evidence of a sustained increase in vascular smooth muscle tone in coronary artery stenoses. Z Kardiol 72 (Suppl 3), pp 87—91
40. Rafflenbeul W, Bossaller C, Lichtlen PR (1985) Intravenous infusion in Nifedipine in patients with unstable angina pectoris. In: PR Lichtlen (ed), Recent aspects in calcium-antagonism, Schattauer, Stuttgart, pp 129—136
41. Sherman CT, Litvack F, Grundfest W et al. (1986) Coronary angioscopy in patients with unstable angina pectoris. N Engl J Med 315: 913—919
42. Telford AM, Wilson C (1985) Trial of heparin versus atenolol in prevention of myocardial infarction in intermediate coronary syndrome. Lancet 1, 1225—1231
43. Winniford MD, Gabliani G, Johnson SM, Mauritson DR, Fulton KL, Hillis LD (1984) Concomitant calcium antagonist plus isosorbide dinitrate therapy for markedly active variant angina. Am Heart J 108, 1269—1273
44. Yasue H, Omoe S, Takizawa A, Nagao M, Hyon H, Nishida S, Horie M (1981) Comparison of coronary arteriographic findings during angina pectoris associated with ST segment elevation or depression. Am J Cardiol 47: 539—546

Authors' address:
Prof. Dr. W. Rafflenbeul
Division of Cardiology
Hannover Medical School
Konstanty-Gutschow-Str. 8
3000 Hannover 61

Variability of myocardial ischemia in chronic stable angina

J. E. Deanfield, D. Spiegelhalter*

The Hospital for Sick Children, Great Ormond Street, London, U.K., and * MRC Biostatistics Unit, Cambridge, U.K.

Introduction

Physicians treating patients with coronary artery disease most commonly use the symptom of angina pectoris as a guide to diagnosis, activity and treatment of ischemic heart disease. However, thousands of people with coronary disease die or sustain myocardial infarctions each year without ever experiencing chest pain. In the Framingham Study, more than 25% of acute myocardial infarctions were unrecognised by the patient or physician and these had the same prognostic impact as those accompanied by classical symptoms (1). Furthermore, the severity of angina pectoris appears to be a poor guide to prognosis (2). It is now clear that transient regional myocardial ischemia may exist in the absence of symptoms in both patients with angina and totally asymptomatic individuals (3, 4). Silent ischemia has been demonstrated during a number of provocative tests in hospital, but this type of brief evaluation may have little relevance to the severity, character and triggers of ischemia during the patient's ordinary daily life. The development of Holter monitoring to detect ST-segment changes occurring during ischemic episodes has provided an unique objective means of evaluating the activity of ischemic heart disease out of hospital. Several studies have shown that silent episodes of ST segment depression may greatly outnumber those accompanied by angina pectoris and occur in previously unsuspected circumstances.

The ability to quantify transient myocardial ischemia during ordinary daily activities is likely to prove valuable for therapeutic and prognostic assessment of patients with coronary artery disease. The objective information which does not depend on symptoms should offer a better means of assessing the effect of treatment and the activity of ischemic heart disease.

Transient myocardial ischemia in patients with angina

A new picture of ischemic heart disease activity is emerging from Holter monitoring studies which challenges a number of conventional beliefs. Studies from several centres have all been remarkably consistent in reporting that episodes of silent ischemia outnumber those accompanied by angina by a ratio of approximately 3 : 1. Not only is transient ischemia frequently silent but it is surprisingly prolonged. In an analysis of 1,934 episodes of transient ST-segment depression recorded in 30 patients with chronic stable angina during 446 days of monitoring, the mean duration of painful episodes was

20.2 ± 18 min and 15.3 ± 16 for painless episodes, with considerable overlap between the two groups (5).

While ST-segment change has been a long accepted standard for evaluating myocardial ischemia in both clinical and experimental studies, there has been considerable doubt about the reliability of the signal when recorded out of hospital in ambulant patients. Certainly, early Holter devices were capable of distorting the ST-T wave, thus leading to an erroneous diagnosis of ischemic changes. The technical problems of poor low frequency response and phase shifts have been largely overcome with improvements in amplitude modulated devices and the development of frequency modulated systems. Multiple studies have demonstrated the ability of several Holter systems to reproduce accurately the ST segment changes seen during exercise testing (8, 9). Further concern has centred on conflicting reports of the incidence of STT wave changes in subjects with no evidence of coronary artery disease. Tzivoni and Stern found no "false positives" among 33 normal ambulant and 42 sleeping subjects, whereas Armstrong reported a 30% incidence of ST-segment depression in 50 asymptomatic men (10, 11). In an attempt to resolve this problem we have studied 80 asymptomatic subjects, evenly distributed amongst four decades older than 20 years, and 20 patients with atypical chest pain but normal coronary arteriograms, exercise tests and tests for coronary spasm. Using frequency modulated recorders only a 2% incidence of 0.1 mV ST-segment depression was found in the normal volunteers and no episodes of ST-segment depression in the 20 patients with normal coronary arteriograms (12). A non-invasive reference technique has been developed using a short lived isotope rubidium 82 and positron tomography to examine directly the relationship between symptoms, ST-segment changes and underlying disturbances of regional myocardial perfusion. Disturbances of perfusion were consistently found during silent transient ST-segment depression after a number of ordinary daily activities such as mental stress, cigarette smoking, cold, as well as during episodes occurring without apparent provocation in patients with chronic stable angina (13, 14). In patients who underwent more than one provocative test, the same myocardial segment showed disturbed perfusion regardless of the type of provocation (15). All of this suggests that in defined populations of patients with angina and coronary disease, transient ST-segment depression can be used as a reliable marker of underlying ischemia irrespective of whether or not it is accompanied by chest pain.

Dynamic nature of ischemia

Holter monitoring provides an opportunity to study the variability of ischemia throughout the day and to follow disease activity over much longer periods. We have found a significant circadian variability in the activity of ischemia with markedly increased numbers of episodes of both symptomatic and silent ischemia in the morning (6—10 a.m.) (16). This has been confirmed in subsequent studies by Rocco and colleagues and parallels the circadian variability for important cardiovascular complications such as acute myocardial infarction and possibly sudden death (17, 18). Interestingly, Campbell and colleagues have demonstrated a similar circadian variation in totally asymptomatic individuals with coronary artery disease and positive exercise tests (19). This surge in ischemic activity in the early morning provides a challenge for design of drug treatment regimes.

Longitudinal studies in patients have demonstrated pronounced day to day differences in both the frequency and duration of ST segment episodes and the proportion accompanied by chest pain. In a study of patients with chronic stable angina who underwent serial ambulatory monitoring and exercise testing, there was additional long term variability in the episodes of ischemia recorded during ordinary daily life with both exacerbations and remissions (5). This dynamic nature of disease activity was not reflected in either the reported symptoms or in the results of exercise testing in the hospital which stayed "stable". Silent exacerbations may precede important clinical events such as acute myocardial infarction. This has now been well documented in two separate reports (5, 20).

A quantitative assessment of the natural variability during daily activity must be obtained if Holter monitoring is to be used to assess the response to therapeutic interventions both in the management of individual patients and in clinical trials. We have performed four consecutive days of frequency modulated Holter monitoring in 36 patients with chronic stable angina and repeated 2 to 4 day periods of monitoring on two to eight further occasions per patient over 18 months. All recordings were performed off anti-anginal therapy. Analysis of variance demonstrated important components of variation due to change in the number of episodes from day to day and week to week, and even greater variability in the duration of ST-segment depression per 24 hours. (A product of variable numbers of episodes and variable individual episode length). Little additional variation was seen over intervals up to 4 months from that occurring from week to week.

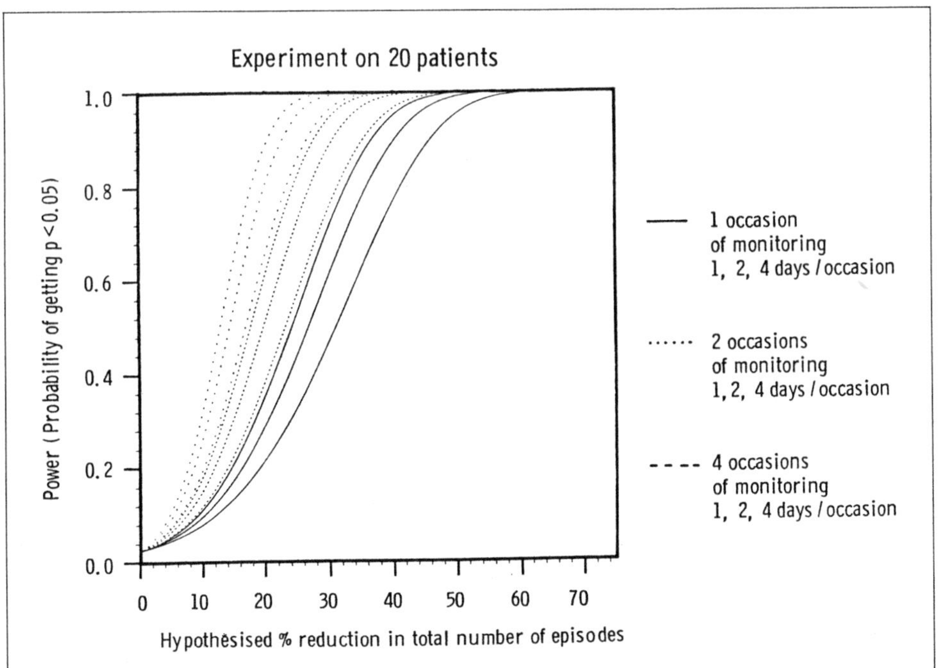

Fig. 1. Relationship of monitoring technique, statistical power and hypothesized reduction in the total number of ST-segment episodes for a trial of 20 patients (see text).

A power function analysis (Fig. 1) permits the rational design of trials by relating the amount of monitoring, number of patients and required reduction in ischemic activity. Increasing the number of days monitoring per occasion and, even more importantly, increasing the number of occasions monitored, greatly increases the chance of detecting significant change as the result of a intervention. A practical trial design on 20 patients using 48 h of monitoring on two occasions would require less than 30% reduction in the number of ischemic episodes to have 80% power of reaching statistical significance. For the individual patient, an 81% reduction in the total number of episodes is required to detect significant effect if a single day of monitoring is used. This can be reduced to 46% by 4 days of monitoring on four occasions. These data emphasize the importance of developing new easier methods for acquisition and analysis of ST-segment information from ambulatory devices if the technique is to be used in routine clinical practice.

New technology

Currently available Holter systems for ST analysis have been based on cassette tapes capable of recording 24 h of electrocardiographic signals. These are tedious to use, firstly because of the limited time period during which data is acquired and secondly because of the need for separate replay and analysis. Recently microprocessor base devices have appeared which are capable of recording and analysing the ST segment change in real time. One such device (Monitor 1, Q med) has been validated in clinical studies and shows great promise for longterm ambulatory monitoring (21). The device has the additional capability of interacting with the patient by the use of an audible tone when preselected criteria for ST change have been reached. This may be useful for correlation of electrocardiographic changes with activities and minor symptoms as well as offering the opportunity to treat silent episodes.

Conclusion

ST-segment Holter monitoring has revealed a number of unsuspected features of ischemic heart disease activity out of hospital. These are likely to affect not only our pathophysiological concepts of the disease but also the way in which patients are followed and treated. It is clear that despite "stable symptoms" myocardial ischemia out of hospital may be highly variable. This variability must be considered when using Holter monitoring for individual patient assessment and design of rational clinical trials. Prolonged monitoring of patients should become feasible with newer real time recording devices.

References

1. Kannel WB (1986) Silent Myocardial Ischemia and Infarction: Insights from the Framingham Study. Cardiology Clinics — Vol. 4, pp 583—591
2. Hultgren HN, Peduzzi P (1984) Relation of Severity of Symptoms to Prognosis in Stable Angina Pectoris. Am J Cardiol 54: 988—993

3. Chierchia S, Lazzari M, Freedman B, et al (1983) Impairment of Myocardial Perfusion and Function Painless Myocardial Ischemia. J Am Coll Cardiol 1: 924—930
4. Cohn P (1986) Silent Myocardial Ischemia: Dimensions of the problem in patients with and without angina. Am J Med 80 (Suppl. 4C): 3—8
5. Deanfield JE, Selwyn AP, Chierchia SL et al (1983) Myocardial ischemia during daily life in patients with stable angina: Its relation to symptoms and heart rate changes. Lancet 1: 753—758
6. Schang SJ, and Pepine CJ (1977) Transient asymptomatic ST-segment depression during daily activity. Am J Cardiol 39: 396—402
7. Cecchi AC, Dovelline EV, Marchi F, et al (1983) Silent myocardial ischemia during ambulatory electrocardiographic monitoring in patients with effort angina. J Am Coll Cardiol 1: 934: 939
8. Tzivoni D, Behorin J, Gavish A, et al (1985) Holter recording during treadmill testing in assessing myocardial ischemic changes. Am J Cardiol, 55: 1200—1203
9. Wolf F, Tzivoni D, and Stern S (1974) Comparison of exercise tests and 24-hour ambulatory electrocardiographic monitoring in detection of ST-T changes. Br Heart J 36: 90—95
10. Tzivoni D, Stern Z Keren A, et al (1980) Electrocardiographic characteristics of neurocirculatory asthenia during every day activities. Br Heart J 44: 426—432
11. Armstrong WF, Jordan JW, Morris SM et al (1982) Prevalence and magnitude of S-T segment and T wave abnormalities in normal men during continuous ambulatory electrocardiography. Am J Cardiol 49: 1638—1642
12. Deanfield JE, Ribiero P, Oakley K et al (1984) Analysis of ST-segment changes in normal subjects: Implications for ambulatory monitoring in angina pectoris. Am J Cardiol 54: 1321—1325
13. Deanfield JE, Kensett M, Wilson RA et al (1984) Silent myocardial ischemia due to mental stress. Lancet 2: 1001—1005
14. Deanfield JE, Shea MJ, Wilson R et al (1985) Direct effect of cigarette smoking causes s ilent ischemia in patients with angina pectoris. (Abstract.) J Am Coll Cardiol 5: 506
15. Deanfield JE, Shea M, Ribiero P, et al (1984) Transient ST-segment depression as a marker of myocardial ischemia during daily life. Am J Cardiol, 54: 1195—1200
16. Deanfield JE, Shea MJ, Selwyn AP (1985) Clinical Evaluation of Transient Myocardial Ischemia during Daily Life. Am J Medicine. Vol 79: 18—24
17. Rocco MB, Barry J, Campbell S, et al (1986) Circadian variation of transient myocardial ischemia (Abstract) J Am Coll Cardiol, 7: 191
18. Muller JE, Stone PH, Turi ZG et al (1985) Circadian variation in the frequency of onset of acute myocardial infarction. N Engl J Med 313: 1315—1322
19. Campbell S, Barry J, Rebecca GS et al (1986) Active ischemia during daily life in asymptomatic patients with positives exercise tests and coronary artery disease. Am J Cardiol 57: 1010—1016
20. Pepine CJ (1978) Aymptomatic myocardial ischema during daily activities. Observations in persons with and without coronary artery disease. In Stern S (ed): Ambulatory ECG Monitoring. Chicago, Year Book Medical Publishers, pp 107—119
21. Levin RI, Cohen D, Frisbie W, Selwyn AP, Barry J, Deanfield JE, Keller B, Campbell D (1986) Potential for Real-Time Processing of the Continuously Monitored Electrocardiogram in the Detection, Quantitation, and Intervention of Silent Myocardial Ischemia. Cardiology Clinics, Vol 4: 735—744

Authors' address:
J. E. Deanfield, M.D.
The Hospital for Sick Children
Great Ormond Street
London WCIN 3JH
UK

Discussion on Management

(Chairmen: A. Resnekov, H. Roskamm)

The first point of the discussion concerned the functional improvement achieved by coronary bypass surgery in the patients that Roskamm had studied. In those patients there was a considerable decrease in pulmonary capillary wedge pressure, which, however, still remained on an increased level. As a reason for this, some degree of interstitial fibrosis was discussed as leading to abnormalities in diastolic function, although there may have been good recovery of systolic function.

Krucoff challenged the hypothesis that a high number of ischemic episodes during a Holter monitoring has quantitative implications for prognosis and that reduction of episodes would actually improve prognosis. For exercise-induced ischemia, however, large studies like the CASS, MRFIT and LRC trials have, as Roskamm pointed out, demonstrated a very substantial impact on prognosis. Therefore Roskamm would draw a line from severe ischemia to bad prognosis and take this as an indication for treatment. Deanfield added that even in the treatment of angina pectoris and the treatment of ischemia demonstrated by exercise tests, an improved prognosis is not documented in large trials. Holter monitoring represents just another method of studying ischemia and possible treatment effects. The advantage of Holter monitoring is that it can detect ischemia out of hospital during everyday activities of the patient. Deanfield agreed that there is no evidence available showing an improved prognosis by improving the amount of ischemia on Holter monitoring, but he also pointed to the strong correlation between ischemia seen on Holter monitoring and ischemia documented by PET scanning in Selwyn studies. This would at least support treatment for a reduction in ischemic episodes as the right directional approach. Lichtlen mentioned that for all studies of medical treatment of coronary heart disease, the much decreased yearly mortality would have to be taken in account. Old studies had shown a yearly mortality of angina pectoris in the range of 10–15%, while today this figure would be much less.

Asked about the meaning of a persistent thallium defect, Rutishauser mentioned that, as in the study of Höfling, and in his PTCA experience, there can be marked improvement in systolic and diastolic function after dilatation or reopening of highly stenotic vessels. Regarding persistent thallium defects, Berman commented on his experience with late redistribution images. He pointed out that even after 24 h or up to 72 h, repeated imaging can be done in thallium scintigraphy. Late redistribution may be shown in some patients who, after 4 h, show a defect that is considered persistent. Therefore Berman cautioned against interpretation of a nonreversible thallium defect as a scar. Whether rubidium 82 would be a better agent for defining myocardial variability seems questionable, according to Berman's experience, as rubidium has such a rapid half-life of only 75 s.

The importance of angina equivalents was pointed out by Rutishauser, who mentioned intense dyspnea not explained by lung findings as one symptom that should make physicians aware of the possibility of ischemia. As Chierchia had shown in earlier reports, the LVEDP rises with every transient ischemic episode without a great difference between silent and symptomatic episodes. Another symptom which can be taken as equivalent to angina would come, not from the backward failure, but from the forward failure of the ischemic heart: fatigue. Undue fatigue can be, in some patients, a rather severe symptom accompanying silent ischemia.

Asked on which type of ECG abnormalities in the post PTCA period he would base therapeutic decisions, Höfling defined ST elevations occuring in the same distribution as had been observed during ballon occlusion, as strong and alarming evidence of coronary occlusion. Of course, these ECG changes have to be persistent before a new intervention, either reopening in the catheterization laboratory or coronary bypass surgery, would be applied. Rutishauser would proceed in a similar way and send any patients with high-grade ECG changes back to the catheterization laboratory. Rutishauser mentioned, regarding monitoring during PTCA, the possible advantages of recording an epicardial ECG over the guide wire. However there were several reservations about this method: Höfling mentioned that changes due to side branch occlusion could be overlooked and that the most important monitoring period was at a time when the guide wire had just been pulled back. Lichtlen reported experience that a guide wire advanced far distally into the inferior wall might miss some ischemia that could be detected on surface ECG. Krucoff mentioned that the degrees of voltage change on epicardial ECG are by no means standardized. Distante recommended echocardiography as a superior means to detect problems in the post PTCA period, but the ease of ECG and pressure monitoring on the CCU was held against that. As a general approach for defining a given patient situation in silent ischemia, Distante proposed Holter monitoring for information about disease activity and a quantitative approach to coronary angiography for defining the fixed impairment of coronary flow. To these two methods, Distante would add the dipyridamol echo test for the detection of asynergy as a consequence of regionally reduced coronary reserve.

Asked by Rafflenbeul about the dose scheme during his mononitrate study, Roskamm pointed out that in this study, a 12 h time span was allowed enable the drug levels to come down and prevent development of tolerance. From his limited experience, it seemed that although the drug levels must have fallen below the threshold of tolerance, there still seemed to be an effect on the ischemic episodes.

Fox again raised the fundamental question of whether silent ischemia should be treated with drugs or other interventions, based on present evidence. Resnekov shared his concerns and called for carefully conducted randomized trials with the endpoint of an improvement in prognosis. He emphasized that the mistakes made during the early days of bypass surgery or PTCA without well-defined indications for treatment, should not be repeated in the treatment of silent ischemia. He rated the question of treatment as undecided before results of randomized trials become available. This view was somewhat opposed by Roskamm, who stated that from his experience and the evidence of the literature he would treat a patient who showed severe ischemia on low exercise levels (e.g. 3 mm ST depression on 50 W). He would not, however, treat patients who showed a very good exercise tolerance, even if some silent ischemia was demonstrable. Roskamm would follow the same guide lines as for patients with angina and have a coronary angiogram performed in severe cases to assist further decision making.

The last part of the discussion centered around the variability of Holter monitoring. Steinbeck questioned how it could be that in patients with many episodes, there was the same percentage of standard deviation as in patients with few episodes per 24 h. Deanfield reported that in the very high numbers there was a slight decrease of the standard deviation, but that basically the percentage of standard deviation for the number of episodes remained constant. This distribution allowed the further calculations he had applied to determine the number of days of monitoring and the number of occasions necessary to demonstrate treatment effects, and be sure that an effect observed was not due to variability. Mathes added that for standard exercise tests also, a fair degree of variability was known. Deanfield, however, referred to his own studies showing that the variability of exercise tests was much less than that of repeated Holter monitorings, and therefore he had diagnosed stable angina pectoris in his patients.

Clinical significance of silent myocardial ischemia

A. Maseri

Royal Postgraduate Medical School, Hammersmith Hospital,
London, England

The growing awareness of the possible occurrence of painless myocardial ischemia is beginning to influence our clinical practice. However, while in some quarters physicians are still perplexed by this entity and are inclined to disregard it, in others, the pendulum is swinging too far in the opposite direction, particularly in terms of diagnosis.

The spectrum of patients

Some patients may only have painless ischemic episodes, are therefore totally asymptomatic and come to medical attention by chance. They should not be confused with patients who, although having coronary atherosclerotic obstructions, do not have any episodes of ischemia either: (1) because the obstructions are not critical, or are compensated by collaterals, or (2) because they have no tendency to develop transient impairment of coronary flow. A minority of patients have only painful ischemic episodes. The large majority of patients have both painless and painful episodes in variable proportion, which can vary greatly even in the same patient, depending not only on the duration of the episodes but also on a variable transmission or perception of painful stimuli. Usually, but not always, the patients with frequent painful ischemic episodes also have frequent painless ones. Conversely, those with rare painful episodes also have rare painless ones. The prevalence of individuals with silent ischemic-like ST segment changes in the population appears to be low when the criteria for positivity are strict.

The causes of silent ischemia

There is no evidence whatsoever to suggest that the mechanisms of ischemia can influence the presence or the absence of pain: painless ischemia can be caused by thrombosis, as in acute myocardial infarction, by spasm, as in variant angina, and by excessive increase of demand, as in chronic stable angina.

The prognosis of silent ischemia

It appears reasonable to assume that for a comparable severity and duration of ischemia, the prognostic significance of painless episodes should be similar to that of painful episodes, as it is actually ischemia which causes both necrosis and arrhythmias. The available information seems to support this proposition. Hence prognosis depends on *the causes of ischemia and on the general setting in which it occurs* rather than on the presence or absence of pain. Indeed the presence of pain has potentially useful and potentially dangerous effects:

- On the one hand, pain alerts patients to stop activities and to seek medical attention; on the other it causes anxiety, increases sympathetic tone, heart work, and may favour the onset of arrhythmias.
- Conversely, in the absence of pain patients are not alerted to stop activities and to seek medical attention.

A reasonable current practice

If I am asked today how I deal with silent ischemia in my clinical practice, I would say that I consider it reasonable to go out looking for it only in individuals suspected to be at very high risk of coronary artery disease. For this purpose, exercise stress testing is more practical than Holter monitoring. However, Holter monitoring can give valuable information on the frequency and severity of silent ischemia in patients with a positive exercise test and no pain.

Until more information is available I am inclined to manage patients with unequivocally documented silent ischemia in the same way as those with painful ischemia, depending on the setting in which ischemia occurs, on its causes, severity and frequency.

Author's address:
A. Maseri M.D., F.R.C.P.
Cardiovascular unit
Royal Postgraduate Medical School,
Hammersmith Hospital,
Ducane Road,
London W12 OHS, England

GPSR Compliance

The European Union's (EU) General Product Safety Regulation (GPSR) is a set of rules that requires consumer products to be safe and our obligations to ensure this.

If you have any concerns about our products, you can contact us on ProductSafety@springernature.com

In case Publisher is established outside the EU, the EU authorized representative is:

Springer Nature Customer Service Center GmbH
Europaplatz 3
69115 Heidelberg, Germany

Batch number: 10577969

Printed by Printforce, the Netherlands